METHODS IN MOLECULAR BIOLOGY™

For other titles published in this series, go to
www.springer.com/series/7651

METHODS IN MOLECULAR BIOLOGY™

G Protein-Coupled Receptors in Drug Discovery

Edited by

Wayne R. Leifert

CSIRO Human Nutrition, Adelaide, SA, Australia

Humana Press

Editor
Wayne R. Leifert
CSIRO Human Nutrition
Kintore Ave.
Adelaide SA 5000
Australia
wayne.leifert@csiro.au

ISBN 978-1-60327-316-9 e-ISBN 978-1-60327-317-6
DOI 10.1007/978-1-60327-317-6
Springer Dordrecht Heidelberg London New York

Library of Congress Control Number: 2009921196

Printed on acid-free paper

Springer is part of Springer Science+Business Media (www.springer.com)

Preface

The G protein-coupled receptors (GPCRs) and associated peripheral G proteins underpin a multitude of physiological processes. The GPCRs represent one of the largest superfamilies in the human genome and are a significant target for bioactive and drug discovery programs. It is estimated that greater than 50% of all drugs, including those in development, currently target GPCRs. Many of the characterized GPCRs have known ligands; however, approximately 20% of GPCRs are described as orphan GPCRs, apparent GPCRs that share the generic high-level structure characteristic of GPCRs but whose endogenous ligand is not known. Therefore, it is expected that the field of GPCR drug discovery and development will greatly expand in the coming years with emphasis on new generations of drugs against GPCRs with unique therapeutic uses which may include drugs such as allosteric regulators, inverse agonists, and identification of orphan GPCR ligands.

As we learn more about the molecular signaling cascades following GPCR activation, we acquire a better appreciation of the complexity of cell signaling and as a result, also acquire a vast array of new molecular methods to investigate these and other processes. The general aim of this book is to provide researchers with a range of protocols that may be useful in their GPCR drug discovery programs. It is also the basis for the development of future assays in this field. Therefore, the range of topics covered and the appropriate methodological approaches in GPCR drug discovery are reflected in this book. It is interesting to note that future directions in drug discovery will require input and collaboration from a plethora of fields of research. As such, this book will likely be of interest to scientists involved in such fields as molecular biology, pharmacology, biochemistry, cellular signaling, and bio-nanotechnology.

With the fine contributions by my "GPCR" colleagues, it has been possible to collate a book that begins with a series of current review articles relevant to the area of high-throughput GPCR screening, with discussion on GPCR structure and GPCR signaling. Importantly, the following chapters are a compendium of detailed laboratory protocol papers, some of which have been used by researchers for many years, while others are recently developed methods and are generating much interest as the next generation of methodological approaches to GPCR research. I sincerely thank the authors who gratefully contributed to this book.

Wayne R. Leifert

Contents

Contributors

RUBEN ABAGYAN • *The Scripps Research Institute, La Jolla, CA, USA*

MAHINDA Y. ABEYWARDENA • *CSIRO Human Nutrition, Adelaide, SA, Australia*

AMANDA L. ALOIA • *School of Biology, Flinders University, Bedford Park, SA, Australia*

ROBERT S. AMES • *Molecular Discovery Research, Biological Reagents and Assay Development, GlaxoSmithKline R&D, King of Prussia, PA, USA*

MICHAEL P. BOKOCH • *Department of Molecular and Cellular Physiology, Stanford University School of Medicine, Stanford, CA, USA*

JOE BRADLEY • *High Throughput Screening Centre of Emphasis, Pfizer Global Research and Development, Sandwich, UK*

HANS BRÄUNER-OSBORNE • *Department of Medicinal Chemistry, Faculty of Pharmaceutical Sciences, University of Copenhagen, Copenhagen, Denmark*

STEPHEN J. BROUGH • *Department of Screening and Compound Profiling, GlaxoSmithKline, Essex, UK*

ANDREW J. BROWN • *Department of Screening and Compound Profiling, GlaxoSmithKline, Hertfordshire, UK*

OLGATINA BUCCO • *Neubody Pty Ltd, Thebarton, SA, Australia*

MELANIE C. BURGER • *Department of Chemistry, McGill University, Montreal, QC, Canada; Department of Chemistry, University of Calgary, Calgary, AB, Canada*

ARTHUR CHRISTOPOULOS • *Monash Institute of Pharmaceutical Sciences and Department of Pharmacology, Monash University, Clayton, Victoria, Australia*

TAMARA COOPER • *School of Molecular and Biomedical Sciences, University of Adelaide, SA, Australia*

DAVID T. CRAMB • *Department of Chemistry, University of Calgary, Calgary, AB, Canada*

ELIZABETH A. DAVENPORT • *Molecular Discovery Research, Biological Reagents and Assay Development, GlaxoSmithKline R&D, Collegeville, PA, USA*

EMILIO DIEZ • *Department of Screening and Compound Profiling, Molecular Discovery Research, GlaxoSmithKline, Madrid, Spain*

SIMON J. DOWELL • *Department of Biological Reagent and Assay Development, GlaxoSmithKline, Hertfordshire, UK*

RICHARD M. EGLEN • *Bio-discovery, PerkinElmer Life and Analytical Sciences, Waltham, MA, USA*

YE FANG • *Biochemical Technologies, Science and Technology Division, Corning Incorporated, Corning, NY, USA*

ANN M. FERRIE • *Biochemical Technologies, Science and Technology Division, Corning Incorporated, Corning, NY, USA*

MAITE DE LOS FRAILES • *Department of Screening and Compound Profiling, Molecular Discovery Research, GlaxoSmithKline, Madrid, Spain*

SIMON P. FRICKER • *Genzyme Corporation, Framingham, MA, USA*
JUAN JOSÉ FUNG • *Department of Molecular and Cellular Physiology, Stanford University School of Medicine, Stanford, CA, USA*
RICHARD V. GLATZ • *SARDI Entomology, Adelaide, SA, Australia*
SÉBASTIEN GRANIER • *Department of Molecular and Cellular Physiology, Stanford University School of Medicine, Stanford, CA, USA; INSERM, U661, CNRS, UMR 5203, Université Montpellier, Institut de Génomique Fonctionnelle, Montpellier, France*
HANSPETER GUBLER • *NIBR IT and Automation Services, Novartis Institutes for BioMedical Research (NIBR), Basel, Switzerland*
NATHAN E. HALL • *Monash Institute of Pharmaceutical Sciences and Department of Pharmacology, Monash University, Clayton, Victoria, Australia*
KASPER B. HANSEN • *Department of Medicinal Chemistry, Faculty of Pharmaceutical Sciences, University of Copenhagen, Copenhagen, Denmark*
KALEECKAL G. HARIKUMAR • *Department of Molecular Pharmacology and Experimental Therapeutics, Mayo Clinic, Scottsdale, AZ, USA*
STEPHEN J. HILL • *Institute of Cell Signalling, Queen's Medical Centre, Nottingham, UK*
SAMUEL KIM • *Department of Chemistry, Stanford University School of Medicine, Stanford, CA, USA*
BRIAN KOBILKA • *Department of Molecular and Cellular Physiology, Stanford University School of Medicine, Stanford, CA, USA*
MARTINA KOCAN • *Laboratory for Molecular Endocrinology, Western Australian Institute for Medical Research and Centre for Medical Research, University of Western Australia, Perth, Australia*
JEAN LABRECQUE • *AnorMED Corp., Langley, BC, Canada*
JOYDEEP LAHIRI • *Biochemical Technologies, Science and Technology Division, Corning Incorporated, Corning, NY, USA*
POLO H.C. LAM • *Molsoft LLC, La Jolla, CA, USA*
WAYNE R. LEIFERT • *CSIRO Human Nutrition, Adelaide, SA, Australia*
KENNETH LUNDSTROM • *PanTherapeutics, Lutry, Switzerland*
DAVID MCLOUGHLIN • *High Throughput Screening Centre of Emphasis, Pfizer Global Research and Development, Sandwich, UK*
EDWARD J. MCMURCHIE • *CSIRO Molecular and Health Technologies, Adelaide, SA, Australia*
LAURENCE J. MILLER • *Department of Molecular Pharmacology and Experimental Therapeutics, Mayo Clinic, Scottsdale, AZ, USA*
PARVATHI NUTHULAGANTI • *Molecular Discovery Research, Biological Reagents and Assay Development, GlaxoSmithKline R&D, King of Prussia, PA, USA*
CHARLES PARNOT • *Department of Molecular and Cellular Physiology, Stanford University School of Medicine, Stanford, CA, USA*
GLEN S. PATTEN • *CSIRO Human Nutrition, Adelaide, SA, Australia*
KEVIN D.G. PFLEGER • *Laboratory for Molecular Endocrinology, Western Australian Institute for Medical Research and Centre for Medical Research, University of Western Australia, Perth, Australia*
VENKATA R.P. RATNALA • *Vertex Pharmaceuticals, Inc., Cambridge, MA, USA*
TERRY REISINE • *Independent consultant, Los Angeles, CA, USA*

DANIEL J. RODRIGUES • *High Throughput Screening Centre of Emphasis, Pfizer Global Research and Development, Sandwich, UK*

PATRICK M. SEXTON • *Monash Institute of Pharmaceutical Sciences and Department of Pharmacology, Monash University, Clayton, Victoria, Australia*

PARITA SHAH • *Department of Screening and Compound Profiling, GlaxoSmithKline, Essex, UK*

JOHN SIMMS • *Monash Institute of Pharmaceutical Sciences and Department of Pharmacology, Monash University, Clayton, Victoria, Australia*

JODY L. SWIFT • *Department of Chemistry, McGill University, Montreal, QC, Canada; Department of Chemistry, University of Calgary, Calgary, AB, Canada*

WALTER G. THOMAS • *School of Biomedical Sciences, The University of Queensland, Brisbane, Queensland, Australia*

ELIZABETH TRAN • *Biochemical Technologies, Science and Technology Division, Corning Incorporated, Corning, NY, USA*

CHRISTINE WILLIAMS • *Director HTS CoE, Pfizer Global Research and Development, Sandwich, Kent, UK*

REBECCA S.Y. WONG • *Genzyme Corporation, Cambridge, MA, USA*

Chapter 1

New Insights into GPCR Function: Implications for HTS

Richard M. Eglen and Terry Reisine

Summary

G protein-coupled receptors (GPCRs) are a large family of proteins that represent targets for approximately 40% of all approved drugs. They possess unique structural motifs that allow them to interact with a diverse series of extracellular ligands, as well as intracellular signaling proteins, such as G proteins, RAMPs, arrestins, and indeed other receptors. Extensive efforts are under way to discover new generations of drugs against GPCRs with unique targeted therapeutic uses, including "designer" drugs such as allosteric regulators, inverse agonists, and drugs targeting hetero-oligomeric complexes. This has been facilitated by the development of new screening technologies to identify novel drugs against both known and orphan GPCRs.

Key words: G protein-coupled receptors, G proteins, Second messengers, High-throughput screening assays, Allosteric regulators, Inverse agonists.

1. Introduction

G protein-coupled receptors (GPCRs) provide much of the diversity in cell-to-cell communication in the human body. These cell surface proteins bind almost all of the known neurotransmitters and hormones that are released synaptically or secreted into the circulatory system *(1)*. The ligand–GPCR binding reaction initiates a cascade of intracellular events in the target cell, including changes in levels of second messengers, ionic conductance, and other signaling events altering cellular activity. Although GPCRs are responsible for normal physiology in the body, dysfunctional GPCR activity can cause abnormal cell function and is involved in the etiology of numerous diseases and disorders. GPCRs have thus historically served a fundamental role in modern pharmacological research and have been targets for many drugs developed by the

Wayne R. Leifert (ed.), *G Protein-Coupled Receptors in Drug Discovery, vol. 552*

Book doi: 10.1007/978-1-60327-317-6_1

pharmaceutical industry to treat various medical indications. By one estimate *(2)*, over 40% of marketed drugs target GPCRs *(3)*. When one considers that the human genome expresses genes for between 800 and 1000 different GPCRs *(4)* and marketed drugs target less than 50 GPCRs, it is evident that the field of GPCR drug discovery and development will grow in the years ahead.

The primary approach used to discover GPCR drugs today involves the use of automated high-throughput screening (HTS) assays since approaches employing crystallography and rational medicinal chemistry – the basis of much of the drug design and discovery against soluble enzymes – cannot be easily employed to discover drugs against GPCRs. Generally, GPCRs resist purification in native, functional conformations and purification is a prerequisite for crystallographic analysis. Over the last decade, HTS technologies to discover GPCR drugs have greatly expanded such that they can be readily adapted to automated fluid dispensing systems and microtiter plate detectors. They are also more sophisticated in terms of measuring the response of the GPCR in a cellular context. Indeed, cell-based assays have become necessary as numerous GPCRs have no known endogenous ligand and are thus considered "orphan" in nature. Furthermore, the possibility of developing drugs targeting GPCRs, but acting through unique mechanisms, such as inverse agonists, allosteric modulators, and drugs interacting with GPCR heterodimers all require novel HTS technologies.

2. GPCR Structure and Function

The GPCR protein family possesses novel structural motifs rendering them unique amongst the various protein superfamilies in the human genome *(5)*. GPCRs are single-chain polypeptides consisting of approximately 300 amino acids, with alternating regions of hydrophilicity and hydrophobicity. Being integral cell membrane proteins, the hydrophobic regions define the transmembrane regions of the receptors. The amino and carboxyl termini and the intervening extra- and intracellular loops are generally more hydrophilic. The pattern of alternating hydrophilicity and hydrophobicity with the amino terminus orientated to the extracellular milieu while the carboxyl tail faces the cell cytoplasm, thus defining the archetypal seven-transmembrane (7-TM) structure of GPCRs.

The hydrophobic, transmembrane regions provide the structural scaffold to confine the receptors to their functional conformations. The hydrophilic regions including the extracellular and intracellular loops and the carboxyl terminus provide contact regions for ligand binding and guanine nucleotide-binding protein (G protein) coupling, respectively. Rather than being static, GPCRs undergo subtle conformational changes in these transmembrane regions when ligands bind to the extracellular domains, flexing intracellular domains to contact G proteins and thus initiate signal transduction.

3. Ligand Binding Domains

GPCRs are classified on the nature of the ligands to which they interact *(6)*. Class 1 includes rhodopsin-like receptors (for which the β-adrenergic receptor is prototypical). Ligands that activate these receptors include biogenic amines, chemokines, prostanoids, and neuropeptides. Class 2 includes the secretin-like receptors and are activated by ligands such as secretin, parathyroid hormone, glucagon, calcitonin gene-related peptide, adrenomedullin, and calcitonin. Class 3 includes metabotropic glutamate receptor-like and calcium-sensing receptors.

Much of what is known about the nature of ligand binding to GPCRs derives from seminal studies conducted on the β-adrenergic receptor; a receptor that binds small molecule ligands in a unique hydrophobic extracellular pocket *(7–9)*. As the endogenous ligands (in the case of the β-adrenergic receptor, the endogenous ligands are epinephrine and norepinephrine) are small, they insert into these binding pockets and interact with sites deep within the core of the receptor structure to induce activation. GPCRs recognizing larger endogenous ligands, such as peptides, bind their ligands differently *(10)*. Here, peptides interact with recognition sites in the extracellular loops of receptors as well as with residues in the hydrophobic pocket *(11–14)*. Targeting of recognition sites to GPCR extracellular loops is critical for creating high affinity of GPCRs for peptides which are too large to intrude entirely into hydrophobic pockets that bind small molecules. Clearly, ligands binding to extracellular loops are expected to induce different conformational changes in the receptor upon binding than small molecules that interact only with residues deep within the receptor core. Interestingly, the multiplicity of recognition sites in peptide receptors may provide the basis for the diversity of ligand interaction with these GPCRs such that different ligands acting on the same receptor can elicit different functions *(10, 11)*.

The ligands referred to as partial agonists, inverse agonists, and allosteric regulators are currently important novel classes of drugs, capable of inducing desired pharmacological effects distinct from classical agonists. These ligands may induce different conformational changes in GPCRs than classical full agonists and, as a consequence, produce unique pharmacological actions. By implication, screening technologies to monitor these diverse activation processes and conformational changes could be useful for discovery of these novel types of GPCR drugs in addition to identifying classical acting drugs.

4. GPCRs and G Proteins

The intracellular domains of GPCRs contain multiple contact regions responsible for receptor coupling to signal transduction systems. The regions most prominent in GPCRs for coupling are the second and third intracellular loops as well as the C-terminal tail. Predominant amongst the intracellular effector molecules contacted by these regions are the G proteins which link GPCRs to second messenger systems, such as adenylyl cyclase, phospholipases, and ionic conductance channels *(15, 16)*.

G proteins interact with cell surface receptors and exhibit inherent GTPase catalytic activity *(17)*. The G protein superfamily consists of heterotrimeric complexes of distinct α, β, and γ subunits. There are thought to be 18 Gα, 5 Gβ, and 11 Gγ subunits, collectively capable of creating a very large number of distinct heterotrimeric complexes *(18)*. These different heterotrimers have significant specificity with regards to both the GPCRs they interact with and the cellular effector systems that they regulate *(17, 19, 20)*. The α subunit of G proteins contains the GTPase catalytic activity as well as many of the receptor contact sites *(17)*. Agonist binding to the GPCR promotes a conformational change that induces coupling with the G protein. The GPCR–G protein interaction accelerates catalysis of guanosine triphosphate (GTP) to guanosine diphosphate (GDP), providing energy needed for dissociation of the α from the βγ subunits (βγ are tightly associated and do not easily dissociate). The free α and βγ subunits then interact with second messenger systems and ionic conductance channels as well as other cellular effectors.

The diversity of GPCR–G protein association has interesting implications with regards to drug discovery. Thus, if drugs can be identified to change the pattern of GPCR–G protein associations or cause a GPCR to preferentially associate with one G protein and not others, then it would be possible to shift the pharmacological profile and functions of a given receptor. This could be used to diminish side effects associated with activation of a given receptor while maintaining desired therapeutic actions or produce new drug effects via a given GPCR. Since GPCR associations with individual G proteins would require a unique structural basis due to the conformation generated by agonist binding, then developing drugs that reproduce that given conformation could direct GPCRs to couple to selective G proteins. This may be accomplished by either finding drugs that bind in a unique manner to the ligand binding domain or identifying allosteric regulators.

Allosteric regulators interact with GPCRs at sites topographically distinct from the classical ligand binding domains *(21–24)*. G proteins act upon allosteric sites to affect GPCR conformation and drugs targeting these unique GPCR–G protein contact sites could prevent coupling of the receptor with some G proteins but not others. Such allosteric regulators could be specific for targeting GPCRs and produce selective therapeutic properties. For example, targeting somatostatin type II receptors (SSTR2) in islet beta cells to couple to $G\alpha_q$ and not couple to $G\alpha_i$ could result in a receptor that stimulates Ca^{2+} mobilization to increase insulin release instead of a receptor that normally inhibits insulin release *(12)*. Such allosteric regulators of the SSTR2 could be used to treat diabetes.

Allosteric regulators are of interest because they can be highly selective for a given GPCR and because they bind to unique structural pockets in the receptor that make contact with the G protein. They are also limited in their maximal effect on a receptor and therefore cannot excessively stimulate or inhibit the receptor as they only act in the presence of endogenous ligands or agonists *(24)*. Importantly, they can be used to modulate the maximal effectiveness of agonists at that receptor and in effect can tone down the receptor activation. This can be useful in prolonging the activation of the receptor and delaying desensitization. It will be of interest to determine whether such regulators can also be used to switch dual acting receptors such as the β_2-adrenergic receptor from one that stimulates to one that inhibits adenylyl cyclase. Since the inhibitory effects are cardioprotective, there may be instances where allosteric regulators could have therapeutic value in diminishing cardiac damage due to excessive stimulation or, in the case of early stages of heart failure, block the inhibitory effects of β_2-adrenergic receptors to facilitate cardiac output.

5. GPCR Mutations, Disease, and Novel Drug Discovery

While GPCRs are critical for mediating the normal functions of neurotransmitters and hormones, they also play a role in a number of diseases. Loss-of-function mutations in GPCRs are involved in a number of diseases of the endocrine system *(25–27)*. For example, loss-of-function mutation of the TSH receptor causes congenital hypothyroidism *(28)*. Mutations of the endothelin type B receptor can result in Hirschsprung disease, a congenital disorder involving bowel obstruction *(29)* and loss of function of parathyroid hormone (PTH) receptors causes Blomstrand chondrodysplasia, a disorder associated with abnormal breast and bone development *(30)*. Furthermore, homozygous loss-of-function mutations in the type 5 chemokine receptor provides resistance to HIV infection because this receptor is critical for the infectivity of this virus *(31)*. This loss-of-function mutation is the basis of the rational for developing some chemokine receptor antagonists to prevent HIV infection.

In addition to loss-of-function mutations, gain-of-function mutations in GPCRs also cause disease. In most cases the gain of function is related to conversion of the wild-type receptor that is dependent on agonist stimulation to a constitutively active receptor that is not dependent on activating ligand. Gain-of-function disorders include constitutively active rhodopsin which can cause night blindness *(32)*; constitutively active PTH-related receptor which causes Jansen-type metaphyseal chondrodysplasia *(33)*; constitutively active thyroid-stimulating hormone (TSH) and follicle-stimulating hormone (FSH) receptors causing congenital hyperthyroidism *(34)* and familial male precocious puberty *(35)*; and mutations in the calcium-sensing GPCR that cause hypocalciuric hypercalcemia and neonatal hyperparathyroidism *(36)*. For these diseases, developing inverse agonists could be useful as therapeutics since they would be predicted to selectively block the actions of the constitutively active receptor.

While direct links between cause and effect have not been made, it is possible that subtle mutations in GPCRs or changes in their expression could be responsible for variations in drug sensitivities among different human populations. Such mutations might not only cause variations in effectiveness or potency of GPCR-directed drugs but also affect drugs that are indirectly active via GPCRs such as neurotransmitter uptake inhibitors including those used to treat depression, since changes in sensitivity could alter how the endogenous transmitters activate GPCRs as well as drugs.

6. GPCR Pharmacology

The fact that a significant proportion of approved drugs target GPCRs suggests that approaches to discover GPCR drugs have historically been successful. These methods have advanced and become more sophisticated with the growing need to target more novel receptors and to discover drugs acting in unique ways to affect GPCR signaling. Classical drugs targeting GPCRs generally come under two categories: agonists, which mimic the actions of endogenous transmitters and hormones to stimulate GPCRs, and antagonists, which have no intrinsic activity but which block activation of the GPCRs by agonists. This somewhat rigid pharmacological terminology has evolved over the years to embrace a wide spectrum of differently acting drugs *(37)*.

For example, agonists can be distinguished as full agonists, partial agonists, and inverse agonists, each with their own sets of advantages and disadvantages as therapeutics. A full agonist produces the same maximal effect as the endogenous neurotransmitter or hormone. Partial agonists bind to GPCRs in a manner that produces less of an effect than full agonists and partial agonists can antagonize full agonists. As a consequence, partial agonists exhibit duality in that they bind to GPCRs in a manner similar to both an agonist and an antagonist.

Partial agonists are therapeutically important because of their dual nature. For example, the μ-opiate receptor partial agonist buprenorphine is less effective than morphine in stimulating the μ-opiate receptor and antagonizes the actions of morphine at this receptor *(14)*. It was approved in 2002 by the Food and Drug Administration (FDA) for treatment of opiate addiction because it blocks the actions of morphine and heroin at the μ-opiate receptor to allow for the addictive drugs to be tapered off while producing some stimulation itself thereby preventing a full-blown withdrawal reaction.

While drugs acting as full and partial agonists have been known for many years, inverse agonists have been identified more recently in the last decade. Like partial agonists, inverse agonists are able to block the effects of full agonists at GPCRs. However, the unique property of these ligands is that they induce opposite effects on the same GPCR as full agonists. Thus, whereas norepinephrine or isoproterenol will stimulate the β-adrenergic receptor to increase adenylyl cyclase activity, inverse agonists would bind to this receptor to decrease adenylyl cyclase activity. The inherent activity of an inverse agonist is dependent on the receptor having some level of constitutive basal activity *(38)*. In fact, most recombinant GPCRs overexpressed in cell lines produce constitutive basal activity which is caused in part by the generation of homodimers. The homodimers are forced to form because of the exaggerated number of receptors expressed in the cell under artificial conditions. Under these conditions, compounds that might otherwise be considered neutral antagonists produce inverse agonism. Inverse agonists may also be useful in treating pathological conditions where GPCRs undergo constitutive activity *in vivo* either because mutations cause the constitutive activity or because the receptors become overexpressed due to some disease process.

7. Technologies for GPCR Compound Screening and Drug Discovery

The approaches that have been used to discover drugs against GPCRs involve either biochemical approaches, such as ligand binding assays using cell membrane preparations, or cell-based technologies which measure functional consequences of receptor activation. Ligand binding technologies have been one of the linchpins in the GPCR drug discovery process *(39)* and most FDA-approved GPCR drugs were discovered using this approach. However, ligand binding technologies are less used in GPCR screening partly since the waste disposal costs are high as well as the fact that they require the use of a high-affinity, selective ligands that can be chemically radiolabeled and for many receptors such ligands are not available.

An alternative approach to ligand binding assays that has been employed for drug discovery measures the activation of GPCRs by the ability of agonist to stimulate GPCR–G protein association. This approach measures the ability of an agonist to promote the binding of radiolabeled non-hydrolyzable GTP analogues, such as ^{35}S-GTPγS to G proteins coupled to a receptor as a measure of GPCR activation *(40)*. Such binding can be detected using a scintillation proximity assay (SPA) format and is easily adaptable for HTS *(41, 42)*. Furthermore, non-radioactive alternatives exist to measure GTPγS binding such as the DELFIA Eu-GTPγS. These non-isotopic ligands with the advantage of reduced cost due to a lack of radioactive waste have also been adapted for HTS. The GTPγS binding approach can be used to identify full agonists, partial agonists, and inverse agonists as well as allosteric regulators. Importantly, novel technologies using GPCR–Gα fusion proteins eliminate the problem of whether the target cells expressing the recombinant GPCR under study have the appropriate endogenous G proteins that couples with the GPCR or whether the ratio of expression of GPCR to G protein is unnatural since by nature the stoichiometry of GPCR to G proteins in the fusion protein is 1:1 *(43–45)*.

Although assays measuring binding of ligands to GPCRs have been used historically to identify GPCR drugs, most current technologies used for GPCR drug discovery are cell based *(46)*. The primary readout of such assays is accumulation of second messenger levels in response to GPCR activation. The second messengers most commonly measured are cAMP, inositol phosphates, and Ca^{2+} *(47–50)*. Assays measuring cellular levels of cAMP are dependent on the activity of adenylyl cyclase and detect GPCRs coupled to the G proteins, $G\alpha_s$, and $G\alpha_i$. Many commercial assays are available to measure this cAMP response including radioimmunoassay approaches, TR-FRET, and β-gal enzyme fragment complementation (EFC) technology *(3)*.

Activation of GPCRs coupled to G_q and G_o is generally measured by detecting cellular levels of Ins P3, the end product of activation of phosphoinositide phospholipase C *(3)*. Non-isotopic assays are primarily used to measure Ins P3 levels for drug screening include PerkinElmer's AlphaScreen technology *(3)*. Because activation of the Ins P3 pathways leads to changes in stored Ca^{2+} one can measure intracellular Ca^{2+} changes in response to GPCR stimulation using a commonly employed fluorometric imaging plate reader (FLIPR) or functional drug screening system (FDSS) which use Fluo-3, Fluo-4, or Calcium 3 dyes and the assays are easily set up for HTS *(51–54)*. In parallel, there has been rapid adoption of cell-based assays employing photoproteins, such as aequorin or Photina, that generate a luminescent signal upon elevations in the level of intracellular Ca^{2+} *(55)*. These techniques have the advantage that large signal to background ratios are generated, especially if the photoproteins are targeted to discrete cellular sites such as the mitochondria which are directly apposed to Ca^{2+} release sites in the endoplasmic reticulum. The great sensitivity makes these assays particularly useful for the detection of allosteric regulators which generally are difficult to detect with less sensitive cell-based assays.

In addition to direct measurements of second messengers, reporter gene assays can be used to detect the consequence of changes in second messengers *(47–49)*. These HTS assays employ constructs consisting of second messenger response elements such as the cAMP-response element (CRE) or the calcium-sensitive activator protein 1 (AP1) or nuclear factor of activated T-cell (NFAT) elements linked to genes that encode for enzymes, such as luciferase or β lactamase, that act to catalyze the formation of luminescent or fluorescent products. Like the photoprotein assays, this technology is highly sensitive to changes in GPCR-mediated changes in second messengers and is easily adapted to HTS format.

In general, the portfolio of G proteins normally coupled to a target GPCR determines whether one employs the cAMP versus the Ins P3/Ca^{2+} assays in the measurement of GPCR activation. However, more generalized assays which can be used as universal GPCR screening technologies have also been developed. One screening assay detects GPCR activity as measured by mitogen-activated protein (MAP) kinase stimulation, since the MAP kinases are believed to be a point of convergence of the vast majority of GPCRs in regulating cell function. A commercially available assay to measure the activity of one of the MAP kinases, extracellular signal-regulated kinase (ERK), is the AlphaScreen SureFire ERK (PerkinElmer). This is a cell-based, homogenous, non-radioactive assay that measures phosphorylated ERK1 and ERK2 *(56)*. Another universal GPCR assay is based on the use of β-arrestin translocation in response to agonist stimulation *(57, 58)*. The technology was originally designed to measure β-arrestin translocation using confocal microscopy but has been modified to be detected by bioluminescence resonance energy transfer (BRET) *(59–61)*. More recently, Wehrman et al. *(62)* have developed an EFC assay to measure β-arrestin translocation in an assay format adapted for HTS (DiscoveRx). Like the MAP kinase assays, this EFC GPCR-based assay is employed for HTS of both known and orphan GPCRs for agonists, inverse agonists, and antagonist identification.

8. Conclusions

The central role of GPCRs in human physiology and their extensive diversity in function have made the GPCR family one of the prime targets for drug discovery. Many GPCRs have discrete biological roles indicating that drugs targeting those proteins are likely to produce specific therapeutic effects. Importantly, has been known from years of pharmaceutical development that GPCR-directed drugs provide good therapeutics and can treat numerous diseases and disorders for which there are few, if any, alternatives.

Advances made in the GPCR research field in the last decade have heightened interest in discovering new GPCR drugs. For example, the finding that some recently de-orphanized GPCRs have powerful biological functions has led to major attempts to better understand the roles of the hundreds of remaining orphan GPCRs, thereby identifying those receptors with the potential to be targets for novel therapeutics. These receptors thus represent a relatively unexplored field of drug discovery and yet may have high value for the pharmaceutical industry partly because of the large number of targets available as well as the unique functions they probably mediate.

The identification of drugs targeting orphan GPCRs, as well as inverse agonists, allosteric regulators, pharmacological chaperones, and hetero-oligomers, while providing important new directions for drug discovery, has also directed the industry to develop novel technologies for HTS. This is necessary since classical drug discovery approaches cannot be easily used to identify drugs targeting orphan GPCRs or identify pharmacological chaperones; certainly they cannot be easily used to identify hetero-oligomer-selective drugs. Historically, the industry has streamlined cell-based assay approaches to measure second messenger accumulation or MAP kinase activity to discover drugs against most if not all known GPCRs. However, novel technologies measuring protein–protein interactions have only been more recently developed. Collectively, these approaches can be used for discovery of almost any type of compound against almost any GPCR in the human genome.

Many of these approaches have now been incorporated into HTS formats and are consequently becoming more commonly employed for drug discovery. As important, novel technologies that measure subtle conformational changes in GPCRs are also emerging using physical techniques *(63, 64)* including dielectric spectroscopy, optical surface plasmon resonance biosensing, isothermal titration calorimetry, second harmonic generation, and differential scanning calorimetry. All of these techniques can be employed to identify allosteric regulators, as well as agonists acting at the same receptor yet producing different functional responses.

When such technologies are optimized for HTS purposes, one anticipates that they will provide a foundation for the development of new generations of drugs, potentially with therapeutic properties beyond these GPCR drugs presently available.

References

1. Limbird, L. (1995) *Cell Surface Receptors: A Short Course on Theory and Method*, 2nd ed. M. Nijhoff, Boston.
2. Wilson, S., and Bergsma, D. (2000) Orphan GPCRs: novel drug targets for the pharmaceutical industry. *Drug Des. Discov.* **17**, 105.
3. Eglen, R.M. (2005) Functional G protein-coupled receptor assays for primary and secondary screening. *Comb. Chem. High Throughput Screen.* **8**, 311–318.
4. Venter, J.C., et al. (2001) The sequence of the human genome. *Science* **291**, 1304–1351.
5. Dohlman, H.G., Throner, J., Caron, M.G., and Lefkowitz, R. (1991) Model systems for the study of seven-transmembrane-segment receptors. *Ann. Rev. Biochem.* **60**, 653–688.
6. Pierce, K.L., Premont, R.T., and Lefkowitz R.J. (2002) Seven-transmembrane receptors. *Nat. Rev. Mol. Cell Biol.* **3**, 639–650.
7. Lefkowitz, R.J., Hoffman, B., and Taylor, P. (1996) Neurotransmission. In: *Goodman & Gilman's The Pharmacological Basis of Therapeutics*, 9th ed. Hardman, J.G., and Limbird, L.E. (eds.), McGraw-Hill, NewYork, pp. 105–139.
8. Ostrowski, J., Kjelsberg, M.A., Caron, M.G., and Lefkowitz, R.J. (1992) Mutagenesis of the β2-adrenergic receptor: how structure elucidates function. *Ann. Rev. Pharmacol. Toxicol.* **32**, 167–183.
9. Strader, C.D., Fong, T.M., Tota, M.R., Underwood, D., and Dixon, R.A. (1994) Structure and function of G protein-coupled receptors. *Ann. Rev. Biochem.* **63**, 101–132.
10. Gurrath, M. (2001) Peptide-binding G protein-coupled receptors: new opportunities for drug design. *Curr. Med. Chem.* **8**, 1605–1648.
11. Blake, A.D., Bot, G., and Reisine, T. (1996) Structure-function analysis of the cloned opiate receptors: peptide and small molecule interactions. *Chem. Biol.* **3**, 967–972.
12. Reisine, T., and Bell, G.I. (1995) Molecular biology of somatostatin receptors. *Endocr. Rev.* **16**, 427–442.
13. Reisine, T. (2002) Pharmacogenomics of opioid systems. In: *Pharmacogenomics: The Search for Individualized Therapies.* Licinio, J. and Wong, M. (eds.). Wiley-VCH, Weinheim, Germany, pp. 461–487.
14. Reisine, T. and Pasternak, G. (1996) Opioid analgesics and antagonists. In: *Goodman & Gilman's The Pharmacological Basis of Therapeutics*, 9th ed. Hardman, J.G., and Limbird, L.E. (eds.), McGraw-Hill, NewYork, pp. 521–555.
15. Granier, S., Kim, S., Shafer, A.M., Ratnala, V.R., Fung, J.J., Zare, R.N., and Kobilka, B.K. (2007) Structure and conformational changes in the C-terminal domain of the β_2-adrenoceptor: insights from fluorescence resonance energy tranfer studies. *J. Biol. Chem.* **282**, 13895–13905.
16. Pitcher, J., Freedman, N., and Lefkowitz, R.J. (1998) G protein-coupled receptor kinases. *Ann. Rev. Biochem.* **67**, 653–692.
17. Ross, E.M. (1996) Pharmacodynamics. In: *Goodman & Gilman's The Pharmacological Basis of Therapeutics*, 9th ed.

Hardman, J.G., and Limbird, L.E. (eds.), McGraw-Hill, NewYork, pp. 29–41.

18. Simon, M., Strathman, M., and Gautam, N. (1991) Diversity of G proteins in signal transduction. *Science* **252**, 802–808.
19. Dessauer, C.W., Posner, B.A., and Gilman, A.G. (1996) Visualizing signal transduction: receptors, G proteins and adenylate cyclases. *Clin. Sci.* **91**, 527–537.
20. Clapham, D.E., and Neer, E. (1993) New roles for G protein βγ-dimers in transmembrane signaling. *Nature* **365**, 403–406.
21. Christopoulos, A., and Kenakin, T. (2002) G Protein-coupled receptor allosterism and complexing. *Pharmacol. Rev.* **54**, 323-374.
22. Christopoulos, A. (2002) Allosteric binding sites on cell-surface receptors: novel targets for drug discovery. *Nat. Rev. Drug Discov.* **1**, 198–210.
23. Christopoulos, A., Sorman, J.L., Mitchelson, F., and El-Fakahany, E. (1999) Characterization of the subtype selectivity of the allosteric modulator heptane-1,7-bis-(dimethyl-3'-pthalimidopropyl) ammonium bromide at cloned muscarinic acetylcholine receptors. *Biochem. Pharmacol.* **57**, 171–179.
24. May, L.T., Avlani, V.A., Sexton, P.M., and Christopoulos, A. (2004) Allosteric modulation of G protein-coupled receptors. *Curr. Pharm. Des.* **10**, 2003–2013.
25. Spiegel, A.M. (1996) Defects in G protein-coupled signal transduction in human disease. *Ann. Rev. Physiol.* **58**, 143–170.
26. Spiegel, A.M., and Weinstein, L. (2004) Inherited diseases involving G proteins and GPCRs. *Annu. Rev. Med.* **55**, 27–39.
27. Lee, A., et al. (2003) Distribution analysis of non-synonymous polymorphisms within the G protein-coupled receptor gene family. *Genomics* **81**, 245–248.
28. Jordan, N., et al. (2003) The W546X mutation of the thyrotropin receptor gene: potential major contributor to thyroid dysfunction in a Caucasian population. *J. Clin. Endocrinol. Metab.* **88**, 1002–1005.
29. Carrasquillo, M.M., McCallion, A.S., Puffenberger, E.G., Kashuk, C.S., Nouri, N., and Chakravarti, A. (2002) Genome-wide association study and mouse model identify interaction between RET and EDNRB pathways in Hirschsprung disease. *Nat. Genet.* **32**, 237–244.
30. Wysolmerski, J.J., Cormier, S., Philbrick, W.M., et al. (2001) Absence of functional type 1 parathyroid hormone (PTH)/PTH-related protein receptors in humans is associated with abnormal breast development and tooth impaction. *J. Clin. Endocrinol. Metab.* **86**, 1487–1488.
31. Liu, R., et al. (1996) Homozygous defect in HIV-1 coreceptor accounts for resistance of some multiply exposed individuals to HIV-1 infection. *Cell* **86**, 367–377.
32. Berson, E.L. (2002) Retinitis pigmentosa and allied diseases. In: *Principles and Practice of Ophthalmology*, Albert, D.M., Jakobiec, F.A., Azar, D.T., and Gragoudas, E.S., (eds.), Saunders, Philadelphia, pp. 2262–2290.
33. Calvi, L.M., and Schipani, E. (2000) The PTH/PTHrP receptor in Jansen's metaphyseal chondrodysplasia. *J. Endocrinol. Invest.* **23**, 545–554.
34. Corvilain, B., Van Sande, J., Dumont, J.E., and Vassert, G. (2001) Somatic and germline mutations of the TSH receptor and thyroid diseases. *Clin. Endocrinol.* **55**, 143–158.
35. Themmen, A.P., and Verhoef-Post, M. (2002) LH receptor defects. *Semin. Reprod. Med.* **20**, 199–204.
36. Hu, J., and Spiegel, A.M. (2003) Naturally occurring mutations of the extracellular Ca^{++} sensing receptor: implications for understanding its structure and function. *Trends Endocrinol. Metab.* **14**, 282–288.
37. Kenakin, T., Bond, R., and Bonner, T. (1992) Definition of pharmacological receptors. *Pharmacol. Rev.* **44**, 351–362.
38. Dinger, M.C., Bader, J.E., Kobor, A.D., Kretzschmar, A.K., and Beck-Sickinger, AG. (2003) Homodimerization of Neuropeptide Y receptors investigated by fluorescence resonance energy transfer in living cells. *J. Biol. Chem.* **278**, 10562–10571.
39. Bylund, D., Deupree, J.D., and Toews, M.L. (2004) Radioligand-binding methods for membrane preparations and intact cells. *Methods Mol. Biol.* **259**, 1–28.
40. Ferrer, M., et al. (2003) A fully automated [35S]GTPgammaS scintillation proximity assay for the high-throughput screening of Gi-linked G protein-coupled receptors. *Assay Drug Develop. Tech.* **1**, 261–273.
41. De Lapp, N. W. (2004) The antibody-capture [(35)S]GTPgammaS scintillation proximity assay: a powerful emerging technique for analysis of GPCR pharmacology. *Trend in Pharmacol. Sci.* **25**, 400–401.
42. Harrison, C., and Traynor, J.R. (2003) The [35S]GTPgammaS binding assay: approaches and applications in pharmacology. *Life Sci.* **74**, 489–508.

43. Milligan, G., and Bouvier, M. (2005) MINIREVIEW: methods to monitor the quaternary structure of G protein-coupled receptors. *FEBS J.* **272**, 2914–2925.
44. Milligan, G., Feng, G.J., Ward, R.J., Sartania, N., Ramsay, D., McLean, A.J., and Carrillo J.J. (2004) G protein-coupled receptor fusion proteins in drug discovery. *Curr. Pharm. Des.* **10**, 1989–2001.
45. Pascal, G., and Milligan, G. (2005) Functional complementation and the analysis of opioid receptor homodimerization. *Mol. Pharmacol.* **68**, 905–915,
46. Rees, S. (2002) Functional assay systems for drug discovery at G protein-coupled receptors and ion channels. *Receptors Channels* **8**, 257–259.
47. Kunapuli, P., et al. (2003) Development of an intact cell reporter gene beta-lactamase assay for G protein-coupled receptors for high-throughput screening. *Anal. Biochem.* **314**, 16–29.
48. Kornienko, O., Lacson, P., Kunapuli, P., Schneewels, J., Hoffman, I., Smith, T., Alberts, M., Inglese, J., and Strulovici, B. (2004) Miniaturization of whole live cell-based GPCR assays using microdispensing and detection systems. *J. Biomol. Screen.* **9**, 186–195.
49. Williams, C. (2004) cAMP detection methods in HTS: selecting the best from the rest. *Nat. Rev. Drug Discov.* **3**, 125–135.
50. Goetz, A.S., Liacos, J., Yingling, J., and Ignar, D.M. (1999) A combination assay for simultaneous assessment of multiple signaling pathways. *J. Pharmacol. Toxicol. Methods* **42**, 225–235.
51. Kassack, M.U., Hoefgen, B., Lehmann, J., Eckstein, N., Quillan, J.M., and Sadee, W. (2002) Functional screening of G protein-coupled receptors by measuring intracellular calcium with a fluorescence microplate reader. *J. Biomol. Screen.* 7, 233–246.
52. Zhang, Y., Kowal, D., Kramer, A., and Dunlop, J. (2003) Evaluation of FLIPR Calcium 3 Assay Kit – a new no-wash fluorescence calcium indicator reagent. *J. Biomol. Screening* **8**, 571–577.
53. Dupriez, V., Maes, K., Le Poul, E., Burgeon, E., and Detheux, M. (2002) Aequorin-based functional assays for G protein-coupled receptors, ion channels, and tyrosine kinase receptors. *Receptors Channels* **8**, 319–330.
54. Le Poul, E., Hisada, S., Miziguchi, Y., Dupriez, V.J., Burgeon, E., and Detheux, M. (2002) Adaptation of aequorin functional assay to high throughput screening. *J. Biomol. Screen.* 7, 57–65.
55. Bovolenta, S., Foti, M., Lohmer, S., and Corazza, S. (2007) Development of a Ca^{2+}-activated photoprotein, photina, and its application to high-throughput screening. *J. Biomol. Screen.* **12**, 694–704.
56. Leroy, D., Missotten, M., Waltzinger, C., Matrin, T., and Scheer, A. (2007) G protein-coupled receptor-mediated ERK 1/2 phosphorylation: towards a generic sensor of GPCR activation. *J. Recept. Signal Transduct. Res.* **27**, 83–97.
57. Barak, L.S., Ferguson, S.S., Zhang, J., and Caron, M.G. (1997) A beta-arrestin/GFP biosensor for detecting GPCR activation. *J. Biol. Chem.* **272**, 27497–27500.
58. Kim, S., et al. (2001) Differential regulation of dopamine D2 and D3 receptors by G protein-coupled receptor kinases and beta-arrestins. *J. Biol. Chem.* **276**, 37409–37414.
59. Bertrand, L., et al. (2002) The BRET2/arrestin assay in stable recombinant cells: a platform to screen for compounds that interact with G protein-coupled receptors (GPCRS). *J. Recept. Signal Transduct. Res.* **22**, 533–541.
60. Heding, A. (2004) Use of BRET 7TM receptor/beta arrestin assay in drug discovery and screening. *Expert Rev. Mol. Diagn.* **3**, 403–411.
61. Vrecl, M., Jorgensen, R., Pogacnik, A., and Heding, A. (2004) Development of a BRET2 screening assay using beta-arrestin 2 mutants *J. Biomol. Screen.* **4**, 322–333.
62. Wehrman, T.S., Casipit, C.L., Gewertz, N.M., and Blau, H.M. (2005) Enzymatic detection of protein translocation. *Nat. Methods* **2**, 521–527.
63. Cooper, M.A. (2006) Non-optical screening platforms: the next wave in label-free screening? *Drug Discov. Today* **11**, 1068–1074.
64. Cooper, M.A. (2006) Optical biosensors: where next and how soon? *Drug Discov. Today* **11**, 1061–1067.

Chapter 2

Screening Technologies for G Protein-Coupled Receptors: From HTS to uHTS

Maite de los Frailes and Emilio Diez

Summary

The discovery of drugs for G protein-coupled receptors (GPCRs) has traditionally been very successful, even before the structural nature of these molecular targets was elucidated. Over the years, this family of proteins has become more important in the understanding and treatment of different human pathologies, representing today close to 30% of the molecular targets of all marketed drugs. The sequencing of the human genome unveiled the existence of many new GPCRs and this has increased even more the interest of this family of proteins as potential drug targets. Today the search for compounds that interfere or modulate the function of GPCRs is one of the major focuses of pharmaceutical companies. The understanding of the molecular events that take place upon receptor activation, together with the need of testing large chemical libraries, has resulted in the development of a variety of methods and technologies to measure the activity of these receptors. In this chapter we will review most of the assay technologies currently in use for "*in vitro*" pharmacological screening, their evolution, their capabilities, and their limitations.

Key words: GPCR (G protein-coupled receptor), HTS (high-throughput screening), uHTS (ultra-high-throughput screening).

1. Introduction

G protein-coupled receptors (GPCRs), also known as seven-transmembrane receptors, are one of the largest families of proteins in the human genome *(1–4)*. They are present in the surface of the cellular membranes and act as receptors for a large variety of extracellular signals including paracrine and endocrine communications, as well as sensors for the external environment. From their ligand point of view, GPCRs include receptors for low-molecular

Wayne R. Leifert (ed.), *G Protein-Coupled Receptors in Drug Discovery, vol. 552*

Book doi: 10.1007/978-1-60327-317-6_2

weight chemicals (such as biogenic monoamines, lipids, purines, and small peptides), proteins, calcium ions, and also they have an important function as sensors for odorants, taste molecules, and photons in the case of the rhodopsin receptor.

According to the International Union of Pharmacology, Human GPCRs can be classified into three main families *(5)*: Class 1, the largest, includes receptors for amines, chemo-peptides, lipids, nucleotides, and a large proportion of odorant, taste, and light receptors. Class 2 includes receptors for neuropeptides and peptidic hormones such as vasoactive intestinal peptide, glucagon, calcitonin, parathyroid hormone, and so on. Class 3, known as the metabotropic glutamate-like subfamily, includes the calcium, GABA, and glutamate receptors among others. GPCRs have traditionally been very good targets for drug discovery and many drugs of the available pharmacopoeia act through modulation of specific GPCRs *(6–8)*. The drug discovery success demonstrated in the past has made this family of proteins one of the most valuable and attractive class in drug discovery efforts. However, this assessment is only partially true since drugs have been discovered almost exclusively for members of the class 1 subfamily. Class 2 and 3 subfamilies have proven to be very difficult pharmacological targets. The reasons for the different success rates is not completely clear, but it is likely a combination of factors including the nature of the ligand–receptor binding region, the design of the screening assays and the use of recombinant versus native systems.

Upon stimulation of GPCRs by the appropriate ligand, this in turn mediates the activation of the intracellular signal transduction machinery. There are two different mechanisms involved in signal transduction: activation of G proteins and activation of the β-arrestin pathways. On the one hand, ligand binding stabilizes the conformation of the receptor in a state that allows for the interaction of its C-terminal domain with the heterotrimeric G protein complex in an activated state. It is in that state that the Gα subunit is able to hydrolyze GTP and to interact with the effector molecule(s) (e.g., adenylate cyclase and/or phospholipase C) *(9)*.On the other hand, the receptor stimulates the activation of G protein-coupled receptor kinases (GRKs), the receptor is then phosphorylated and able to bind β-arrestin. Translocation and binding of β-arrestin to the receptor inhibit the GTPase activity thus inactivating this signal transduction pathway and driving the receptor to internalization. Moreover, the binding of β-arrestin results in a series of G protein independent intracellular events *(10)*.

Drug discovery for GPCRs started even before the structure and biochemical processes triggered by these receptors were well understood, and the techniques employed to discover drugs were based mainly on traditional pharmacological experiments and radioligand binding assays. As the understanding of the molecular events involved in GPCR's function increases, the number of techniques to study the pharmacology of the receptors has also expanded. In this review we will describe some of these technologies (**Fig. 1**). The intention is to give not only a historical perspective but more importantly to provide information on the technical capabilities and limitations of the different type of assays.

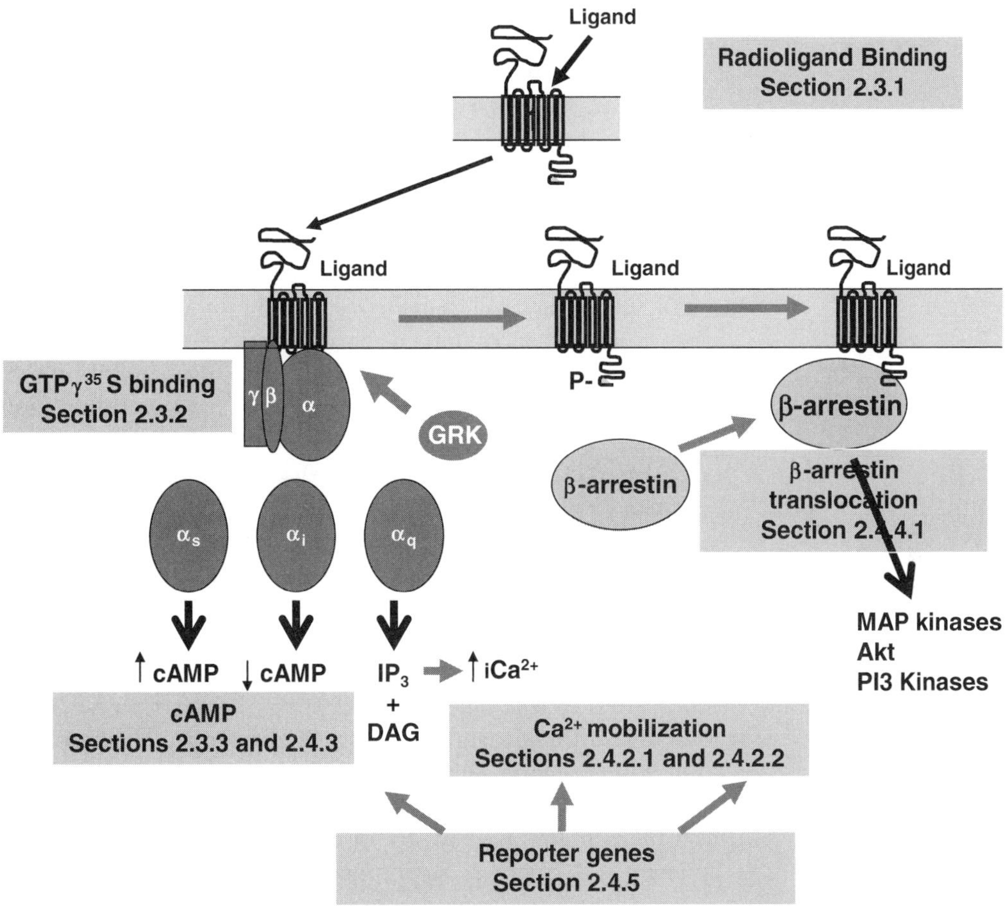

Fig. 1. **Screening technologies utilized in uHTS for GPCRs.** "*In vitro*" pharmacological activity of GPCRs can be measured at different levels during receptor activation. The initial binding of the ligand can be monitored by different methods, but prevalent technologies in uHTS are based on the use of radioactive ligands. Upon receptor activation, a series of conformational changes trigger the interaction of the receptor with various intracellular proteins, including heterotrimeric G protein complexes and β-arrestins. The activation of these pathways results in the generation of intracellular second messengers (e.g., cAMP, iCa, and protein kinases) and eventually in major cellular events. Today there are a variety of uHTS methodologies that can be used to monitor; for example, cAMP, intracellular Ca, and β-arrestin translocation, among others. Some of these methods can be carried out with membrane preparations and others require the use of intact cells. Different sections in this chapter describe the use of these technologies in different scenarios.

2. Screening GPCRs: From HTS to uHTS

2.1. The uHTS "Revolution"

The need to screen a large number of targets against extensive small molecule libraries has led to the demand for an increase in both the sensitivity and the throughput of the assays. Over the past few years high-throughput screening (HTS) technologies to support GPCR drug discovery have greatly expanded. These new technologies can be adapted to automated liquid dispensing systems and high-density plate readers, typically able to process a 384- or 1536-well plate in a few seconds or minutes *(11)*. From the screening platforms of the 90 s capable of testing hundreds or thousands of compounds per day, the technology has now evolved to ultra-HTS (uHTS) methods with capacity for testing hundreds of thousands of samples per day. This evolution has been supported by technological developments in three major fields: (1) detection systems and assay methods, (2) liquid handling devices and robotics, and (3) process flow and information management.

From conventional photoconductive and photo-emissive devices in traditional radioactivity and fluorescence readers, charge-coupled devices (CCDs) have been developed and incorporated into the new generation of "imagers," in substitution of the standard cameras based on vacuum-tube technology. Very high-resolution CCD chips are combined with telecentric lens and supported by electronics and software packages to allow for 384 or 1536 individual experiments being viewed simultaneously *(12)*.

Technological development of detection systems has been complemented by advances in liquid handling devices that can achieve robust high-speed dispensation of compounds and assay reagents in very low volumes. Syringe-solenoid and piezoelectric dispensers *(13)* and acoustic-based dispensers *(14)* are all non-contact liquid handling devices that can dispense drops in the nanoliter range, in a robust and efficient manner for either reformatting compounds or adding assay reagents. Finally, assay plate technology has also undergone a revolution, from the traditional 96-well plate format to the currently used 384- and 1536- (or even 3456-) well plates.

The possibility of exploring novel mechanisms of action such as partial agonists, inverse agonists, or allosteric regulators, in addition to the classical full agonists and competitive antagonists has required innovative HTS protocols and technologies *(15)*. The use of fully automated screening platforms has become the standard approach for the effective screening of large collections of compounds on selected GPCRs of interest. In the new century, uHTS is a reality in automated drug discovery laboratories, specially for GPCRs, where a myriad of uHTS assay formats and technologies are now available.

2.2. Assay Requirements for GPCR uHTS

An appropriate assay for uHTS would have to meet at least the following criteria: statistically robust and reproducible, low compound interference (simple and easy discrimination of false positives), amenable to automation and to the use of screening platforms (low volume 384- or 1536-well plates compatible, short incubation time, reagent stability, and low cost), feasibility for data annotation and storage, and the most important of all, appropriate "*in vitro*" pharmacology and physiological relevance.

The technologies used for screening GPCRs are based on both biochemical and cell-based assays. Although the convenience of ligand binding versus functional assays is always important to consider, in general cell-based assays are of greater physiological relevance than cell-free systems. More than 50% of HTS utilized in early drug discovery are cellular assays, with a clear trend to increase, especially for GPCRs *(16)*. In the following sections we will describe the most commonly used GPCR uHTS assays, those that have been implemented in hit identification programmes and are leading to the discovery of both classical and new generation of GPCR-based medicines.

2.3. Membrane-Based Assays

In "ligand binding assays" a compound has to compete with a high-affinity ligand for the binding to a particular receptor, the target of interest. They were first developed in the early 1970s and have been used for decades. Many drugs in the market were initially discovered 30 years ago using this technology, which is still present in the HTS assay portfolio. In most cases the technology uses radioactive ligands that selectively bind with high affinity to one particular receptor in a cell membrane preparation *(17)*. Maintained in the portfolio for more than 30 years, ligand binding is probably the methodology that has undergone more technological changes to evolve from "low-to-medium-to-high-to-ultra-high-throughput screening." From high volume (5 mL) washing protocols to homogeneous low volume ($<$10 μl) assays.

2.3.1. Radioligand Binding Assays

A plethora of GPCR high-affinity radiolabeled agonists and antagonists are commercially available for a variety of receptors. In general, antagonists are more broadly used as their binding to the receptor is usually less influenced by external factors such as concentration of ions. Main radioisotopes used are tritium (^{3}H) and iodine-125 (^{125}I). ^{125}I-labeled ligands have usually higher specific activity, which can increase assay sensitivity and allows less biological material to be used, usually membrane preparations from cells where the receptor of interest has been overexpressed. A clear disadvantage of iodinated ligands is their shorter half-life. They have to be used before extensive radioactivity decay. Also, the logistic to prevent human exposure to radioactivity is more complicated for ^{125}I- than for ^{3}H-ligands.

Radioligand binding technology can clearly show whether a ligand directly interacts with a GPCR, but it cannot define whether the compound is an agonist or an antagonist. Secondary evaluation of compounds is therefore required in functional assays that vary depending on the intracellular signaling pathway triggered by the receptor of interest.

Traditional radioligand binding assays were based on the separation of bound and free ligand by multiple washing and filtration steps. Although they are usually very robust assays, the throughput of these methods is low and the amount of radioactive waste generated is very high. The development of non-separation assays constituted a key milestone in HTS for GPCRs. Radioactive homogeneous assays were developed by different groups, always following the principle of "scintillation proximity." One of the components (usually the receptor) is immobilized on a solid support. The interaction between a radiolabeled molecule and its receptor is only detected when the label is in close proximity to the scintillant containing solid support. The most extensively used technique uses scintillant-coated beads and is known as SPA (trademark, GE) *(18–22)*. The bead is composed of a matrix whose outer surface has been modified by a coating of wheat germ agglutinin (WGA) to enable cellular membranes to bind. SPA binding assays are designed as "mix, equilibrate, and measure" format. In a typical SPA radioligand binding assay, membrane preparation (usually 0.5–3 μg/well) containing the GPCR receptor of interest is incubated with high specific activity (80–200 Ci/m*M*) radioligand, in the presence or absence of test compounds followed by an additional incubation with SPA beads previously coated (4–16 h at 4°C) with WGA. Non-specific binding is determined in the presence of an excess (>100 K_d) of unlabeled specific ligand. The radioactive energy released by the immobilized radioligand excites the scintillant-SPA bead, resulting in the emission of detectable light. Energy released from unbound radioligand is not close enough to the SPA bead and is dissipated in the assay medium; hence no light is emitted. Plates can be centrifuged or allowed to settle prior to counting to eliminate potential non-specific signals (excitation of bead fluor by unbound isotope).

There are some critical factors to develop an optimal SPA-binding assay. First, membranes and radioligand concentration have to be in the appropriated range to maintain the pharmacology and allow for a good signal-to-background (S/B) ratio; for example, ligand depletion could be observed when an excess of membrane is present since this could facilitate non-specific binding. Second, a high concentration of WGA-SPA beads could result in an increase in signal primarily owing to an increase in non-proximity effects (random collisions of the radioactive elements with the scintillant-WGA-bead, independent of receptor). Thirdly, the equilibrium time. Although ligand–receptor pair dependent, the association of radioligand with membranes is usually relatively rapid. A significant signal can be detected within 5 min of adding radioligand and the equilibrium is reached typically in about 30 min. Once full equilibrium is reached, the signal is usually stable for hours and overnight incubations are sometimes required to improve assay quality.

Test compounds competing with the radioligand for receptor binding sites will result in a reduced signal. The SPA format eliminates the requirement of separation steps and can effectively measure equilibrium binding characteristics. Equilibrium dissociation constants, K_d and B_{max}, can easily be estimated by non-linear regression analysis from saturation binding experiments run with fixed concentrations of membranes and increasing concentrations of radioligand. Apparent K_i estimation and Schild analysis can also be carried out using SPA technology. With regard to automation and throughput, SPA can be easily automated and has demonstrated to provide enough quality in 1536-well plates and throughputs of more that 150,000 wells/analyst/day. **Table 1** summarizes assay parameters of a real uHTS campaign carried out at GSK using SPA *(23)*.

The use of fluorescent ligands in ligand binding assays would help to reduce the disadvantages associated with the use of radioactivity. However, fluoro-ligands have not been extensively used for drug discovery of GPCRs owing to the difficulty of tagging the ligands without affecting pharmacology of the receptors.

Table 1
Example of a radioligand binding uHTS campaign: summary of assay parameters

Radioligand binding SPA assay	Plate type	Final assay volume	Average Z′	S/B	Compounds tested	Wells/ day	Cell type	Reader
D2 inhibitors	1536	10 μL	0.75	3.8	872 K	150 K	CHO-hD2 R	ViewLux

The program was specifically looking for partial agonists. In the radioligand binding assay, primary hits are visualized just as inhibitors, independently of their pharmacological mechanism of action. Secondary evaluation of hits was necessary to further define type of action upon receptor binding (functional cAMP assay). Z′ is a statistical parameter that accounts for assay quality and reliability. It is reflective of both the assay signal rate (S/B) and the data variation associated with the signal measurement (coefficient of variation). The Z′ value ranges from 0 to 1 and it is generally accepted that Z′> 0.4 provides a robust, reliable, and discriminative assay *(23)*.

2.3.2. GTPγS Binding Assays

In spite of the high sensitivity of radioligand binding assays, they do not provide information on the functional effect of the compounds identified. That limitation has been overcome during the last decade or so, with the design of functional assays for uHTS. One of the most commonly used functional assays is based on the binding of GTP to Gα subunits. Upon receptor activation, the Gα subunit exchanges GDP to GTP, triggering the intrinsic GTPase activity while it cycles the Gα protein back to the GDP-bound basal state. This nucleotide exchange can be monitored by measuring the binding of guanosine 5′-γ thiotriphosphate (GTPγS), an analogue of GTP that is resistant to GTPase activity. The standard GTPγS binding assay is performed with the radioactive GTPγ^{35}S, so that the level of receptor activation of the receptor can be followed by the increase of radioactivity bound to the cellular membrane *(24)*.

Biological material used is usually a preparation of membranes from cells overexpressing the target receptor. In the traditional format, binding of GTPγ^{35}S was measured by separating the membrane-bound fraction from the free nucleotide by filtration. Radioactivity was then quantified on filters after addition of scintillation liquid. In the most recent non-separation protocols, the receptor membranes are immobilized on SPA beads (or on the surface of "Flash plates") typically through WGA. This homogeneous protocol has made the technology suitable for uHTS and allowed for miniaturization to 384- or even 1536-well plates *(25–27)*. The technology is mainly utilized for Gi-coupled receptors, as the assay renders poor S/B ratios for other G proteins. This is based on the fact that the Gi family have higher rates of basal nucleotide exchange than the other G proteins.

A critical factor in the development of GTPγ^{35}S binding assays is to minimize the basal binding of GTPγ^{35}S to membranes in the absence of ligand. This background is due to Gα protein constitutive activity and can be decreased by using micromolar concentrations of GDP in the assay *(24, 28)*.

The GTPase activation by GPCRs is a very early process in the signal transduction cascade, which makes the technology less sensitive to interferences due to signal amplification or regulation by cellular processes that characterize other technologies based on more distal events (e.g., reporter gene assays). GTPγ^{35}S binding assays can be used for screening GPCRs when looking for classical agonists and antagonists. In addition the technology has demonstrated to allow the identification of molecules with alternative mechanisms of action, such as inverse agonists (compounds suppressing basal signaling activity of the receptor) and neutral antagonists (antagonists with no intrinsic activity, that do not affect basal signaling) *(29)*. **Table 2** shows a summary of the results obtained during a real GTPγ^{35}S binding uHTS campaign in 1536-well plates.

2.3.3. cAMP Membrane-Based Assays

Some technologies (e.g., LANCE^{TM} cAMP assay; Perkin Elmer, Waltham MA 02451 USA) allow the realization of functional cAMP assays using membrane preparation from cells overexpressing the target receptor. However, this assay format cannot easily

Table 2
Summary of uHTS parameters for a GTPγS^{35} binding assay

GTPγS^{35} *binding*	Plate type	Final assay volume	Median Z′	S/ B	Compouds tested	Wells/ day	Cell type	Reader
μ-Opioid receptor antagonists	1536	5 μL	0.55	2.8	1.7 M	188 K	CHO-μ-opioid receptor	ViewLux

More than 150,000 wells/day were tested in a 5 μL final assay volume. The low S/B ratio is a characteristic of GTPγS^{35} binding assays. However, the assay was very robust with Z′> 0.5 in 1536-well assay format due to low variability.

detect inhibition of adenylyl cyclase via Gα_i. Detection of steady-state levels of cAMP is generally measured in intact cells as it will be described in cell-based assays section below.

2.4. Cell-Based Functional Assays

Compound attrition during the process of drug development is due to a variety of factors including toxicity issues and lack of information on the effect the compound would have on the entire biological system. Traditional end-point biochemical assays do not necessarily provide enough information to predict future failures. On the opposite side, high content analysis assays can deliver massive amounts of biological data, but are less feasible for HTS and in most cases throughput is not enough to screen big libraries of compounds. Halfway between these two extremes are the assays that detect second messengers in a cellular environment. These types of assays meet the requirements of high throughput and high information, whilst also maintaining the specificity, sensitivity, reproducibility, and robustness of biochemical or membrane-based assays. After years of experience, we are now able to develop cell-based assays that can meet all the requirements of uHTS campaigns, including automation feasibility. Two relevant examples for GPCRs are those assays based on changes of intracellular levels of cAMP and calcium upon receptor activation. Until very recently, most cell-based HTS assays were developed with stable cell lines. Critical factors to achieve an appropriate assay performance are the level of receptor expression and the stability of the functional signal over the time. The highest expression level may not always correlate with the most representative biological response, especially for GPCRs where the level and efficiency of G protein coupling is critical to generate an appropriated functional response *(30)*.

More recently, transient transfections have been used and this trend is clearly increasing. The old dogma that transient transfection induces more assay variability is currently being broken. New technologies that support very efficient gene delivery (e.g., BacMam) and high expression without gene integration into the host genome are now available and are being used more and more to develop screening assays *(31)*.

2.4.1. Some Considerations on Assay Modes: Agonists, Antagonist, and Allosteric Modulators

The identification of allosteric ligands, which bind to sites topographically distinct from the classical orthosteric binding site, offers new opportunities for drug discovery *(32)*. Allosteric modulators have a number of advantages over orthosteric drugs, including enhanced selectivity and saturability. Because of their ability to modulate receptor conformation in the presence of an endogenous agonist, allosteric modulators can fine-tune classical pharmacological responses, altering both affinity and efficacy.

Families B and C of GPCRs have historically been considered as low tractable targets from the point of view of drug discovery. However, many of these receptors are highly validated for different therapeutic applications. Metabotropic glutamate receptors are one clear example; various members of the family have very characteristic brain distribution patterns and have been associated with different central nervous system pathologies, so that specific agonist or antagonists are critical for the development of safe drugs. Owing to the highly conserved orthosteric ligand binding domain within the family, specificity has been very difficult to achieve. However, in the past few years, allosteric modulation has proved to be a very good alternative to gain selectivity in drug action for these types of receptors *(33)*. In order to support this novel approach, most of the assays utilized in the discovery phase had to be re-engineered. In addition to metabotropic receptors, similar approaches have been applied to members of the family B of GPCRs, such as PTH or GLP-1. In the next sections, we will describe some examples of assays specifically designed for the identification of allosteric modulators of GPCRs using different assay technologies such as $[Ca^{2+}]_i$ mobilization and gene reporter assays. The results show how these novel designs can be applied to various uHTS programs.

2.4.2. Calcium Mobilization Assays

Gq and Go coupled receptors regulate intracellular calcium concentrations either through phospholipase C activation (IP_3-mediated calcium release from the endoplasmic reticulum) or through the regulation of voltage-sensitive ion channels (e.g., M3 receptor). The two main technologies to quantify intracellular Ca^{2+} in uHTS mode use Ca^{2+}-sensitive dyes (fluorescent assays) or photoproteins (luminescence assays) sensible to calcium.

2.4.2.1. Fluorescence Probes for Calcium Assays (FLIPR™)

The use of calcium-sensitive dyes (mainly Fluo-4) which increase their quantum yield upon binding of calcium is by far the most common protocol. The cells are incubated with the fluorescent dye in the presence of probenecid, an anion exchange protein inhibitor, which acts to prevent dye leakage. In recently developed non-washing protocols, extracellular dye is quenched by the addition of quenching dyes such as brilliant black, which has made the technology fully compatible with automated HTS platforms *(34)*.

One of the most commonly used instruments for calcium-based HTS is FLIPR™(Fluorometric Imaging Plate Reader; Molecular Devices Corp., Sunnyvale, CA, USA). With its CCD camera, FLIPR collects data at a sufficient rate (usually every second) to follow the magnitude and time course of fluorescent intracellular signaling events. The reader has been available for some years in 384-well format and more recently also in 1536-well mode. The instrument is based on a semi-confocal technology that uses an argon-ion laser for excitation and an optical configuration to record signals only from the cell monolayer at the bottom of the plate. This characteristic is responsible for the main limitation of the technology: the need of using adherent cells that have to be seeded in assay plates several hours before the assay starts (usually overnight incubations at 37°C).

Although it could be target and cell line-dependent, the FLIPR assays usually have a high S/B ratio, making them particularly useful for detecting allosteric regulators. Dual readout protocols can also be easily developed so that both agonists and antagonists (or agonists and positive allosteric modulators) of the same receptor can be detected in a single HTS assay.

For Gq receptors that do not couple efficiently to the calcium signaling pathway, or for Gi-coupled receptors, co-expression of Gα15/16 or various mutant forms of G proteins (e.g., Gqi5) is frequently used. These "promiscuous" G proteins have been demonstrated to improve the receptor coupling to the Ca^{2+} pathway and to provide a more effective response in FLIPR assays *(35, 36)*.

FLIPR has been extensively used for screening GPCRs in most pharmaceutical companies for more than 10 years and it is still considered the golden technology for GPCR drug discovery. The kinetic information gathered from each well may be used to simply identify primary hits in HTS mode, or may be analyzed in more detail to discriminate false and true positives, to mechanistic studies, or for specificity assessment to ensure receptor-mediated activity. Specificity studies are usually run as part of the HTS campaign when dose–response experiments with selected hits are carried out. In agonist mode, compounds are run in parallel against the target of interest and also in the parental cell line that does not express the target receptor. When searching for antagonist activity the specificity assay is carried out in the same HTS cell line with activation of an endogenous receptor.

In spite of the limitation of working with adherent cells and the complexity of multiple liquid handling steps, the technology can be fully automated and has demonstrated to achieve the throughput required to be considered an uHTS technology. An integrated system of two readers in an automated platform that can work unattended overnight, can manage 100,000 wells/day, in a dual assay, which means more than 200,000 kinetic profiles. **Table 3** summarizes some characteristics of a real dual-FLIPR uHTS campaign.

Table 3
Assay parameters from a typical FLIPR assay searching for both agonists and antagonists of the receptor for different hit identification programs

Fluorescence intracellular calcium (FLIPR)	Plate type	Assay volume	Median Z′	Average Z′	S/B	Compounds tested	Wells/day	Cell type	Reader
Ghrelin agonists	384	30 µL	0.60	0.57	6–8	1.1 M	131 K	HEK293-BacMam-Ghrelin	FLIPR
Ghrelin antagonists	384	30 µL	0.74	0.70	6–8	688 K	131 K	HEK293-BacMam-Ghrelin	FLIPR

The protocol is designed as a "dual assay" which allows the detection of both types of molecules in the same well.

2.4.2.2. Bioluminescence Calcium Assays (Photoproteins)

Bioluminescent proteins such as aequorin can be used to monitor intracellular calcium. Aequorin was initially cloned from *Aequorea victoria*. It is composed of two different units, the apoprotein apoaequorin (22 kDa) and the prosthetic group coelenterazine (472 Da), a molecule belonging to the luciferin family. In the presence of molecular oxygen, the two components of aequorin reconstitute spontaneously, giving the functional protein. There are several *EF-hand* domains in the structure of aequorin that function as binding sites for Ca^{2+} ions. Upon Ca^{+2} binding, a conformational change is induced in the coelenterazine molecule resulting in its oxidized form, coelenteramide and CO_2. As the excited coelenteramide relaxes to the ground state, blue light (490 nm) is emitted that can be easily detected with a luminometer. The intensity of light emitted is proportional to the intracellular concentration of calcium *(37)*.

Apoaequorin can easily be expressed in mammalian cells. Coelenterazine is a hydrophobic molecule and therefore is easily taken up across the plasma membrane. Therefore, coelenterazine is added to the culture medium and the cells generate a functional protein that can be used to measure Ca^{2+} concentration. Aequorin has a number of advantages over other Ca^{2+} indicators: it has a low leakage rate from cells and lacks phenomena of intracellular compartmentalization or sequestration. The bioluminescence does not require light excitation like fluorescent probes and does not induce auto-fluorescence, photo-bleaching or exhibit biological degradation problems *(38)*. For uHTS, the main advantage of aequorin over the fluorescent calcium assays is the feasibility of working with cells in suspension, thus making the technology more amenable to 1536-well format. The main disadvantage compared with FLIPR assays is the incapacity of the technology to provide dual protocols in the same well as those described above for FLIPR when searching for agonists and antagonists, or agonists and positive allosteric modulators on the same assay. This is partly due to liquid handling limitations of current readers. **Table 4** summarizes basic assay parameters from an aequorin-based uHTS campaign.

Table 4
Example of an aequorin-calcium uHTS campaign

Aequorin Calcium assay	Plate type	Assay volume	Median Z′	Average Z′	S/N	Compounds tested	Wells/ day	Cell type	Reader
5HT2a antagonists	1536	6 μL	0.68	0.67	158	1.8 M	200 K	HEK 293-h5HT2a	LumiLux

The possibility of working with suspension cells, enables the performance of 200,000 samples/day, with just one instrument, with an assay robustness and reliability equivalent to the traditional calcium technologies.

2.4.3. cAMP Cell-Based Assays

Adenylyl cyclase can be stimulated (via $G\alpha_s$) or inhibited (via $G\alpha_i$) upon ligand activation of GPCR. Stimulation of cAMP accumulation is generally substantial, allowing for easy assay development of agonists or antagonists to GPCRs coupled to $G\alpha_s$. However, inhibition of cAMP upon $G\alpha_i$-coupled receptor activation is usually of less magnitude, variable and dependent of the basal level of cAMP. Thus, $G\alpha_i$ assays are generally developed using agents, such as forskolin, that activate adenylyl cyclase. Historically, cAMP was measured using radioimmunoassays *(39)* and reporter gene assays using CRE-luc constructs *(40)*. As mentioned above, radioactive methods are not the best option for uHTS from both a logistical and an economic point of view due to the high cost of the reagents, apart from safety issues. Gene reporter assays measure downstream events and therefore require long incubation times (4–6 h) with the compounds which results in a high rate of false positives, especially for assays screening antagonists. More recently, nonradioactive methods to detect cAMP in intact cells have been developed, commercialized and successfully adapted to uHTS, including (amongst others) high-affinity enzyme complementation, luminescence – single oxygen channeling

(ALPHAScreen®), fluorescence polarization, and time-resolved fluorescence resonance energy transfer (TR-FRET). All of the above are based on competition binding assays using specific anti-cAMP monoclonal antibodies in homogeneous ("non-wash") formats *(41)*.

In the enzyme fragment complementation (EFC) cAMP assays, the cAMP from cell lysates competes with the enzyme (β-galactosidase) donor (ED)-cAMP supplied by the kit for binding to the anti-cAMP antibody. Upon antibody binding, the ED fragment cannot bind to the enzyme acceptor (EA). This lack of enzyme complementation results in a decrease of signal. The amount of ED-cAMP available for complementation to EA is proportional to the concentration of "cold" cAMP (produced by cells) available to compete for antibody binding *(42)*. This assay format has been reported to be amenable to miniaturization up to 3456-well format for both agonist and antagonist responses, even for Gi-coupled receptors *(43)*.

ALPHAscreen® is a bead-based assay bringing two small diameter beads (200 nm) into proximity upon specific interaction of two biomolecules (bioluminescence resonance energy transfer-BRET technology). On laser excitation at 680 nm, ambient oxygen is converted to the single state by a photosensitizer in the donor bead. The excited oxygen molecule can diffuse up to 200 nm before rapidly decaying. If the acceptor bead is in close proximity, the singlet oxygen reacts with the chemiluminescencer (a thioxene derivative) in the acceptor bead to generate chemiluminescence at 370 nm. This energy is then transferred to fluorophores in the same bead, shifting the emission wavelength to 520–600 nm. Half-life of the decay is 0.3 s and allows the operation in time-resolved mode *(44)*. In the ALPHAscreen® cAMP assay, the biotinylated cAMP is bound to streptavidin-donor beads and the anti-cAMP antibody to acceptor beads. Free cAMP from cell lysates competes against biotinylated-donor bound cAMP for the binding to the cAMP antibody. It has been demonstrated that ALPHAscreen® technology is highly sensitive. Partial agonists can be displayed as full agonists, not being an inconvenient for HTS, but requiring a secondary assay for hit characterization. For antagonist screens, the technology has the clear advantage of being able to detect inverse agonists in addition to classical competitive antagonists *(45)*.

TR-FRET methods are based on energy transfer from a lanthanide donor (e.g., europium either chelated or encrypted in a carrier molecule) to a fluorophore acceptor such as allophycocyanin (APC or XL665), or to a low molecular weight dye such as Alexa-647 when they are in close proximity (less than 10 nm). Laser light pulses with a wavelength of 337/340 nm excite the Eu-carrier, and the energy emitted is transferred to the acceptor, which has a maximum of excitation at 340 nm, and emits time-resolved light at 665 nm.

There are two main TR-FRET cAMP assays commercially available, LANCE® (PerkinElmer) and HTRF (Cisbio Bioassays, IBA group, Bedford, MA 01730 USA). LANCE®assays are based on the loss of energy transfer when an excess of either endogenous or exogenously added cAMP competes with the biotin-cAMP for the binding to a cAMP antibody. This prevents the energy transfer between the europium streptavidin/biotin–cAMP complex and the Alexa fluorophore-labeled anti-cAMP antibody. In the LANCE® format, the use of a biotinylated cAMP tracer allows the optimization of the europium/Alexa-647 ratio to get maximal sensitivity, while avoiding long-term avidity (signal stability over time, while pharmacology of compounds is kept constant). This feature is a clear advantage for uHTS campaigns, where a high number of plates have to be tested in each run. However, the technology could be sensitive to compounds interfering with the biotin–streptavidin interaction. The S/B ratio is usually low (2–3), but very robust assays can be configured due to the consistency of results.

HTRF® technology has been optimized to obtain a high S/B ratio and can work both with adherent or suspension cells. As in the LANCE® assays, the specific HTRF signal is inversely proportional to the concentration of cAMP in the standard or samples and can be used to measure agonist and antagonists effects on Gs- and Gi-coupled receptors. LANCE® and HTRF®cAMP assays are currently broadly used to uHTS of Gs- and Gi-coupled receptors. The assays are homogeneous and in general exhibit high sensitivity, reproducibility, robustness, precision, dimethyl sulfoxide tolerance, signal stability, and feasibility to miniaturization and automation *(46)*. An example of the quality of an uHTS campaign is summarized in **Table 5**.

Table 5
Summary of a uHTS campaign with LANCE cAMP assay

LANCE cAMP assay	Plate type	Assay volume	Median Z′	Average Z′	S/N	Compounds tested	Wells/day	Cell type	Reader
5HT6 antagonits	1536	8 µL	0.66	0.64	2	1.67 M	200 K	U2Os-BacMam h 5HT6 R	ViewLux

200,000 samples/day were easily run with a single addition protocol using frozen cells (U2OS) transiently transfected with BacMam-h5HT receptor viruses 24 h before testing.

2.4.4. β-Arrestin Activation Assays

Although the molecular events which orchestrate receptor desensitization and internalization are complex and not yet fully elucidated, it is clear that β-arrestins 1 and 2 play a critical role. Activation of GPCRs upon binding of specific agonists leads to second messenger signaling and their stabilized conformation allow them to become substrates for GRKs. After phorphorylation by GRKs, receptors are able to bind β-arrestins, which are recruited from the cytoplasm to the cell membrane. β-Arrestins bind to the receptor and inhibit further G protein signaling which results in receptor desensitization. β-Arrestins also participate in driving receptors to the membrane trafficking machinery, causing receptor internalization from the cell surface and sequestration from G proteins *(47, 48)*. β-Arrestin recruitment is a very generic process in GPCR activation with only a few examples where this has not been demonstrated. In spite of their function as negative regulators of GPCR-mediated signaling, new roles for β-arrestins have been discovered in recent years. They can function as scaffold proteins that interact with several cytosolic proteins and link GPCRs to intracellular signaling pathways such as mitogen-activated protein kinase (MAPK) cascades, ERKs 1 and 2, JNK3, and p38 *(10, 49–51)*.

Classically, it was thought that all signal transduction mechanisms for a particular receptor correlated, that is, ligand binding stimulated or inhibited all receptor functions to an equal extent. We now know this paradigm of "correlated efficacies" is not correct, and that receptor pharmacology is much more complex. The "ligand bias" concept that describes the ability of ligands to selectively stabilize receptor conformations that stimulate or inhibit subsets of receptor activities has recently been demonstrated for β-arrestin signaling *(52)*. There are examples of "perfect bias," where ligands stimulate β-arrestin functions without inducing G proteins signals, or vice versa *(53, 54)*. β-Arrestin-biased ligands might provide opportunities for the development of novel therapies, for example, by blocking G protein pathways while stimulating potentially beneficial β-arrestin signals, such as ERK, Akt, and PI3K, that might be beneficially cytoprotective. For these reasons, there is a recent and growing interest in screening GPCRs looking for β-arrestin ligands. β-Arrestin-based screens may find ligands that other approaches will not identify *(55)*.

As described in this chapter, there are many well-established assays with high sensitivity and specificity that can be used in uHTS campaigns for G protein function. However, there are far fewer methods for assessing β-arrestin efficacy. The most specific is the measurement of the β-arrestin translocation to receptors. This is usually measured via fluorescently tagged β-arrestins monitored with either microscopic imaging of β-arrestin redistribution to activated receptors *(56)* or with FRET or BRET assays that detect the interaction of β-arrestin and the receptors *(57)*. These assays have the clear advantage of being highly specific for both the receptor of interest and the activation of β-arrestin pathway but have usually limited sensitivity. For high content technologies, the need of expensive confocal imaging instrumentation could be an additional limitation. More recently, Wehrman et al. *(58)*

have developed an EFC assay to measure β-arrestin translocation in an assay that is suitable for HTS or even uHTS (described below).

2.4.4.1. Enzyme Fragment Complementation Assay

This approach is based on the use of two complementing fragments of the β-galactosidase (β-gal) enzyme that are expressed within stably transfected cells. The larger portion of β-gal, termed EA for enzyme acceptor, is fused to the C terminus of human β-arrestin 2. The smaller, 4 kDa complementing fragment of β-gal, termed ProLink™tag, is expressed as a fusion protein with the GPCR of interest at the C terminus and has a weaker affinity for EA. Upon GPCR activation, the interaction of β-arrestin with the GPCR forces the interaction of ProLink and EA, thus allowing complementation of the two fragments of β-gal and the formation of a functional enzyme capable of hydrolyzing substrate and generating a chemiluminescent signal. The technology, also known as PathHunter™ – β-arrestin assay, is a novel *cellular* application of the established EFC technology pioneered by DiscoveRx (Caliper Life Sciences, Hopkinton, MA 01748 USA). The assay is extremely sensitive. In **Table 6** we summarize the data obtained from the validation of a HTS β-arrestin EFC translocation assay recently set up in our laboratory.

Table 6
Summary of parameters from a β-arrestin translocation (PathHunter-EFC) assay validation

β-Arrestin translocation EFC assay	Plate type	Assay volume	Median Z′	Average Z′	S/N	Compounds tested	Wells/ day	Cell type	Reader
CCR4 β-arrestin validation-antagonists assay	384	25 μL	0.6	0.58	2–4	9,856	21,504	CHO-PathHunter β-arrestin – CCR4 cells	Viewlux
CCR4 β-arrestin "focussed set" screening	384	25 μL	0.52	0.52	2–4	8,298	20,736	CHO-PathHunter β-arrestin – CCR4 cells	Viewlux

2.4.5. Reporter Gene Assays

Gene reporter systems can be used as indicators of transcriptional activity in cells. Typically, a reporter gene is joined to a promoter sequence in an expression vector that is introduced into cultured cells by standard transfection methods. Stable cell lines that integrate this reporter gene of interest into the chromosome can be selected and propagated by using a selectable marker, included in the transfection vector. These engineered cell lines can be used for drug screening and to monitor the effect of exogenous agents. In general, enzymatic reporters are used for drug discovery as they are quite sensitive due to the small amount of reporter enzyme required to generate the products of the reaction *(59–61)*.

Cell-based reporter gene assays have been extensively used in HTS due to their high sensitivity, robust signal, feasibility of miniaturization, and simplicity of protocols. One of the most common reporters is the bioluminescent enzyme luciferase, derived from the coding sequence of the *luc* gene cloned from the firefly *Photinus pyralis (62)*. The firefly luciferase catalyzes a reaction using D-luciferin and ATP in the presence of oxygen and Mg^{2+}, resulting in light emission. The total amount of light measured during a given time interval is proportional to the amount of luciferase reporter activity in the sample. Light emission is typically quantified over a defined assay period using a luminometer. The very high quantum yield (>88%) of the firefly luciferase reaction makes it the highest sensitive chemoluminescence reaction known in nature (sensitivity in the sub-attomolar range) with a linear dynamic range of 7–8 orders of magnitude. The "flash" nature of this light emission (half-life 2–3 s) was initially the main drawback of the luciferase system. The assay was first improved by including coenzyme A in the reaction, which provides a longer, sustained light reaction with greater sensitivity, and later on by the development of "stabilized" luciferase-detection reagents, which are now commercially available. The extended "glow" reaction of the enhanced luciferase assay allows for accurate measurement of the luminescence reaction for extended periods of time (half-life 4–5 h).

Luciferase assays are ideal for HTS *(63)*. The reporter gene is not endogenously expressed in mammalian cells; the enzymatic assay is highly sensitive, quantitative, rapid, easy, reproducible, and safe.

Usually, commercially available reagents are used, which contain an optimized mixture of luciferin, ATP, Coenzyme A, and cell lysis buffer, specially designed for batch-processing systems using high-density microplates. In uHTS projects, where a large number of processed plates might have to wait in stackers before measurement, a long signal half-life is important, so "glow" reagents are generally used. The primary drawback of the luciferase system is that its substrate luciferin does not enter cells efficiently; thereby a cell lysis step is needed to allow exposure of the enzyme to the substrate, which is clearly associated to one of the main sources of intra-plate variability in luciferase assays. Microplate orbital mixing using commercially available mixers improves assay readouts by increasing maximal signal and minimizing variability, thereby improving assay precision *(64)*. Recent versions of HTS "glow luciferase" reagents have been optimized for reducing the effects of incomplete mixing and capillary action (wicking) often seen in rounded square wells, without decreasing sensitivity.

Different GPCRs signaling pathways can be monitored, but reporters have been mainly and extensively used to measure modulation of Gs–Gi coupling by means of cAMP-responsive elements. For Gi-coupled receptors, forskolin is used to stimulate adenylyl cyclase, which leads to an increase in intracellular cAMP levels and transcriptional activation of the luciferase reporter. The Gi receptor stimulation with a specific ligand (agonist) leads to a reduction of forskolin-stimulated luciferase expression and the resulting luminescence signal due to the negative coupling of the receptor to adenylyl cyclase.

Luciferase assays have been successfully developed, validated, and optimized for their application in automated HTS for a variety of GPCRs, including the "low tractable" families B *(65)* and C *(66)* GPCRs. Assays can be optimized to look for competitive agonists and antagonists as well as positive allosteric modulators.

The potential disadvantages of reporter assays for HTS is the high hit rate in antagonist mode (inhibition assays or "decreasing signal" assays) due to potential cytotoxicity of compounds during the long incubation time (typically from 4 to 16 h). For that reason, reporter assays are more frequently used for agonists than for antagonist screens. As the technology measures downstream events in the receptor signaling pathway, reporter gene assays can also have a high rate of false positives (>1%). This is overcomed by evaluating primary hits in specificity assays (i.e., same cell line used for HTS, bearing the reporter construction but not the overexpressed target) which are usually run in parallel with the primary assay at the steps of dose–response experiments.

Although it can be target and cell line dependent, luciferase reporter assays usually exhibit high S/B ratios (from 5 to 40) and low coefficient of variation leading to very robust assays with high Z' values (typically >0.7). **Table 7** summarizes general features and statistical parameters of a reporter gene assay screening campaign conducted at GSK.

Table 7
A typical GPCR reporter gene assay HTS campaign

Reporter gene assay	Plate type	Assay volume	Median Z'	Average Z'	S/N	Compounds tested	Wells/day	Cell type	Reader
GLP-1 agonists and positive allosteric modulators	384	15 μL	0.72	0.70	59	1.1 M	30 K in both assay modes	CHO/6CRE-Luc GLP1	Leadseeker

Although very sensitive, assay miniaturization beyond 384-well plates is generally difficult as a consequence of evaporation issues due to the long incubation time. Reporter gene assays are usually highly sensitive and very robust. This particular screen was designed to look for positive allosteric modulators as well as agonists, on the same assay. Both types of compounds were identified.

3. Conclusions

The search for drugs that modulate the activity of GPCRs started several decades ago, even before scientists understood the molecular nature of these receptors. Over the years, GPCRs have become one of the most important molecular targets for drug discovery. In this chapter we have covered many types of assays that have been traditionally used by screening groups in the pharmaceutical industry. We have also tried to describe the current trends on GPCR assay technologies and the rationale behind those changes. It is important to mention that the paper has not attempted to cover all assays available and we have focussed on describing those where we have personal experience. It is also important to highlight that the latest technologies developed are based not only on improvements on technological advances, but more importantly based on a better scientific understanding of the molecular mechanism by which GPCRs activate intracellular events. We believe that these scientific advances together with the appropriate development of assays for HTS will result in the discovery of novel classes of drugs with more specific mechanisms of action and will eventually yield better and safer drugs.

Acknowledgments

We thank many of our colleagues at GSK that continuously work in the generation of reagent, the development of assays , and the performance of HTS for GPCRs. The generation of the HTS data, the hits, the leads, and the candidates identified would have been impossible without the coordinated effort of all those scientists in many different GSK locations throughout the world. Specially, we thank Robert Hertzberg and Thomas Meek for their continuous support over the years.

References

1. Venter, J.C., Adams, M.D., Myers, E.W., et al. (2001) The sequence of the human genome. *Science* **291**, 1304–1351.
2. Drews, J. (2000) Drug discovery: a historical perspective. *Science* **287**, 1960–1964.
3. Ma, P., and Zemmel, R. (2002) Value of novelty? *Nat. Rev. Drug Discov.* **1**, 571–572.
4. Overington, J.P., Al-Lazikani, B., and Hopkins, A.L. (2006) How many drug targets are there? *Nat. Rev. Drug Discov.* **5**, 993–996.
5. Foord, S.M., Bonner, T.I., Neubig, R.R., Rosser, E.M., Pin, J.P., Davenport, A.P., Spedding, M., and Harmar, A.J. (2005) International union of pharmacology. XLVI G protein-coupled receptor list. *Pharmacol. Rev.* **57**, 279–288.

6. Neubig, R.R., Spedding, M., Kenakin, T., and Christopoulos, A. (2003) International Union of Pharmacology Committee on Receptor Nomenclature and Drug Classification. XXXVIII Update on terms and symbols in quantitative pharmacology *Pharmacol. Rev.* **55**, 597–606.
7. Jacoby, E., Bouhelal, R., Gerspacher, M., and Seuwen, K. (2006) The 7TM G Protein-Coupled Receptor Target Family. *Chem. Med. Chem.* **1**, 760–782.
8. Wieland, T., and Michel, M. (2005) Can a GDP-liganded G protein be active? *Mol. Pharmacol.* **68**, 559–562.
9. Milligan, G., and Kostenis, E. (2006) Heterotrimeric G proteins: a short history. *Br. J. Pharmacol.* **147**(Suppl 1), S46–S55.
10. Lefkowitz, R.J., and Shenoy, S.K. (2005) Transduction of receptor signals by beta-arrestins. *Science* **308**, 512–517.
11. Hertzberg, R., and Pope, A.J. (2000) High-throughput screening: new technology for the 21st century. *Curr. Opin. Chem. Biol.* **4**, 445–451.
12. Ramm, P. (1999) Imaging systems in assay screening. *Drug Discov. Today* **4**,401–410.
13. Rose, D. (1999) Micro-dispensing technologies in drug discovery. *Drug Discov. Today* **4**, 411–419.
14. Labcyte home page: http://www.labcyte.com/Index.aspx?MenuID=1000143, *Echo R Liquid Handling System.*
15. Eglen, R.M., Bosse, R., and Reisine T. (2007) Emerging concepts of guanine nucleotide-binding protein-coupled receptor (GPCR) function and implications for High Throughput Screening. *Assay and Drug Develop Technol.* **5**, 425–451.
16. Moore, K., and Rees, S. (2001). Cell-based versus isolated target screening: how lucky do you feel? *J. Biomol. Screen.* **6**, 69–74.
17. Cook, N.D. (1996). Scintillation proximity assay: a versatile high-throughput screening technology. *Drug Discov. Today* **1**, 287–294.
18. Kahl, S., Hubbard, F.R., Sittampalam, G.S., and Zock, J. (1997) Validation of a High Throughput Scintillation Proximity Assay for 5-Hydroxytryptamine 1E Receptor Binding Activity. *J. Biomol. Screen.* **2**, 33–40.
19. Bossé, R., Garlick, R., Brown, B., and Menard, L. (1998) Development of Non-separation Binding and Functional Assays for G Protein-Coupled Receptors for High Throughput Screening: Pharmacological Characterization of the Immobilized CCR5 Receptor on FlashPlate. *J. Biomol. Screen.* **3**, 285–292.
20. Green, A., Walls, S., Wise, A., Green, R.H., Martin, A.M., and Marshall, F.H. (2000) Characterization of [^{3}H]-CGP54626A binding to heterodimeric $GABA_B$ receptors stably expressed in mammalian cells. *Br. J. Pharmacol.* **131**, 1766–1774.
21. Bylund, D., Deupree, J.D., and Toews, M.L. (2004) Radioligand-binding methods for membrane preparations and intact cells. *Methods Mol. Biol.* **259**, 1–28.
22. Ahsen, O.V., Schmidt, A., Klotz, M., and Parczyk, K. (2006) Assay Concordance between SPA and TR-FRET in high-throughput screening. *J. Biomol. Screen.* **11**, 606–616.
23. Zhang, J.H. (1999) A simple statistical parameter for use in evaluation and validation of high throughput screening assays. *J. Biomol. Screen.* **4**, 67–73.
24. Harrison, C., and Traynor, J.R. (2003) The [(35)S] GTPgammaS binding assay: approaches and applications in pharmacology. *Life Sciences* **74**, 489–508.
25. Ferrer, M., Kolodin, G.D., Zuck, P., Peltier, R., Berry, K., Mandala, S., Rosen, H., Ota, H., Ozaki, S., Inglese, J., and Strulovice, B. (2003) A Fully Automated [^{35}S-GTPγS] Scintillation proximity sssay for the high-throughput screening of Gi-linked G protein-coupled receptors. *Assay and Drug Develop. Technol.* **1**, 261–273.
26. Johnson, E.N., Shi, X., Cassaday, J., Ferrer, M., Strulovici, B., and Kunapuli, P. (2008) A 1,536-well [(35)S] GTPgammaS scintillation proximity binding assay for ultra-high-throughput screening of an orphan Galphai-coupled GPCR. *Assay and Drug Develop. Technol.* **6**, 327–337.
27. Yan, J.H., Li, Q.Y., Boutin, J.A., Renard, M.P., Ding, Y.X., Hao, X.J., Zhao, W.M., and Wang, M.W. (2008) The high-throughput screening of novel antagonists on melanin-concentrating hormone receptor. *Acta Pharmacol. Sinica* **29**, 752–758.
28. Windh, R.T., and Manning, D.R. (2002) Analysis of G protein activation in Sf9 and mammalian cells by agonist-promoted [^{35}S-GTPγS] binding. *Methods Enzymol.* **344**, 3–14.
29. Wang, D., Raehal, K., Bilski, E., and Sadeée, W. (2001) Inverse agonists and neutral antagonists at μ opioid receptor (MOR): possible role of basal receptor signalling in narcotic dependence. *J. Neurochem.* 77, 1590–1600.

30. Pagliaro, L., and Praestegaard, M. (2001) Transfected cell lines as tools for high throughput screening: a call for standards. *J. Biomol. Screen.* **6**, 133–136.
31. Kost, T., Condreay, J.P, Ames, R.S, Rees, S., and Romanos, M.A. (2007) Implementation of BacMam virus gene delivery technology in a drug discovery setting. *Drug Discov. Today* **12**, 396–403.
32. Soudijn, W., Wijngaarden, I.V., and Ijzerman, A.P. (2004) Allosteric modulation of G protein-coupled receptors: perspectives and recent developments. *Drug Discov. Today* **9**, 752–758.
33. Pinkerton, A.B., Cube, R.V., Hutchinson, J.H., James, J.K, Gardner, M.F., Rowe, B.A., Schaffhauser, H., Rodriguez, D.E., Campbell, U.C., Daggett, L.P., and Vernier, J.-M. (2005) Allosteric potentiators of the metabotropic glutamate receptor 2 (mGlu2). Part 3: Identification and biological activity of indanone containing mGluR2 receptor potentiators. *Bioorganic Med. Chem. Lett.* **15**, 1565–1571.
34. Chambers, C., Smith, F., Williams, C., Marcos, S., Liu, S.M., Hayter, P., Ciaramella, G., Keighley, W., Gribbon, P., and Sewing, A. (2003) Measuring intracellular calcium fluxes in high throughput mode. *Comb. Chem. High Throughput Screen.* **6**, 355–362.
35. Offermanns, S., and Simon, M.I. (1995) G alpha 15 and G alpha 16 couple a wide variety of receptors to phospholipase C. *J. Biol. Chem.* **270**, 15175–15180.
36. Kostensis, E.J. (2002) Potentiation of GPCRs-signalling via membrane targeting of G protein alpha subunits. *Receptors Signal Transduct.* **22**, 267–281.
37. Ungrin, M.D., Singh, L.M., Stocco, R., Sas, D.E., and Abramovitz, M. (1999) An Automated aequorin luminescence-based functional calcium assay for G protein-coupled receptors. *Anal. Biochem.* **272**, 34–42.
38. Le Poul, E., Hisada, S., Mizuguchi, Y., Dupriez, V.J., Burgeon, E., and Detheux, M. (2002) Adaptation of aequorin functional assay to high throughput screening. *J. Biomol. Screen.***7**, 57–65.
39. Kariv, I., Stevens, M.E., Behrens, D.L., and Oldenburg, K.R. (1999) High throughput quantification of cAMP production mediated by activation of seven transmembrane domain receptors. *J. Biomol. Screen.* **4**, 27–32.
40. Kemp, D.M., George, S.E., Kent, T.C., Bungay, P.J., and Naylor, L.H. (2002) The effect of ICRE on screening methods involving CRE-mediated reporter gene expression. *J. Biomol. Screen.* **7**, 141–148.
41. Gabriel, D., Vernier, M., Pfeifer, M.J., Dasen, B., Tenaillon, L., and Bouhelal, R. (2003) High throughput screening technologies for direct cyclic AMP measurement. *Assay Drug Develop. Technol.* **1**, 291–303.
42. Golla, R., and Seethala, R. (2002) A homogeneous enzyme fragment complementation cyclic AMP screen for GPCR agonist. *J. Biomol. Screen.* **7**, 515–525.
43. Weber, M., Muthusubramaniam, L., Murray, J., Hudak, E., Kornienko, O., Johnson, E.N., Strulovici, B., and Kunapuli, P. (2007) Ultra-high-throughput screening for antagonists of a Gi-coupled receptor in a 2.2-μl 3456-well plate format cAMP Assay. *Assay Drug Dev. Technol.* **5**, 117–125.
44. Ullman, E.F., Kirakossiona, H., and Singh, S. (1994) Luminescent oxygen channelling immunoassay: measurement of particle binding kinetics by chemiluminescence. *Proc. Natl. Acad. Sci. USA* **91**, 5426–5430.
45. Elster, L., Elling, C., and Heding, A. (2007) Bioluminescence resonance energy transfer as a screening assay: focus on partial and inverse agonism. *J. Biomol. Screen.* **12**, 41–49.
46. Kasia, P., and Xie, H. (2006) A comparison of PerkinElmer's LANCE cAMP assay performance to that of state of the art competitive technologies. *PE- Application Notes.* http://las.perkinelmer.com/content/Application Notes/APP LANCEcAMPComparison.pdf 1–8.
47. Claing, A., Laporte, S.A, Caron, M.G., and Lefkowitz, R.J. (2002). Endocytosis of G protein-coupled receptors: roles of G protein-coupled receptor kinases and β-arrestin proteins. *Prog. Neurobiol.* **66**, 61–79.
48. Reiter, E., and Lefkowitz, R.J. (2006). GRKs and beta-arrestins: roles in receptor silencing, trafficking and signalling. *Trends Endocrinol. Metab.* **17**, 159–165.
49. Ahn, S., Nelson, C., Garrison, T.R., Miller, W.E., and Lefkowitz, R.L. (2002) Desensitization, internalization, and signalling functions of β-arrestins demonstrated by RNA interference. *Proc. Natl. Acad. Sci. USA* **18**, 1740–1744.
50. Ren, X-R., Reiter E., Ahn, S., Kim, J., Chen, W., and Lefkowitz, R.J. (2004) Different G protein-coupled receptor kinases govern G protein and beta-arrestin-mediated signalling of V2 vasopressin receptor. *Proc. Natl. Acad. Sci. USA* **102**, 1448–1453.
51. Kang, J., Shi, Y., Xiang, B., Qu, B., Su, W., Zhu, M., Zhang, M., Bao, G., Wang, F., and

Zhang, X. (2005). A nuclear function of β-arrestin 1 in GPCR signalling regulation of histone acetylation and gene transcription. *Cell* **123**, 833–847.

52. Violin, J.D., and Lefkowith, R.J. (2007) β-arrestin-biased ligands at seven-transmembrane receptors. *Trends Pharmacol. Sci.* **28**, 417–422.
53. Wei, H., Ahn, S., Shenoy, S.K., Hunyady, L., Luttrell, L.M., and Lefkowitz, R. J. (2003) Independent beta-arrestin 2 and G protein-mediated pathways for angiotensin II activation of extracellular signal-regulated kinases 1 and 2. *Proc. Natl. Acad. Sci. USA* **100**, 10782–10787.
54. Kohout, T.A., Nicholas, S.L., Perry, S.J., Reinhart, G., Junger, S., and Struthers R.S. (2004) Differential desensitization, receptor phosphorylation, beta-arrestin recruitment, and ERK1/2 activation by the two endogenous ligands for the CC chemokine receptor 7. *J. Biol. Chem.* **279**, 23214–23222.
55. Bruns, R., Chhum, S., Dinh, A.T., Doerr, H., Dunn, N.R., Ly, Y.T., Mitman, C.L., Rickards, H.D., Sol, C., Wan, E.W., and Raffa, R.B. (2006) A potential novel strategy to separate therapeutic- and side-effects that are mediated via the same receptor: β-arrestin 2/G protein coupling antagonists. *J. Clin. Pharm. Ther.* **31**, 119–128.
56. Conway, B.R., Minor, L.M., Xu, J.Z., Gunnet, J.W., DeBiasio, R., Dándrea, M.R., Rubin, R., Debiasio, R., Giuliano, K., Zhou, L., and Demarest, K.T. (1999) Quantification of G protein receptor internalization using G protein-coupled receptor-green fluorescent protein conjugates with the ArrayScan^{TM} high-content screening systems. *J. Biomol. Screen.* **4**, 75–86.
57. Bertrand, L., Parent, S., Caron, M., Legault, M., Joly, E.N., Angers, S., Bouvier, M., Brown, M., Benoit, H., Houle, B., and Ménard, L. (2002) The BRET2/arrestin assay in stable recombinant cells: a platform to screen for compounds that interact with G protein-coupled receptors (GPCRs). *J. Receptor Signal Transduct. Res.* **22**, 533–541.
58. Wehrman, T.S., Casipit, C.L., Gewertz, N.M., and Blau, H.M. (2005) Enzymatic detection of protein translocation. *Nat. Methods* **2**, 521–527.
59. de Wet, J.R., Wood, K.V., deLuca, M., Helinski, D.R., and Subramini, S. (1987) Firefly luciferase gene: structure and expression in mammalian cells. *Mol. Cell. Biol.* **7**, 725–737.
60. Wilson, T., and Hastings, J.W. (1998). Bioluminescence. *Annu. Rev. Cell. Dev. Biol.* **14**, 197–230.
61. Athwal, G.K., El-Kholy, E.O., and Cass, A.E.G. (1991) *Amplified Bioluminescence Assays.* In: Bioluminescence and Chemiluminescence Current Status. Stanley, P.E., and Kricka, L.J. (eds.), pp. 67–70.
62. Wood, K.V. (1998) The chemistry of bioluminescence reporter assays. *Promega Notes* **65**, 14–20.
63. Kent, T.C., Thompson, K.S., and Naylor, L.H. (2005) Development of a generic dual-reporter gene assay for screening G protein-coupled receptors. *J. Biomol. Screen.* **10**, 437–447.
64. Hancock, M., Medina, M.N., Smith, B.M., and Orth, A.P. (2007) Microplate orbital mixing improves high-throughput cell-based assay readouts. *J. Biomol. Screen.* **12**, 140–144.
65. Chen, D., Liao, J., Li, N., Zhou, C., Wang, G., Zhang, R., Zhang, S., Lin, L., Chen, K., Xie, X., Nan, F., Young, A., and Wang, M.W. (2007) A nonpeptidic agonist of glucagon-like peptide 1 receptors with efficacy in diabetic db/db mice. *Proc. Natl. Acad. Sci. USA* **104**, 943–948.
66. Terstapen, G.S., Giacometti, A., Ballini, E., and Aldegheri, L. (2000) Development of a functional reporter gene HTS assay for the identification of mGluR7 modulators. *J. Biomol. Screen.* **5**, 255–261.

Chapter 3

GPCR Signaling: Understanding the Pathway to Successful Drug Discovery

Christine Williams and Stephen J. Hill

Summary

Modulators of G protein-coupled receptors (GPCRs) form a key area for the pharmaceutical industry, representing ~27% of all Food and Drug Administration (FDA)-approved drugs. Consequently, there are a wide variety of *in vitro* plate-based screening technologies that enable the measurement of compound affinity, potency, and efficacy for almost every type of GPCR. However, to maximize success it is prudent to ensure that (i) the most suitable assay formats are identified, (ii) they are configured optimally to detect the desired compound activity, and (iii) that they form a basis for predicting clinical effects. To achieve this, an understanding of the pathways and mechanisms of receptor activation relevant to the disease mechanism, as well as the benefits and/or limitations of the specific techniques, is key.

Key words: Signaling, G protein, G protein-coupled receptor, Screen, Drug discovery.

1. Introduction

There are a variety of receptor and ligand types, with receptors ranging in structure from single transmembrane to multiple transmembrane regions and ligands ranging from small amino acids to larger peptide or protein molecules. Since the pioneering work of Langley *(1)* and Ehrlich *(2)* at the beginning of the twentieth century, receptors and especially G protein-coupled receptors (GPCRs) have grown to be one of the most important areas of research in the pharmaceutical industry, representing a significant portion of approved drugs *(3)*. However, one of the key challenges faced in this context is how to respond to the increasing complexity of GPCR pharmacology in order to identify novel drugs with the desired pharmacological profile *(4)*. There are a number of

Wayne R. Leifert (ed.), *G Protein-Coupled Receptors in Drug Discovery, vol. 552*

Book doi: 10.1007/978-1-60327-317-6_3

levels of complexity in GPCR pharmacology that are important in this respect. For example, ligand effects were historically categorized into two main forms: (i) agonists and partial agonists which bind and promote a positive conformational change that results in G protein activation and (ii) neutral antagonists which bind but do not in themselves cause any modulation of receptor function. However, over the last two decades, it has become apparent that this is insufficient to describe GPCR molecular pharmacology and evidence supporting the existence of inverse agonists (which bind to the receptor and negatively modulate constitutive receptor function) *(5)*, as well as allosteric ligands (which are distinct in that they evoke their effects indirectly via a discrete binding pocket and that can cause a variety of effects, i.e., positive, negative or modulatory) *(6)* is now readily available. Furthermore, receptor dimerization, agonist dependent trafficking, and G protein-independent signaling are all areas that have emerged in recent years *(7, 8)* that highlight the considerations that must be addressed. Whilst these factors may provide real opportunities for cell and tissue-specific therapeutics, they clearly present the pharmaceutical industry with a practical challenge in deciding the best screening strategy. Therefore, in this overview, we discuss some of the issues that need to be addressed in a successful drug discovery program aimed at GPCR targets.

2. GPCR Signal Transduction

2.1. G Protein-Mediated Signaling

Classical GPCR pharmacology indicates that receptor activation occurs via agonist-induced conformational changes in the receptor which, upon interaction with a heterotrimeric G protein (composed of α, β, and γ subunits), initiates a cascade of events known as the G protein cycle (**Fig. 1**). Upon agonist binding to the receptor, the inactive α subunit, which is associated with the βγ subunits, is activated through exchange of GDP for GTP at the guanine nucleotide binding site *(9)*. This results in dissociation of the active α subunit from the receptor and the βγ subunits and enables interaction with specific effector proteins (as indicated below). Intrinsic GTPase activity within the α subunit then hydrolyzes GTP to GDP, converting the α subunit back to an inactive conformation that dissociates from the effector protein and reassociates with the βγ subunits.

There are four major types of G protein that can be identified by a preferential interaction with different signaling effector molecules (**Fig. 2**) *(10)*. Upon activation, Gs and Gi/o G proteins are characterized as resulting in an increase or decrease in cAMP, respectively. This is achieved through modulation of the adenylyl

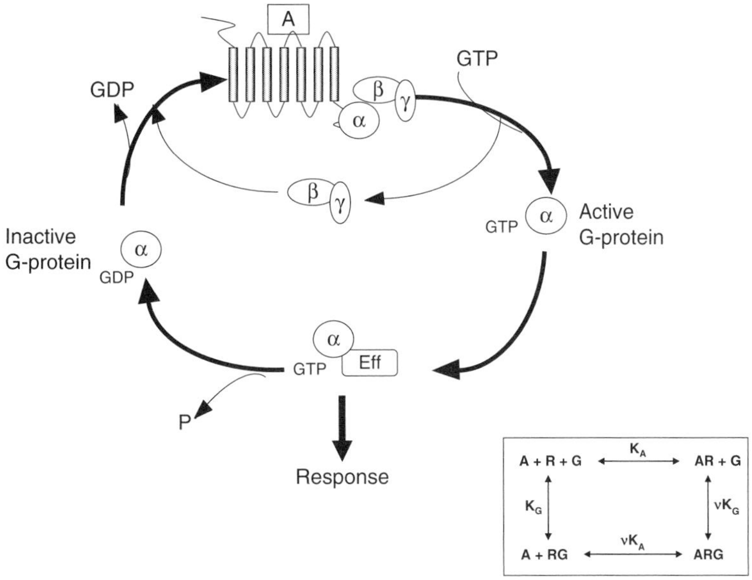

Fig. 1. The G protein cycle. Following agonist binding to a GPCR, a cascade of events known as the G protein cycle is initiated. This process involves changes in the conformation of the receptor and interaction with a heterotrimeric G protein which consists of three subunits (α, β, γ). In the G protein cycle the α subunit is found in three conformational states: (i) an inactive state with GDP bound, α_{GDP}; (ii) a state where the guanine nucleotide binding site is empty, α; and (iii) an active state with GTP bound, α_{GTP}. The binding of an agonist causes a conformational change in the receptor which facilitates interaction with the G protein and thereby promotes formation of a ternary complex. Subsequently, GTP is bound to the empty guanine nucleotide binding site of the α subunit, causing dissociation of the α subunit from the agonist-occupied receptor and the βγ subunits. The α subunit, in the active state, now interacts with specific effector proteins which results in changes in the concentration of intracellular signaling molecules (e.g., cAMP and Ca^{2+}). The intrinsic GTPase activity of the α subunit hydrolyzes GTP to GDP, resulting in a conformational change in the α subunit such that the α subunit dissociates from the effector protein. The inactive α subunit now reassociates with the βγ subunits and the cycle is repeated if an appropriate agonist-occupied receptor is encountered. Formation of the ternary complex can be explained by the equilibrium constants K_A (which describes binding of agonist to receptor) and K_G (the association of free receptor with G protein) and ν (the cooperativity factor describing the allosteric effect of G protein-induced conformational changes on the agonist binding equilibrium).

cyclase family of enzymes, which convert adenosine triphosphate (ATP) to cAMP and inorganic pyrophosphate. Further regulation of these enzymes is achieved via Ca^{2+} and calmodulin and sequestration of active $G_{\alpha s}$ molecules by the $\beta\gamma_i$ dimers. In addition to adenylyl cyclase regulation, Go G proteins have also been reported to modulate ion channel activity. In contrast, the Gq G proteins modulate the enzyme phospholipase C β (PLCβ) which regulates intracellular signaling molecules such as phosphatidyl inositol biphosphate (PIP2), inositol triphosphate (IP3), and intracellular Ca^{2+}. Finally, the G12/13 G proteins are primarily involved in Rho-mediated responses, although they have also been linked to the Gq pathway. Once produced, these signal transduction molecules are able to bind to protein kinases within the cell, initiating phosphorylation events that regulate target enzymes (such as mitogen-activated protein kinase, MAPK) and eventually the

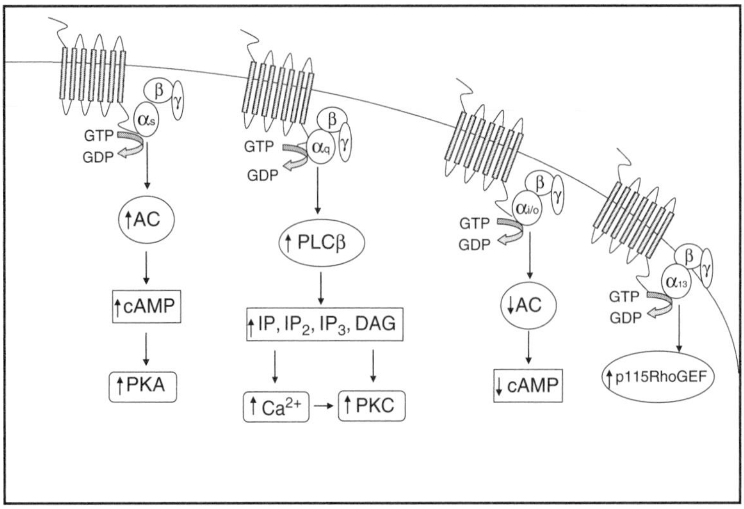

Fig. 2. Typical G protein-mediated receptor signaling events. Upon activation GPCRs can initiate a diverse range of signaling cascades. These are predominated by, but not limited to, heterotrimeric G protein-mediated events. An active agonist/receptor complex is able to interact with these G proteins and facilitate their activation via exchange of GDP for GTP at the α subunit. Following G protein activation, the dissociated α subunit and βγ dimers modulate activity of effector proteins that control the level of intracellular signaling molecules. These second messengers modulate protein kinases and transcription factors, which ultimately result in the observed functional response of the cell. The Gs and Gi/o G proteins are generally characterized by a positive or negative effect, respectively, on adenylyl cyclase and cAMP. The Gq G proteins are associated with a positive effect on phospholipase C β (PLCβ) and subsequent levels of phosphatidyl inositol biphosphate (PIP2), inositol triphosphate (IP3), and Ca^{2+}. In contrast the G12/13 G proteins are less well characterized but are often associated with a positive effect on Rho-mediated events.

physiological response of the cell. Whilst many receptors are typically characterized as interacting with one preferred type of G protein, it is generally accepted that many GPCRs can activate multiple G proteins, leading to agonist-dependent trafficking *(11)*.

Like all signaling events, receptor activation cascades are tightly regulated to prevent acute and chronic overstimulation. These events are mediated by PKA and PKC (often termed heterologous desensitization) or specific G protein-coupled receptor kinases (GRKs) and β-arrestin (often termed homologous desensitization) *(12, 13)*. In both cases, the kinase phosphorylates key intracellular residues of the receptor, which either directly or indirectly prevents interaction with the G protein. In general, these phosphorylated receptor complexes are internalized via clathrin-coated vesicles and through acidic endosomes, where the receptor is dephosphorylated by phosphatases, thereby enabling re-sensitization. The receptor is then either recycled to the cell surface or degraded in lysosomes. However, there is now emerging evidence that some GRKs may achieve desensitization via a phosphorylation-independent event and that some GRK-mediated desensitization is agonist independent *(14, 15)*, providing further complexity to this regulatory event.

2.2. G Protein-Independent Signaling

In addition to the events described above, it is becoming clear that GPCRs can elicit downstream signaling responses that are mediated independent of heterotrimeric G proteins *(16–18)*. Although β-arrestin has classically been associated with the desensitization and internalization of GPCRs, it is becoming clear that this GPCR-interacting protein may have an important role in orchestrating both the location of receptors within particular signaling domains of a cell and their ability to trigger a range of different responses. For example, there is an increasing body of evidence to suggest that the activation of the p42/44 MAP kinase pathway can be achieved via a β-arrestin mediated response, independent of any G proteins *(16, 19–22)*. However, this phenomenon is not limited to β-arrestin and there are more examples emerging in which GPCR-interacting proteins are directly mediating signaling events. For example, Homer has been demonstrated to have an important role in clustering metabotropic glutamate receptors at the postsynaptic density in neurons of the central nervous system and to orchestrate signaling to a range of signaling proteins such as the inositol-1,4,5-trisphosphate receptor *(23)*. Similar roles are played for a range of GPCRs by other scaffolding proteins such as post-synaptic density-95 (PSD-95), caveolin-1, A-kinase-anchoring proteins, and the Na/K exchange protein *(7, 24–27)*.

3. Signaling in the Context of Screen Design

Receptor-mediated events within the cell are clearly complex, with the possibility of any given receptor evoking multiple effects via a combination of G protein and non-G protein-mediated events (**Fig. 3**). This complexity and the potential impact on clinical relevance is nicely illustrated by the human β2-adrenoceptor, which signals through either cyclic AMP accumulation or ERK1/2 phosphorylation *(19, 20, 28)*. At this receptor, the prototypical β-blocker propranolol can act as an inverse agonist on Gs-mediated cyclic AMP accumulation but as an agonist of β-arrestin-mediated ERK1/2 phosphorylation *(19, 20)*. Furthermore, evidence is now accumulating to suggest that antagonist affinities may also vary depending upon the agonist and signaling response used to screen for them *(29, 30)*. Therefore, while measuring these receptor ligand binding and subsequent signal transduction events can be achieved through a variety of label (radiometric, absorbent, fluorescent, and luminescent) and label-free methods *(4, 31)* designing a screen cascade that predicts from *in vitro* plate-based data, *in vitro* tissue-based data, through *in vivo* data to clinical effects requires a full understanding of the pharmacological mechanisms. Recent advancements in systems biology,

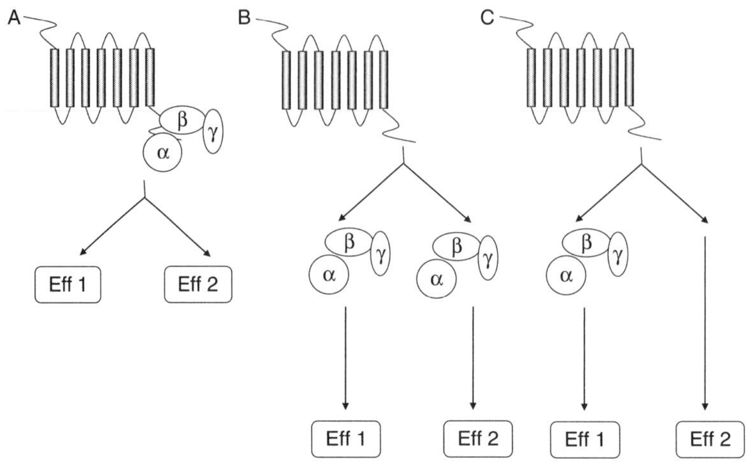

Fig. 3. An illustration of the complexity of GPCR signaling. (**A**) Agonist-induced conformational changes in the receptor result in the activation of a single class of G protein that can modulate the function of two different effectors. (**B**) Agonist-induced conformational changes in the receptor result in the activation of two different species of G protein, which in turn modulate the function of distinct effectors. (**C**) Agonist-induced conformational changes in the receptor result in the activation of a single class of G protein-mediated event and a distinct effect that is not mediated via any G proteins.

the physicochemical modeling of cell signaling pathways and the industry focus on biomarker development are encouraging in this respect *(32–34)*. In addition, analysis of genetic polymorphisms in the population may also provide some indication of pharmacological relevance *(35, 36)*. Although it is rarely possible to fully define the target and the appropriate signaling pathway in the absence of clinical data, there are simple parameters that can be evaluated during screen design, in conjunction with the available information, in order to maximize the chances of success.

3.1. Choosing a Screening Approach

If the receptor is known to activate a number of G proteins and the disease-specific mechanism is not clear, a screening approach that detects multiple pathways can be applied. For example, the temporal difference in a calcium mobilization assay and a cAMP reporter gene assay enables sequential analysis of a phospholipase C- and adenylyl cyclase-mediated signal *(37)*, or the use of some label-free technologies *(38)* can enable parallel signaling analysis. There are hurdles to be considered in either of these cases, namely the potential for additional screening work and the additional complexity in terms of prioritizing compounds for chemistry follow-up. Furthermore, label-free screening is not yet compatible with the level of throughput required for primary screening in most large pharmaceutical companies and the potential for false positives to interfere with medicinal chemistry design is an issue that is as yet to be clarified. However, despite these factors such an approach is worth considering as it does increase the likelihood that chemical start points with the appropriate pharmacology will be identified.

In contrast, when the signaling pathway is understood the situation is clearer with an assay technology that utilizes the appropriate end point being preferable. Surprisingly, this is not always the approach applied in the industry as many screens are prosecuted in a standardized format and/or Gi-coupled targets are deliberately switched to an alternative pathway that facilitates screening without the need for forskolin (required to stimulate the system such that agonist effects can be observed) *(39, 40)*. Such an approach can prove successful, but needs to be employed with caution. Not only could the use of "promiscuous" G proteins lead to a very poor signal window, these approaches may result in chemistry efforts to optimize potential drug candidates with inappropriate clinical pharmacology.

3.2. The Impact of Assay and Reagent Choice

Understanding how the tools employed influence the appropriate detection of any desired pharmacological response is critical. Whilst a full review of all of the relevant considerations and their impact on the pharmacology obtained is beyond the scope of this chapter, two key factors worth highlighting are the cell line and the assay type. For example, in a recombinant receptor system the balance of receptor to signaling molecules and how this equates to receptor occupancy and saturation of the signaling cascade can influence the data obtained. Put simply, a "full" agonist doesn't necessarily need to occupy all receptors to evoke a maximal functional response if all the signaling capacity is saturated before "all" the receptors are occupied. In contrast, for a partial agonist (by default) all the receptors will be occupied and "all" the signaling capacity will still not be achieved. Therefore, if the receptor expression and/or your signaling capacity is too low partial agonists will generally appear as antagonists. However, it is not just partial versus full agonism that is influenced by receptor expression levels. Many receptors will demonstrate constitutive activity when overexpressed and whilst this may be beneficial in terms of observing inverse agonism, it can complicate agonist characterization through the appearance of protean agonism (where an agonist in a quiescent system appears as an inverse agonist in another, as it evokes a conformational change less active than the constitutively active one). A receptor well characterized in this respect is the H3 receptor *(41)*. The combination of constitutive activity, receptor splice variants, and species variations has made preclinical evaluation of H3 ligand pharmacology particularly challenging *(42)*.

The assay of choice can also influence the data observed, for example assays that detect effects lower down the signal transduction cascade have increased potential to identify partial agonists as full, or increase the potency of full agonists, due to amplification of the response *(43)*. A good example of this is the evaluation of the calcitonin C1a-like receptor using a cAMP accumulation assay versus a luciferase reporter gene system *(44)*. Furthermore, some technologies demonstrate a non-linear relationship between receptor activation and signal detection which mask differences in the level of response. This was clearly highlighted by Allen et al. *(45)* when investigating a fluorescence polarization cAMP accumulation assay. Therefore, taking all of these factors into consideration, it is prudent to design the reagent and assay in parallel or employ native/primary cell types in order to ensure that the appropriate pharmacology is identified.

In addition to the effect of receptor expression levels and assay type on observed pharmacology, there is also the influence of the ligand choice. As indicated in the introduction ligands can be classified as being agonists, antagonists, and inverse agonists when acting at the same site as the endogenous hormone or neurotransmitter (i.e., the orthosteric site). However, there is an increasing evidence that GPCRs possess more than one binding site and that drugs acting at a site distinct from the orthosteric site (i.e., at an allosteric site) can influence both the binding of ligands to the orthosteric site as well as triggering intracellular signaling directly from the allosteric site *(46)*. For example, when considering the human β1-adrenoceptor, CGP12177 acts as a neutral antagonist of the orthosteric site but at higher concentrations can trigger intracellular signaling via a secondary site or conformation that is relatively resistant to antagonism by other β-blockers *(30, 47)*. These allosteric effects are not limited to receptor ligands, as the G protein itself can be considered as an allosteric regulator of the orthosteric ligand binding site of the GPCR. The binding affinity of the G protein for the activated receptor (R^*) and its cooperativity factor (ν; the term that describes how effectively G protein binding increases agonist binding to the orthosteric site of the GPCR as a consequence of a G protein-induced conformational change; **Fig. 4**) will determine ultimately the potency of the final measured response. Since G protein binding will alter the conformation of the orthosteric binding site, the effect will not be identical for every agonist. Furthermore, if the GPCR binds to a different G protein in another cell or microdomain within an individual cell, then this has the potential to change the agonist affinity and/or efficacy leading to agonist trafficking *(7)*. Good examples of this are the 5-HT_{2C} receptor *(48)* and the calcium sensing receptor *(49)*.

3.3. The Impact of Kinetics

An appreciation of the impact of assay kinetics on the pharmacological profile obtained is also important. Ensuring that the standard incubation times recommended in manufacturer instructions are appropriate can prove key in determining compound potencies *(50)*. Furthermore, assay kinetics can be particularly important in transient assay formats where antagonists with slow on-rates may appear less potent than predicted (unless a pre-incubation step is included) and may appear non-competitive in Schild analysis *(51, 52)*. Discrepancies due to kinetics may be

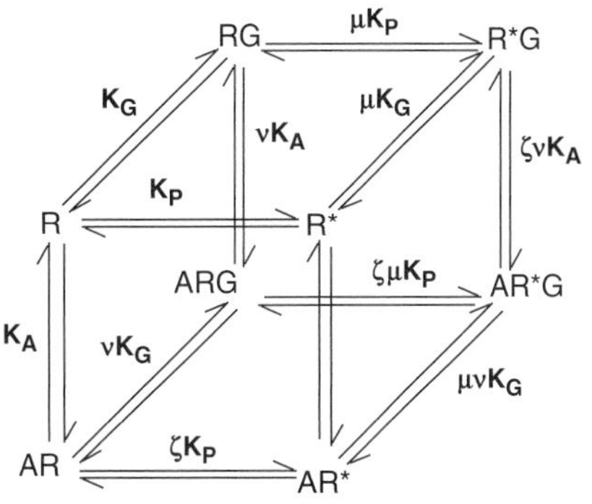

Fig. 4. The eight basic receptor states of a GPCR according to the cubic ternary complex model. The equilibrium constants K_A, K_G, and K_P define the equilibria between agonist and receptor (K_A), receptor and G protein (K_G), or inactive (R) and active (R*) receptors (K_P). The thermodynamic constants μ, ν, and ζ characterize the role played by the different species involved in the equilibrium. The constant ζ determines whether a ligand is an agonist ($\zeta>1$), antagonist ($\zeta=1$), or inverse agonist ($\zeta<1$). The constant μ plays a similar role to ζ and relates to the effect of the G protein being bound. Increasing μ has the effect of making G proteins prefer to bind to R*. The constant ν indicates the effect that R binding to G has on the agonist binding equilibrium. Increasing ν corresponds to an increased ligand preference for binding to a G protein-coupled receptor. Similarly, an increase in ν makes agonist-bound receptors more likely to bind to G proteins.

limited in reporter gene assays, where long incubation times (>4 h) are required for the gene transcription event. This is particularly important when considering how predictive *in vitro* data is in terms of exposure in the clinical setting. Monaghan et al. *(53)* highlighted the importance of this point with their work on the V2 receptor compound, SK&F 101926, which demonstrated that the *in vitro* and *in vivo* studies carried out did not predict for the human clinical data obtained with this compound. In addition, recent work on both the human β1- and β2-adrenoceptors has highlighted substantial stimulation of gene expression (~ 60% of the maximum achieved with a full agonist) for a range of β-blockers that are currently used in clinical practice *(20, 47, 54)*. This effect may be particularly relevant when one considers that these drugs are designed to maintain prolonged receptor occupancy during 24 h once-a-day dosing practice.

4. Conclusions

Drug discovery teams can no longer afford to apply one method to their GPCR screening, or make do with reagents they find "off the shelf." To ensure success is maximized they need to employ *in silico* tools to help identify appropriate targets and mechanisms, they need to carefully consider the pharmacological response they desire and to tailor-make a screen cascade that considers not just the target, but the signaling cascade(s) and level of response.

References

1. Langley, J.N. (1906) On nerve endings and on special excitable substances in cells. *Proc. Roy. Soc.* **B78**, 170–194.
2. Ehrlich, P. (1913) Chemotherapeutics: scientific principles, methods and results. *Lancet* **2**, 445–451.
3. Overington, J.P., Al-Lazikani, B., and Hopkins, A.L. (2006) How many drug targets are there? *Nat. Rev. Drug. Discov.* **5**, 993–996.
4. McLoughlin, D.J., Bertelli, F., and Williams, C. (2007) The A, B, C's of G protein-coupled receptor pharmacology in assay development for HTS. *Expert Opin. Drug Discov.* **2**, 1–17.
5. Kenakin, T. (2004) Efficacy as a vector: the relative prevalence and paucity of inverse agonism. *Mol. Pharmacol.* **65**, 2–11.
6. Christopolous, A. (2002) Allosteric binding sites on cell-surface receptors: novel targets for drug discovery. *Nat. Rev. Drug Discov.* **1**, 198–210.
7. Hill, S.J. (2006) G protein-coupled receptors: past, present and future. *Br. J. Pharmacol.* **147**, S27–S37.
8. Schulte, G., and Levy, F.O. (2007) Novel aspects of G protein-coupled receptor signalling – different ways to achieve specificity. *Acta Physiol.* **190**, 33–38.
9. Leifert, W.R., Aloia, A.L., Bucco, O., and McMurchie, E.J. (2005) GPCR-induced dissociation of G protein subunits in early stage signal transduction. *Mol. Memb. Biol.* **22**, 507–517.
10. Cabera-Vera, T.M., Vanhauwe, J., Thomas, T.O., et al. (2003) Insights into G protein structure, function and regulation. *Endocr. Rev.* **24**, 765–781.
11. Hermans, E. (2003) Biochemical and pharmacological control of the multiplicity of coupling at G protein-coupled receptors. *Pharmacol. Ther.* **99**, 24–44.
12. Moore, C.A.C., Milano, S.K., and Benovic, J.L. (2007) Regulation of receptor trafficking by GRKs and arrestins. *Annu. Rev. Physiol.* **69**, 19.1–19.32.
13. Lefkowitz, R.J. (1998) G protein-coupled receptors: III. New Roles for receptor kinases and β-arrestins in receptor signalling and desensitization. *J. Biol. Chem.* **273**, 18677–18680.
14. Ferguson, S.S.G. (2007) Phosphorylation-independent attenuation of GPCR signalling. *Trends Pharmacol. Sci.* **28**, 173–179.
15. Barak, L.S., Wilbanks, A.M., and Caron, M.G. Constitutive desensitization: a new paradigm for G protein-coupled receptor regulation. *Assay Drug Dev. Tech.* (2003) **1**(2), 339–346.
16. Seta, K., Nanamori, M., Modrall, J.G., Neubig, R.R., and Sadoshima J (2002) AT1 receptor mutant lacking heterotrimeric G protein coupling activates the Src-Ras-ERK pathway without nuclear translocation of ERKs. *J. Biol. Chem.* **277**, 9268–9277.
17. Luttrell, L.M., Roudabush, F.L., Choy, E.W., Miller, W.E., Field, M.E., Pierce, K., and Lefkowitz, R.J. (2001) Activation and targetting of extracellular-signal-regulated kinases by β-arrestin scaffolds. *Proc. Natl. Acad. Sci. USA* **98**, 2449–2454.
18. Wei, H., Ahn, S., Shenoy, S.K., Karnik, S.S., Hunyadi, L., Luttrell, L.M., and Lefkowitz, R.J. (2003) Independent β-arrestin-2 and G protein-mediated pathways for angiotensin II activation of extracellular signal regulated kinases 1 and 2. *Proc. Natl. Acad. Sci. USA* **100**, 10782–10787.
19. Azzi, M., Charest, P.G., Angers, S., Rousseau, G., Kahout, T., Bouvier, M., and Pineyro, G. (2003) Beta-arrestin-mediated activation of MAPK by inverse agonists reveals distinct active conformations for G protein-coupled receptors. *Proc. Natl. Acad. Sci. USA* **100**, 11406–11411.
20. Baker, J.G., Hall, I.P., and Hill, S.J. (2003) Agonist and inverse agonist actions of β-blockers at the human β2-adrenoceptor provide evidence for agonist-directed signalling. *Mol. Pharmacol.* **63**, 1357–1369.
21. Gesty-Palmer, D., Chen, M., Reiter, E., Ahn, S., Nelson, C.D., Wang, S., Eckhardt, A.E., Cowan, C.L., Spurney, R.F., Luttrell, L.M., and Lefkowitz, R.J. (2006) Distinct beta-arrestin- and G protein-dependent pathways for parathyroid hormone receptor-stimulated ERK1/2 activation. *J. Biol. Chem.* **281**, 10856–10864.

22. Wisler, J.W., DeWire, S.M., Whalen, E.J., Wiolin, J.D., Drake, M.T., Ahn, S., Shenoy, S.K., and Lefkowitz, R.J. (2007) A unique mechanism of beta-blocker action: carvedilol stimulates beta-arrestin signalling. *Proc. Natl. Acad. Sci. USA* **104**, 16657–16662.
23. Duncan, R.S., Sung-Yong, H., and Koulen, P. (2005) Effects of Vesl/Homer proteins on intracellular signalling. *Exp. Biol. Med.* **230**, 527–535.
24. Gines, S., Ciruela, F., Burgueno, J., Casado, V., Canela, E.I., Mallol, J., Lluis, C., and Franco, R. (2001) Involvement of caveolin in ligand-induced recruitment and internalization of A_1 adenosine receptor and adenosine deaminase in an epithelial cell line. *Mol. Pharmacol.* **59**, 1314–1323.
25. Fraser, J.D., Cong, M., Kim, J., Rollins, E.N., Daaka, Y., Lefkowitz, R.J., and Scott, J.D. (2000) Assembly of an A kinase-anchoring protein-β2-adrenergic receptor complex facilitates receptor phosphorylation and signalling. *Curr. Biol.* **10**, 409–412.
26. Ostrom, R.S., and Insel, P.A. (2004) The evolving role of lipid rafts and caveolae in G protein-coupled receptor signalling: implications for molecular pharmacology. *Br. J. Pharmacol.* **143**, 235–245.
27. Hall, R.A., Premont, R.T., Chow, C.W., Blitzer, J.T., Pitcher, J.A., Claing, A., Stoffel, R.H., Barak, L.S., Shenolikar, S., Weinman, E.J., Grinstein, S., and Lefowitz, R.J. (1998). The β2-adrenergic receptor interacts with the Na^+/H^+ exchanger regulatory factor to control Na^+/H^+ exchange. *Nature* **392**, 626–630.
28. Galendrin, S., and Bouvier, M. (2006) Distinct signalling profiles of the β1 and β2 adrenergic receptor ligands toward adenylyl cyclase and mitogen-activated protein kinase reveals the pleuridimensionality of efficacy. *Mol. Pharmacol.* **70**, 1575–1584.
29. Baker, J.G., Hall, I.P., and Hill, S.J. (2003) Influence of agonist efficacy and receptor phosphorylation on antagonist affinity measurements: differences between second messenger and reporter gene responses. *Mol. Pharmacol.* **64**, 679–688.
30. Baker, J.G., and Hill, S.J. (2007) Multiple GPCR conformations and signalling pathways: implications for antagonist affinity estimates. *Trends Pharmacol. Sci.* **28**, 374–381.
31. Thomsen, W., Frazer, J., and Unett, D. (2005) Functional assays for screening GPCR targets. *Curr. Opin. Biotechnol.* **16**, 655–665.
32. Maruyama, M.R., Bornheimer, S.J., Venkatasubramanian, V., and Subramaniam, S. (2005) Reduced-order modelling of biochemical networks: application to the GTPase-cycle signalling module. *Syst. Biol.* **152**, 229–242.
33. Zhang, Y., and Rundell, A. (2006) Comparative study of parameter sensitivity analyses of the TCR-activated ERK-MAPK signalling pathway. *Syst. Biol.* **153**, 201–211.
34. Zolg, J.W., and Langen, H. (2004) How industry is approaching the search for new diagnostic markers and biomarkers. *Mol. Cell. Proteomics* **3**, 345–354.
35. Penny, M.A., and McHale, D. (2005) Pharmacogenomics and the drug discovery pipeline: when should it be implemented? *Am. J. Pharmacogenomics* **5**, 53–62.
36. Johnson, J.A., and Lima, J.J. (2003) Drug receptor/effector polymorphisms and pharmacogenetics: current status and challenges. *Pharmacogenetics* **13**, 525–534.
37. Goetz, A.S., et al. (1999) A combination assay for simultaneous assessment of multiple signalling pathways. *J. Pharmacol. Toxicol.Methods* **42**(4), 225–235.
38. Fang, Y., and Ferrie, A.M. (2008) Label-free optical biosensor for ligand-directed functional selectivity acting on beta(2) adrenoceptor in living cells. *FEBS Lett.* **582**, 558–564.
39. Kostenis, E. (2006) G proteins in drug screening: from analysis of receptor-G protein specificity to manipulation of GPCR-mediated signalling pathways. *Curr. Pharm. Des.* **12**, 1703–1715.
40. Milligan, G., and Rees, S. (1999) Chimeric Gα proteins: their potential use in drug discovery. *Trends Pharmacol. Sci.* **20**, 118-124.
41. Gbahou, F. Rouleau, A., Morisset, S., et al. (2003) Protean agonism at histamine H3 receptors *in vitro* and *in vivo*. *Proc. Natl. Acad. Sci. USA* **100**, 11086–11091.
42. Hancock, A.A. (2006) The challenge of drug discovery of a GPCR target: analaysis of preclinical pharmacology of histamine H3 antagonists/inverse agonists. *Biochem. Pharmacol.* **71**, 1103–1113.
43. Williams, C. (2004) cAMP detection methods in HTS: selecting the best from the rest. *Nat. Rev. Drug Discov.* **3**, 125–135.
44. George, S.E., Bungay, P.J., and Naylor, L.H. (1997) Evaluation of a CRE-directed luciferase reporter gene assay as an alternative to measuring cAMP accumulation. *J. Biomol. Screen.* **2**, 235–240.

45. Allen, M., Hall, D., Collins, B., and Moore, K. (2002) A homogeneous high throughput nonradioactive method for measurement of functional activity of Gs-coupled receptors in membranes. *J. Biomol. Screen.* 7, 35–44.
46. Leach, K., Sexton, P.M., and Christopoulos, A. (2007) Allosteric GPCR modulators: taking advantage of permissive receptor pharmacology. *Trends Pharmacol. Sci.* **28**, 382–389.
47. Baker, J.G., Hall, I.P., and Hill, S.J. (2003) Agonist actions of "β-blockers" provide evidence for two agonist activation sites on the human β1-adrenoceptor. *Mol. Pharmacol.* **63**, 1312–1321.
48. Berg, K.A., Maayani, S., Goldfarb, J., Scaramellini, C., Leff, P., and Clarke, W.P. (1998) Effect pathway-dependent relative efficacy at serotonin type 2A and 2C receptors: Evidence for agonist-directed trafficking of receptor stimulus. *Mol. Pharmacol.* **54**, 94–104.
49. Makita, N., Sato, J., Manaka, K., Shoji, Y., Oishi, A., Hashimoto, M., Fujita, T., and Iira, T. (2007) An acquired hypocalcemia autoantibody induces allosteric transition among active Ca-sensing receptor conformations. *Proc. Natl. Acad. Sci. USA* **104**, 5443–5448.
50. Williams, C., and Sewing, A. (2005) G protein-coupled receptor assays: to measure affinity or efficacy that is the question. *Comb. Chem. High Throughput Screen.* **8**, 285–292.
51. Christopoulos, A., Parsons, A.M., Lew, M.J., and El-Fakahany, E.E. (1999) The assessment of antagonist potency under conditions of transient response kinetics. *Eur. J. Pharmacol.* **382**, 217–227.
52. Sakamoto, A., Yanagisawa M., Tsujimoto G., Nakao K., Toyo-oka, T., and Masaki, T. (1994) Pseudo-noncompetitive antagonism by BQ123 of intracellular calcium transients mediated by human ETA endothelin receptor. *Biochem. Biophys. Res. Comm.* **200**, 679–686.
53. Monaghan, M.L., Diver, T., Huffman, W.F., and Kinter, L.B. (1993) Antagonism of antidiuretic hormone in domestic pigs. *Gen. Pharmacol.* **24**, 1013–1020.
54. Baker, J.G., Hall, I.P., and Hill, S.J. (2004) Temporal characteristics of CRE-mediated gene transcription: requirement for sustained cAMP production. *Mol. Pharmacol.* **65**, 986–998.

Chapter 4

An Overview on GPCRs and Drug Discovery: Structure-Based Drug Design and Structural Biology on GPCRs

Kenneth Lundstrom

Summary

G protein-coupled receptors (GPCRs) represent 50–60% of the current drug targets. There is no doubt that this family of membrane proteins plays a crucial role in drug discovery today. Classically, a number of drugs based on GPCRs have been developed for such different indications as cardiovascular, metabolic, neurodegenerative, psychiatric, and oncologic diseases. Owing to the restricted structural information on GPCRs, only limited exploration of structure-based drug design has been possible. Much effort has been dedicated to structural biology on GPCRs and very recently an X-ray structure of the β2-adrenergic receptor was obtained. This breakthrough will certainly increase the efforts in structural biology on GPCRs and furthermore speed up and facilitate the drug discovery process.

Key words: GPCRs, Drug discovery, Overexpression, Functional receptor, X-ray crystallography, Structure-based drug design.

1. Introduction

The drug discovery process has passed through dramatic changes during the past 20 years. The requirements for drug manufacturing and especially the safety aspects related to the final medicine have become immense. This development has made the drug discovery and development processes both time-consuming and labor intensive. Not surprisingly, development of drugs has become extremely expensive. In addition, the success rate of bringing new successful drugs to the market has been worryingly low. One approach to speed up drug discovery and also to reduce the adverse effects of developed drugs has been to apply structure-based drug design. There are a number of examples of success. For

Wayne R. Leifert (ed.), *G Protein-Coupled Receptors in Drug Discovery, vol. 552*

Book doi: 10.1007/978-1-60327-317-6_4

instance, structural information has played an important role in lead optimization in drug screening programs *(1)*. Furthermore, high-resolution structures of HIV proteinase *(2)* and influenza virus neuraminidase *(3)* have contributed directly to the development of AIDS (Agenerase® and Viracept®) and flu (Relenza®) drugs, respectively. In total, more than 10 drugs can today be considered as designed based on known high-resolution structures of target molecules.

Despite their prominent position as drug targets, very modest progress in structure-based drug design has been observed for membrane proteins. Although some 70% of the current drug targets are membrane proteins, minimal direct efforts in structure-based drug discovery has been conducted on membrane proteins. The simple reason is the very small number of high-resolution structures available for membrane proteins in general and more specifically for drug targets. Among the more than 35,000 structures deposited today in public databases less than 200 exist on membrane proteins *(4)*.

2. GPCRs as Drug Targets

GPCRs represent a broad spectrum of drug targets as they are the mediators for so many essential biological activities. Their function can be triggered by such different components as neurotransmitters, peptides, hormones, chemokines, amino acids, calcium ions, odorants, and even light, which results in signal transduction events on the cell, tissue, organ, and whole organism level to adjust to environmental requirements. Not surprisingly, GPCRs have been targeted for many types of maladies including cardiovascular, metabolic, neurodegenerative, neurological, virological, and tumorigenic diseases.

It is estimated that the human genome contains approximately 800 GPCRs of which a relatively large number is represented by odorant receptors. The ligands for many odorant receptors are still unknown and therefore they are called orphan receptors. Also several non-odorant receptors belong to the group of receptors for which ligands are not available. In total, some 100 GPCRs are classified as orphan receptors and are considered as potentially interesting novel drug targets as described in more detail below *(5)*.

Although GPCR signaling is mediated through G proteins, it has fairly recently become evident that other signaling pathways are possible. For instance, c-Src tyrosine kinase interaction with the proline-rich SH3 domain in the third intracellular loop of the β3-adrenergic receptor activates the extracellular signal-regulated kinase (ERK)–mitogen-activated protein kinase (MAPK) cascade *(6)*. Another example includes the interaction between β-arrestin-1 and c-Src, which facilitates the β2-adrenergic receptor-dependent activation of the ERK–MAPK pathway *(7)*. Moreover, the β-arrestin-1–c-Src interaction plays an important role in glucose transport mediated by endothelin receptors *(8)* and the activation of the STAT (signal transducer and activator of transcription) transcription factor *(9)*. These "alternative" pathways might present interesting opportunities for the development of novel drugs.

Among the 200 top selling drugs today a quarter is based on GPCRs with annual sales exceeding $200 billion worldwide *(10)*. Included in the best-selling GPCR-based drugs are salmeterol, an anti-asthmatic β2-adrenergic agonist; olanzapine, an antipsychotic serotonin 5-HT2/dopamine receptor antagonist; and clopidrogel, an antithrombotic P2Y12 purinergic receptor antagonist *(11)*. Other "blockbuster" drugs targeted to GPCRs are H1-antihistamines (fexofenadine, cetirizine, and desloratadine) and antihypertensive angiotensin II receptor antagonists (losartan, valsartan, cardesartan, and irbesartan).

3. Conventional Drug Discovery Approaches

Before initiation of any drug screening program it is highly recommended to invest resources in target validation *(12)*. In this context, bioinformatics approaches including database mining, comparative homology and species analysis, and *in silico* expression studies are essential. Moreover, localization studies by *in situ* hybridization, RT-PCRs, and microarrays are excellent means for expression comparison in tissues originating from healthy and diseased individuals. Furthermore, it has been demonstrated that mutations in GPCRs can induce disease as is the case for constitutive activity of certain GPCRs *(13)* and it is important to validate the effect of various mutations. Once targets have been defined drug screening can commence.

Typically, classic drug screening programs have relied on pharmacological evaluation of GPCRs by radioligand binding assays *(14)*. In this context, large chemical libraries are screened in binding assays for hits. The advent of recombinant protein expression methods has substantially facilitated the drug screening process as is described in more detail below. Assay development has focused strongly on automation and miniaturization and, for instance, fluorescence intensity, fluorescence polarization, time-resolved fluorescence resonance energy transfer (TR-FRET), and fluorescence macroconfocal technology (FMAT) methods have been utilized for high-throughput screening in 96-, 384-, and 1536-well formats *(15)*. The conventional process involves further chemical modifications of discovered hit molecules on so-called lead compounds. These compounds will be further tested for potency by saturation binding assays, but also for specificity by performing pharmacological evaluation on related receptor families and as well as on receptor subtypes.

Much attention is today paid to the composition of the chemical libraries used for the screening process. The design of chemical libraries has become more and more important and approaches have been taken to generate ligand-based libraries and relying on physicochemical and substructural properties *(16)*. Structure-based library design is described in more detail below.

The majority of drug screening efforts have recently shifted from binding assays to functional determination of receptor coupling to G proteins. The advantage of change in strategy is the possibility to evaluate agonists, antagonists, partial agonists, and inverse agonists. A number of cell-based assays measuring cAMP stimulation, inositol phosphate accumulation, and intracellular Ca^{2+}-release have been established *(17)*. Application of Ca^{2+}-sensitive dyes has allowed fluorescence imaging in automated 384-well format. Other screening approaches include the establishment of stable cell lines for second messenger and reporter gene detection (β-lactamase and luciferase) for detection of transcriptional regulation of promoter elements activated by GPCRs *(18)*. Moreover, transient expression of GPCRs in melanophores from the neural crest of *Xenopus laevis* has allowed monitoring functional activity by measurement of light absorption based on pigment dispersion *(19)*. Today agonist activation and antagonist inhibition has been evaluated for more than 100 GPCRs in the melanophore system. Although application of functional screening assays for GPCRs has broadened the drug discovery process and facilitated finding new drug molecules, a number of other approaches have been taken as presented below.

4. Chemical Libraries and Structure-based Drug Design

Although the first high-resolution structure of a GPCR became available only recently, approaches have previously been made to use structural information in drug design *(20)*. One approach has been two- and three-dimensional mapping of the ligand–GPCR interaction sites applying homology models of rhodopsin and site-directed mutagenesis to determine structure–activity relationships (SARs) for ligands *(16)*. Moreover, structural information on GPCR ligands has presented the basis for design of chemical libraries for screening purposes *(21)*. Pharmacophore-based design of combinatorial libraries was applied to design a novel series of indolyl sulfonamides as selective high-affinity serotonin 5-HT_6 receptor ligands and resulted in the identification of some novel compounds *(22)*. Pharmacophore models have also been used for virtual screening approaches to identify nonpeptidic ligands for peptide-binding GPCRs such as the somatostatin receptor known for its poor bioavailability and low metabolic stability *(23)*. Nonpeptidic antagonists for the urotensin II receptor could be identified based on truncated peptide derivatives of the cyclic 11 amino acid peptide urotensin II *(24)*. Alanine scanning and NMR spectroscopy resulted in the identification of the Trp-Lys-Trp motif in the cyclic part of the human urotensin II. Likewise, when two different pharmacore models were established 172 virtual antagonist hits were identified for the muscarinic M3 receptor leading to three compounds with a novel scaffold *(25)*. Other nonpeptidic GPCR ligands have been designed for opioid *(26)*, thrombin *(27)*, and somatostatin *(28)* receptors.

Moreover, ligand-based three-dimensional quantitative SAR (3D-QSAR) methods have been applied for lead optimization. Using comparative molecular field analysis (CoMFA) for the correlation of the steric and electronic field environment a number of GPCR lead compounds were optimized *(29, 30)*. For instance, successful ligand optimization for dopamine *(31, 32)*, serotonin *(33, 34)*, endothelin *(35)*, and adenosine *(36, 37)* receptors has been reported for CoMFA. Moreover, ligand selectivity has also been addressed by demonstrating side affinities for a series of aryl piperazines active against the serotonin 5-HT1A receptor for the α1-adrenergic receptor *(38)*. When the ligand-based CoMFA method was combined with 3D receptor modeling of serotonin receptor subtypes, the serotonin 5-HT2C/2B indoline urea lead series showed only minor side affinity against the serotonin 5-HT2A receptor *(39, 40)*.

The progress in chemogenomics has also had a big impact on the design of targeted libraries. The PREDICT technology was developed for 3D structure modeling of GPCRs *(41)*. PREDICT does not require a structural template and can be used for any GPCR amino acid sequence. Consequently, PREDICT has been applied for dopamine D2, neurokinin 1, neuropeptide Y1, and chemokine CCR3 receptors and demonstrated good agreement with data from a large number of experiments.

Virtual screening has become important in drug discovery because of potential time and cost reductions. For instance, applying the 2.8 Å-resolution X-ray structure of bovine rhodopsin as a homology model for antagonist screening of three human GPCRs (the dopamine D3 receptor, the muscarinic M1 receptor, and the vasopressin V1a receptor) *(42)* showed that it was possible to distinguish known antagonists from randomly chosen molecules.

Three different docking programs (Dock, FlexX, Gold) were used in combination with seven scoring functions (ChemScore, Dock, FlexX, Fresno, Gold, Pmf, Score). In another approach, PREDICT was applied for virtual screening of several GPCRs resulting in enrichment factors of 9- to 44-fold better than what was obtained from random screening *(43)*. Moreover, a practical scoring function was applied to assess the druggability of compounds, which consisted of 12 metrics taking into account physical, chemical, and structural properties and undesirable functional groups *(44)*. Evaluation of the 12-metric scoring function for 44 different databases including more than 3.8 million commercially available compounds indicated that the majority of compounds that did not show satisfactory druggability had a high molecular weight and high log*P* values and also indicated the presence of reactive functional groups.

5. Novel Approaches Including Dimerization and Orphan GPCRs

In addition to conventional screening of molecules reacting with GPCRs more adventurous approaches have been to target pathways other than those involving G proteins *(20)*. Typically, a number of GPCRs can signal through interaction with arrestins and other cellular proteins. For instance, receptor–protein interaction occurs between the angiotensin 1A receptor and the C terminus of the Janus 2 kinase (JAK2) through activation of the STAT transcription factor *(9)*. Investment in targets for alternative pathways might bring substantial rewards as the signaling through G proteins has been so well documented and fairly few novel discoveries are anticipated. On the other hand, employing combinatorial chemistry and advanced chemical libraries for the screening procedure might be productive *(16)*.

There are two other interesting relatively novel approaches for drug discovery on GPCRs. Approximately a decade ago the existence of GPCR dimers and higher multimers was documented *(45)*. Interestingly, it was demonstrated that $GABA_B$ receptors required both $GABA_B$-r1 and $GABA_B$-r2 subunits in a dimer composition to obtain functional receptors on the plasma membrane *(46)*. Other GPCRs such as taste receptors can also form dimers. Most interestingly, the heterodimeric T1R1+T1R3 combination generates the umami receptor, whereas the T1R2+T1R3 heterodimer defines the sensor for sweet taste *(47, 48)*. Moreover, when the leukotriene BLT1 receptor was expressed in *Escherichia coli* inclusion bodies low-affinity binding homodimers were obtained after refolding, which could be reverted to high-affinity binding after addition of a heterotrimeric Gα12β1γ2 complex to the refolded GPCRs *(49)*. This suggested the requirement of GPCR dimerization.

The biggest impact dimerization can have on drug discovery is most likely on the activation of different signaling pathways, receptor desensitization and sensitization, and modulation of GPCRs *(45, 50)*. For this reason, the number of potential drugs could increase significantly and programs on oligomeric GPCRs could be included in drug screening strategies. The action of drug molecules on additional sites in comparison to monomeric GPCR binding sites would also have an impact on drug design. In this context, novel designs of dimeric ligands with two covalently linked monovalent ligands could possibly more efficiently induce or stabilize dimeric GPCR conformations *(51)*. In order to prevent the potential protein–protein interaction in dimers, enhancement or disruption of oligomerization could be promoted in drug design.

Another approach has been to target orphan GPCRs. By definition, these are receptors for which no ligand has been defined yet. Despite extensive deorphanization programs some 100 orphan GPCRs still exist *(52)*. Orphan receptors are considered as potentially interesting targets as the initiation of several drug discovery programs indicate. In this context, nociceptin/orphanin FQ has been evaluated for pain and anxiety *(53)*, orexin/hypocretin for narcolepsy *(54)* and food intake *(55)*, ghrelin for obesity *(56)*, and metastin for potency in oncology *(57)*. The impact of orphan GPCRs is difficult to evaluate as only few receptors have been deorphanized, so far. One concern has been the relatively low endogenous levels of their ligands and their potential signaling through G protein-independent pathways. Drug development programs on orphan receptors can therefore be considered risky, but the rewards through finding novel treatment for disease, when successful, will also be substantial.

6. Overexpression of GPCRs

To support drug screening activities and structural biology initiatives it is essential to obtain high-level expression of GPCRs. As the seven-transmembrane topology of GPCRs makes the expression more difficult and demanding compared to soluble protein, it is not surprising that more or less every available expression system has been tested *(58)*. Both prokaryotic and eukaryotic expression systems have been used frequently and recently also cell-free *E. coli*- and wheat germ-based systems have been applied. Although cell-free translation has mainly been used for soluble proteins, novel development has also allowed reasonable expression of membrane proteins *(59, 60)*. *E. coli* vectors are the most frequently used prokaryotic vectors. GPCRs have been expressed both in inclusion bodies *(61)* and the plasma membrane *(62)*. The approach of production in inclusion bodies generates relatively high expression level, but the drawback is that extensive refolding exercise is required to restore the GPCR *(63)*. On the other hand, targeting GPCRs to the plasma membrane can generate functional GPCRs. However, the membrane insertion often results in growth regression of bacterial host cells and reduced recombinant protein yields due to the GPCR toxicity. Improved expression has been achieved by introduction of mutations and deletions in the target GPCR and engineering fusions to, for instance, maltose binding protein (MBP) *(64)*. This approach has resulted in production of milligram levels of rat neurotensin receptor in *E. coli* cultured in fermentors *(65)*. In addition to *E. coli*, *Halobacterium salinarum (66)* and *Lactococcus lactis (67)* have been applied for GPCR expression. The yields obtained have so far, however, been relatively modest.

Yeast-based expression of GPCRs has received plenty of attention. The most frequently used yeast hosts are *Saccharomyces cerevisiae (68, 69)* and *Pichia pastoris (70)*. Particularly, the application of *P. pastoris* has resulted in high binding activity (up to 100 pmol/mg) and impressive yields (5 mg/L) of a large number of GPCRs *(71)*. Likewise, Baculovirus vectors carrying GPCRs have been introduced into insect cells resulting in robust expression of functionally active GPCRs *(72)*. Up to 16 GPCRs were expressed from Baculovirus vectors in parallel resulting in 250 pmol/mg receptor *(73)*. The production of GPCRs in insect cells cultured in bioreactors has provided sufficient material for structural studies on GPCRs as described below. Application of mammalian expression systems for the overexpression of GPCRs has been to some extent hampered by time-consuming and expensive procedures and low expression levels. Despite that a mutant HEK293 cell line allowed production of up to 6 mg/L of rhodopsin *(74)*. A number of viral vectors such as adenoviruses, vaccinia viruses, lentiviruses, and alphaviruses have also been used for GPCR expression. Particularly, Semliki Forest virus (SFV) vectors, an alphavirus, have been applied for the expression of more than 100 GPCRs in different cell lines *(75, 76)*. The SFV system has shown high expression levels measured by saturation binding (>100 pmol/mg) and functional coupling to G proteins (intracellular Ca^{2+} release, inositol phosphate accumulation, cAMP stimulation, and GTPγS binding). Furthermore, the system has been scaled up to allow large-scale production in multiple liter volumes in spinner and roller flasks as well as in bioreactors.

7. Structural Biology on GPCRs

Although no high-resolution structure of therapeutically interesting GPCRs had been solved until recently, reasonable information has been available for GPCRs from other structures. Tertiary models of various GPCRs have been built based on the high-resolution structure of bacteriorhodopsin obtained from *Halobacterium salinarium* *(77)*. A further improvement occurred when the three-dimensional structure of bovine rhodopsin became available *(78)* as modeling could switch to this mammalian receptor. However, the real breakthrough was seen very recently when the high-resolution structure of the human β2-adrenergic receptor–lysozyme complex was solved by receptor overexpression in Baculovirus-infected insect cells *(79, 80)*. The fusion protein was bound to the partial inverse agonist carazolol at a 2.4 Å resolution. Despite a similar location of carazolol in the β2-adrenergic receptor and retinal in rhodopsin, structural differences in the ligand-binding site and other regions were observed. This clearly signifies the shortcomings of using rhodopsin as a template for GPCR modeling.

In absence of high-resolution structures, site-directed mutagenesis has been applied to investigate the site(s) of interaction between GPCRs and their ligands. In combination with bioinformatics and modeling, site-directed mutagenesis supported by *in vitro* expression in cells can provide important information on change in binding affinity and functional activity. For instance, mutation of an asparagine residue in the TM2 of the GnRH receptor resulted in complete loss of binding activity *(81)*. However, the presence of a second mutation in the TM7 restored the binding activity, which indicated a close proximity of TM2 and TM7. Studies on the neurokinin-1 receptor (NK1R) showed that three adjacent N-terminal residues (Asn23, Glu24, and Phe25) affected substance P binding *(82)*. Moreover, His108 located on the top of TM3 and Tyr287 on the top of TM7 were shown to interact with substance P *(83)*. Other studies revealed that the binding mode for the nonpeptide antagonist CP 96,345 was different from substance P *(84)* for NK1R and their binding pockets were also different *(85)*. Furthermore, mutant His197 showed a significantly reduced affinity to CP 96,345 *(86)*. For other GPCRs, it was demonstrated by site-directed mutagenesis that ligand binding at the β2-adrenergic receptor occurred mainly within the membrane-spanning regions flanking TMs 3, 5, 6, and 7 *(87)* and that three binding sites for 5-hydroxytryptamine (5-HT), propranolol, and 8-hydroxy-*N,N*-dipropylaminotetralin (8-OH-DPAT) within the highly conserved 7TM domain existed for the serotonin 5-HT1A receptor *(88)*. Overall, based on results obtained from molecular modeling and mutagenesis studies it was suggested that family A receptors might share a common binding pocket *(89, 90)*. However, because the same effect can be obtained by allosteric modulations *(91)* and constitutive signaling *(92)* this view might be oversimplified.

Other approaches to obtain structural information have been to define the proximity and orientation of TM regions by the introduction of histidine zinc (II) binding sites into neurokinin *(93)* and opioid receptors *(94)*. Furthermore, distance constraints and flexibility of extracellular loops could be determined for the muscarinic M3 receptor by engineering of cysteine mutants *(95)*. In another approach, fluorescent unnatural amino acids were introduced at defined sites for determination of distances and tertiary structures by FRET technology *(96)*. Finally, electron paramagnetic resonance (EPR) spectroscopy and cysteine cross-linking has provided information on helix orientation, flexibility of receptor loops, and the conformational changes induced by light *(97)*.

8. Conclusions and Future Prospects

GPCRs will continue to serve as the most important drug targets in modern medicine. Although drug screening on GPCRs is anticipated to constitute a large part of these activities other approaches will be applied. Much attention will be given to the design of larger and more specialized (GPCR-oriented) libraries. The development of sophisticated software programs and the advancement in bioinformatics will further improve the possibilities of increasing virtual screening methods. This will certainly significantly reduce both costs and time in drug development. As most of the conventional approaches for GPCR screening have already been explored and the chances of discovery of novel drug molecules diminish, it will be essential to look for new opportunities. Orphan GPCRs might be interesting targets for further exploration as ligand molecules with novel therapeutic properties might be discovered. Moreover, investigation of non-G protein signaling pathways for GPCRs might reveal novel mechanisms of actions and in that context discovery of novel therapeutic targets. Finally, structure-based drug design has indeed seen a major breakthrough through the determination of the first human GPCR structure. It is anticipated that other GPCR structures will follow shortly, which will certainly open up extensive new possibilities for rational drug design approaches.

References

1. Blundel, T.L. (1996) Structure-based drug design. *Nature* **384S**, 23–26.
2. Stoll, V., Qin, W., Stewart, K.D., Jakob, C., Park, C., Walter, K., Simmer, R.L., Helfrich, R., Bussiere, D., Kao, J., Kempf, D., Sham, H.L., and Norbeck, D.W. (2002) X-ray crystallographic structure of ABT-378 (lopinavir) bound to HIV-1 protease. *Bioorg. Med. Chem.* **10**, 2803–2806.
3. Varghese, J.N. (1999) Development of neuraminidase inhibitors as anti-influenza virus drugs. *Drug Dev. Res.* **46**, 176–196.
4. http://www.mpibp-frankfurt.mpg.de/michel/public/memprotstruct.html
5. Civelli, O., Nothacker, H.P., Saito, Y., Wang, Z., Lin, S.H., and Reinsheid, R.K. (2001) Novel neurotransmitters as natural ligands of orphan G protein-coupled receptors. *Trends Neurosci.* **24**, 230–237.
6. Cao, W., Luttrell, L.M., Medvedev, A.V., Pierce, K.L., Daniel, K.W., Dixon, T.M., Lefkowitz, R.J., and Collins, S. (2000) Direct binding of activated c-Src to the beta 3-adrenergic receptor is required for MAP kinase activation. *J. Biol. Chem.* **275**, 38131–38134.
7. Luttrell, L.M., Ferguson, S.S., Daaka, Y., Miller, W.E., Maudsley, S., Della Rocca, G.J., Lin, F., Kawakatsu, H., Owada, K., Luttrell, D.K., Caron, M.G., and Lefkowitz, R.J. (1999) Beta-arrestin-dependent formation of beta2 adrenergic receptor–Src protein kinase complexes. *Science* **283**, 655–661.
8. Imamura, T., Huang, J., Dalle, S., Ugi, S., Usui, I., Luttrell, L.M., Miller, W.E., Lefkowitz, R.J., and Olefsky, J.M. (2001) Beta-arrestin-mediated recruitment of the Src family kinase Yes mediates endothelin-1-stimulated glucose transport. *J. Biol. Chem.* **276**, 43663–43667.
9. Marrero, M.B., Schieffer, B., Paxton, W.G., Heerdt, L., Berk, B.C., Delafontaine, P., and Bernstein, K.E. (1995) Direct stimulation of Jak/STAT pathway by the angiotensin II AT1 receptor. *Nature* **375**, 247–250.
10. Vanti, W.B., Swaminathan, S., Blevins, R., Bonini, J.A., O'Dowd, B.F., and George, S.R. (2001) Patent status of the therapeutically important G protein-coupled receptors. *Endocr. Rev.* **21**, 90–113.
11. Esbenshade, T.A. (2006) G protein-coupled receptors as targets for drug discovery. In *G Protein-Coupled Receptors in Drug Discovery*. Lundstrom, K. and Chiu, M. (eds.), CRC Press, Boca Raton, FL, USA, pp. 15–36.
12. Lundstrom, K. (2006) Latest development in drug discovery on G protein-coupled receptors. *Curr. Prot. Pept. Sci.* 7, 465–470.
13. Seifert, R., and Wenzel-Seifert, K. (2002) Constitutive activity of G protein-coupled receptors: cause of disease and common property of wild-type receptors. *Naunyn Schmiedebergs Arch. Pharmacol.* **366**, 381–416.
14. Hodgson, J. (1992) Receptor screening and the search for new pharmaceuticals. *Biotechnology* **10**, 973–980.
15. Miraglia, S., Swartzman, E.E., Mellentin-Michelotti, J., Evangelista, L., Smith, C., Gunawan, I.I., Lohman, K., Goldberg, E.M., Manian, B., and Yuan, P.M. (1999) Homogeneous cell- and bead-based assays for high throughput screening using fluorometric microvolume assay technology. *J. Biomol. Screen.* **4**, 193–204.
16. Jimonet, P., and Jager, R. (2004) Strategies for designing GPCR-focused libraries and screening sets. *Curr. Opin. Drug Discov. Develop.* 7, 325–333.
17. Warrior, U., Gopalakrishan, S., Vanhauwe, J., and Burns, D. (2006) High throughput screening assays for G protein-coupled receptors. In *G Protein-Coupled Receptors in Drug Discovery*. Lundstrom, K. and Chiu, M. (eds.), CRC Press, Boca Raton, FL, USA, pp. 158–189.
18. Kunapuli, P., Ransom, R., Murphy, K.L., Pettibone, D., Kerby, J., Grimwood, S., Zuck, P., Hodder, P., Lacson, R., Hoffman, I., Inglese, J., and Strulovici, B. (2003) Development of an intact cell reporter gene beta-lactamase assay for G protein-coupled receptors for high-throughput screening. *Anal. Biochem.* **314**, 16–29.
19. Chen, G., Way, J., Armour, S., Watson, C., Queen, K., Jayawickreme, C.K., Chen, W.J., and Kenakin, T. (2000) Use of constitutive G protein-coupled receptor activity for drug discovery. *Mol. Pharmacol.* **57**, 125–134.
20. Lundstrom, K. (2006) Latest development in drug discovery on G protein-coupled receptors. *Curr. Prot. Peptide Sci.* 7, 465–470.
21. Holenz, J., Merce, R., Diaz, J.L., Guitart, X., Codony, X., Dordal, A., Romero, G., Torrens, A., Mas, J., Andaluz, B., Hernandez, S., Monroy, X., Sanchez, E., Hernandez, E., Perez, R., Cubi, R., Sanfeliu, O., and

Buschmann, H. (2005) Medicinal chemistry driven approaches toward novel and selective serotonin 5-HT6 receptor ligands. *J. Med. Chem.* **48**, 1781–1795.

22. Klabunde, T. and Hessler, G. (2002) Drug design strategies for targeting G protein-coupled receptors. *Chem. Bio. Chem.* **3**, 928–944.
23. Veber, D.F. In *Peptides, Chemistry and Biology: Proceedings of the 12th American Peptide Symposium*. Smith, J.A. and Rivier, J.E. (eds.), ESCOM, Leiden, The Netherlands, pp. 3–14.
24. Flohr, S., Kurz, M., Kostenis, E., Brkovich, A., Fournier, A., and Klabunde, T. (2002) Identification of nonpeptidic urotensin II receptor antagonists by virtual screening based on a pharmacophore model derived from structure–activity relationships and nuclear magnetic resonance studies on urotensin II. *J. Med. Chem.* **45**, 1799–1805.
25. Marriott, D.P., Dougall, I.G., Meghani, P., Liu, Y.-J., and Flower, D.R. (1999) Lead generation using pharmacophore mapping and three-dimensional database searching: application to muscarinic M(3) receptor antagonists. *J. Med. Chem.* **42**, 3210–3216.
26. Alfaro-Lopez, J., Okayama, T., Hosohata, K., Davis, P., Porreca, F., Yamamura, H.I., and Hruby, V.J. (1999) Exploring the structure–activity relationships of [1-(4-tert-butyl-3'-hydroxy)benzhydryl-4-benzylpiperazine] (SL-3111), a high-affinity and selective delta-opioid receptor nonpeptide agonist ligand. *J. Med. Chem.* **42**, 5359–5368.
27. Alexopoulos, K., Panagiotopoulos, D., Mavromoustakos, T., Fatseas, P., Paredes-Carbajal, M.C., Mascher, D., Mihailescu, S., and Matsoukas, J. (2001) Exploring the structure–activity relationships of [1-(4-tert-butyl-3'-hydroxy)benzhydryl-4-benzylpiperazine] (SL-3111), a high-affinity and selective delta-opioid receptor nonpeptide agonist ligand. *J. Med. Chem.* **44**, 328–339.
28. Neelamkavil, S., Arison, B., Birzin, E., Feng, J.J., Chen, K.H., Lin, A., Cheng, F.C., Taylor, L., Thornton, E.R., Smith, A.B. 3rd, and Hirschmann, R. (2005) Replacement of Phe6, Phe7, and Phe11 of D-Trp8-somatostatin-14 with L-pyrazinylalanine. Predicted and observed effects on binding affinities at hSST2 and hSST4. An unexpected effect of the chirality of Trp8 on NMR spectra in methanol. *J. Med. Chem.* **16**, 4025–4030.
29. Cramer, R.D., Patterson, D.E., and Brunce, J.D. (1989) Recent advances in comparative molecular field analysis (CoMFA). *Prog. Clin. Biol. Res.* **291**, 161–165.
30. Kim, K.H., Greco, G., Novellino, E., Silipo, C., and Vittoria A. (1993) Use of the hydrogen bond potential function in a comparative molecular field analysis (CoMFA) on a set of benzodiazepines. *J. Comput. Aided Mol. Des.* 7, 263–280.
31. Salama, I., Hocke, C., Utz, W., Prante, O., Boeckler, F., Hübner, H., Kuwert, T., and Gmeiner, P. (2007) Structure-selectivity investigations of D2-like receptor ligands by CoMFA and CoMSIA guiding the discovery of D3 selective PET radioligands. *J. Med. Chem.* **50**, 489–500.
32. Tropsha, A., and Wang, S.X. (2006) QSAR modeling of GPCR ligands: methodologies and examples of applications. *Ernst. Schering. Found. Symp. Proc.* **2**, 49–73.
33. Gaillard, P., Carrupt, P.-A., Testa, B., and Schambel, P. (1996) Binding of arylpiperazines, (aryloxy)propanolamines, and tetrahydropyridylindoles to the 5-HT1A receptor: contribution of the molecular lipophilicity potential to three-dimensional quantitative structure–affinity relationship models. *J. Med. Chem.* **39**, 126–134.
34. Lopez-Rodriguez, M.L., Murcia, M., Benhamu, B., Viso, A., Campillo, M., and Pardo, L. (2002) Benzimidazole derivatives. 3. 3D-QSAR/CoMFA model and computational simulation for the recognition of 5-HT(4) receptor antagonists. *J. Med. Chem.* **45**, 4806–4815.
35. Wu, C., Decker, E.R., Blok, N., Bui, H., Chen, Q., Raju, B., Bourgoyne, A.R., Knowles, V., Biediger, R.J., Market, R.V., Lin, S., Dupré, B., Kogan, T.P., Holland, G.W., Brock, T.A., and Dixon, R.A. (1999) Endothelin antagonists: substituted mesitylcarboxamides with high potency and selectivity for ET(A) receptors. *J. Med. Chem.* **42**, 4485–4499.
36. Siddiqi, S.M., Pearlstein, R.A., Sanders, L.H., and Jacobsen, K.A. (1995) Comparative molecular field analysis of selective A3 adenosine receptor agonists. *Bioorg. Med. Chem.* **3**, 1331–1343.
37. Rieger, J.M., Brown, M.L., Sullivan, G.W., Linden, J., and Macdonald, T.L. (2001) Design, synthesis, and evaluation of novel A2A adenosine receptor agonists. *J. Med. Chem.* **44**, 531–539.
38. Lopez-Rodriguez, M.L., Rosado, M.L., Benhamu, B., Morcillo, M.J., Fernandez, E., and Schaper, K.J. (1997) Synthesis and structure – activity relationships of a new model of arylpiperazines. 2. Three-dimensional quantitative

structure–activity relationships of hydantoin-phenylpiperazine derivatives with affinity for 5-HT1A and alpha 1 receptors. A comparison of CoMFA models. *J. Med. Chem.* **40**, 1648–1656.

39. Forbes, I.T., Dabbs, S., Duckworth, D.M., Ham, P., Jones, G.E., King, F.D., Saunders, D.V., Blaney, F.E., Naylor, C.B., Baxter, G.S., Blackburn, T.P., Kennett, G.A., and Wood, M.D. (1996) Synthesis, biological activity, and molecular modeling of selective 5-HT(2C/2B) receptor antagonists. *J. Med. Chem.* **39**, 4966–4977.
40. Bromidge, S.M., Dabbs, S., Davies, D.T., Duckworth, D.M., Forbes, I.T., Ham, P., Jones, G.E., King, F.D., Saunders, D.V., Starr, S., Thewlis, K.M., Wyman, P.A., Blaney, F.E., Naylor, C.B., Bailey, F., Blackburn, T.P., Holland, V., Kennett, G.A., Riley, G.J., and Wood, M.D. (1998) Novel and selective 5-HT2C/2B receptor antagonists as potential anxiolytic agents: synthesis, quantitative structure–activity relationships, and molecular modeling of substituted 1-(3-pyridylcarbamoyl)indolines. *J. Med. Chem.* **41**, 1598–1612.
41. Shacham, S., Topf, M., Avisar, N., Glaser, F., Marantz, Y., Bar-Haim, S., Noiman, S., Naor, Z., and Becker, O.M. (2001) Modeling the 3D structure of GPCRs from sequence. *Med. Res. Rev.* **21**, 472–483.
42. Bissantz, C., Bernard, P., Hibert, M., and Rognan D. (2003) Protein-based virtual screening of chemical databases. II. Are homology models of G protein-coupled receptors suitable targets? *Proteins* **50**, 5–25.
43. Shacham, S., Marantz, Y., Bar-Haim, S., Kalid, O., Warshaviak, D., Avisar, N., Inbal, B., Heifetz, A., Fichman, M., Topf, M., Naor, Z., Noiman, S., and Becker, O.M. (2004) PREDICT modeling and *in-silico* screening for G protein-coupled receptors. *Proteins* **57**, 51–86.
44. Sirois, S., Hatzakis, G., Wei, D., Du, Q., and Chou, K.C. (2005) Assessment of chemical libraries for their druggability. *Comput. Biol. Chem.* **29**, 55–67.
45. Milligan, G. (2004) G protein-coupled receptor dimerization: function and ligand pharmacology. *Mol. Pharmacol.* **66**, 1–7.
46. Jones, K.A., Borowsky, B., Tamm, J.A., Craig, D.A., Durkin, M.M., Dai, M., Yao, W.J., Johnson, M., Gunwaldsen, C., Huang, L.Y., Tang, C., Shen, Q., Salon, J.A., Morse, K., Laz, T., Smith, K.E., Nagarathnam, D., Noble, S.A., Branchek, T.A., and Gerald, C. (1998) GABA(B) receptors function as a heteromeric assembly of the subunits GABA(B)R1 and GABA(B)R2. *Nature* **396**, 674–679.
47. Li, X., Staszewski, L., Xu, H., Durick, K., Zoller, M., and Adler, E. (2002) Human receptors for sweet and umami taste. *Proc. Natl. Acad. Sci. USA* **99**, 4692–4696.
48. Zhao, G.Q., Zhang, Y., Hoon, M.A., Chandrashekar, J., Erlenbach, I., Ryba, N.J., and Zuker, C.S. (2003) The receptors for mammalian sweet and umami taste. *Cell* **115**, 255–266.
49. Baneres, J.L., and Parello, J. (2003) Structure-based analysis of GPCR function: evidence for a novel pentameric assembly between the dimeric leukotriene B4 receptor BLT1 and the G protein. *J. Mol. Biol.* **329**, 815–829.
50. Tallman, J. (2000) Dimerization of G protein-coupled receptors: implications for drug design and signaling. *Neuropsychopharmacology* **23**, S1–S2.
51. George, S.R., O'Dowd, B.F., and Lee, S.P. (2002) G protein-coupled receptor oligomerization and its potential for drug discovery. *Nat. Rev. Drug Discov.* **1**, 808–820.
52. Civelli, O. (2005) In *G Protein-coupled Receptors in Drug Discovery.* Lundstrom, K. and Chiu, M.(eds.), CRC Press, Boca Rotan, FL, USA, pp. 337–356.
53. Koster, A., Montkowski, A., Schulz, S., Stube, E.M., Knaudt, K., Jenck, F., Moreau, J.L., Nothacker, H.P., Civelli, O., and Reinscheid, R.K. (1999) Targeted disruption of the orphanin FQ/nociceptin gene increases stress susceptibility and impairs stress adaptation in mice. *Proc. Natl. Acad. Sci. USA* **96**, 10444–10449.
54. Chemelli, R.M., Willie, J.T., Sinton, C.M., Elmquist, J.K., Scammell, T., Lee, C., Richardson, J.A., Williams, S.C., Xiong, Y., Kisanuki, Y., Fitch, T.E., Nakazato, M., Hammer, R.E., Saper, C.B., and Yanagisawa, M. (1999) Narcolepsy in orexin knockout mice: molecular genetics of sleep regulation. *Cell* **98**, 437–451.
55. Sakurai, T., Amemiya, A., Ishii, M., Matsuzaki, I., Chemelli, R.M., Tanaka, H., Williams, S.C., Richardson, J.A., Kozlowski, G.P., Wilson, S., Arch, J.R., Buckingham, R.E., Haynes, A.C., Carr, S.A., Annan, R.S., McNulty, D.E., Liu, W.S., Terrett, J.A., Elshourbagy, N.A., Bergsma, D.J., and Yanagisawa, M. (1998) Orexins and orexin receptors: a family of hypothalamic neuropeptides and G protein-coupled receptors that regulate feeding behavior. *Cell* **92**, 573–585.

56. Nakazato, M., Murakami, N., Date, Y., Kojima, M., Matsuo, H., Kangawa, K., and Matsukura, S. (2001) A role for ghrelin in the central regulation of feeding. *Nature* **409**, 194–198.

57. Ohtaki, T., Shintani, Y., Honda, S., Matsumoto, H., Hori, A., Kanehashi, K., Terao, S., Kumano, S., Takatsu, Y., Masuda, Y., Ishibashi, Y., Watanabe, T., Asada, M., Yamada, T., Suenaga, M., Kitada, C., Usuki, S., Kurokawa, T., Onda, H., Nishimura, O., and Fujino, M. (2001) Metastasis suppressor gene KiSS-1 encodes peptide ligand of a G protein-coupled receptor. *Nature* **411**, 613–617.

58. Lundstrom, K. (2006) Biology of G protein-coupled receptors. In *G Protein-Coupled Receptors in Drug Discovery*. Lundstrom, K. and Chiu, M. (eds.), CRC Press, Boca Raton, FL, USA, pp. 3–14.

59. Spirin, A.S., Baranov, V.I., Ryabova, L.A., Ovodov, S.Y., and Alakhov, Y.B. (1988) A continuous cell-free translation system capable of producing polypeptides in high yield. *Science* **242**, 1162–1164.

60. Klammt, C., Lohr, F., Schafer, B., Haase, W., Dotsch, V., Ruterjans, H., Glaubitz, C., and Bernhard, F. (2004) High level cell-free expression and specific labeling of integral membrane proteins. *Eur. J. Biochem.* **271**, 568–580.

61. Lundstrom, K., Wagner, R., Reinhart, C., Desmyter, A., Cherouati, N., Magnin, T., Zeder-Lutz, G., Courtot, M., Prual, C., André, N., Hassaine, G., Michel, H., Cambillau, C., and Pattus, F. (2006) Structural genomics on membrane proteins: comparison of more than 100 GPCRs in 3 expression systems. *J. Struct. Funct. Genomics* 7, 77–91.

62. Luca, S., White, J.F., Sohal, A.K., Filippov, D.V., van Boom, J.H., Grisshammer, R., and Baldus, M. (2003) The conformation of neurotensin bound to its G protein-coupled receptor. *Proc Natl Acad Sci USA* **100**, 10706–10711.

63. Kiefer, H. (2003) *In vitro* folding of alpha-helical membrane proteins. *Biochim. Biophys. Acta* **1610**, 57–62.

64. Weiss, H.M., and Grisshammer, R. (2002) Purification and characterization of the human adenosine A2a receptor functionally expressed in *Escherichia coli*. *Eur. J. Biochem.* **269**, 82–92.

65. Grisshammer, R., White, J.F., Trinh, L.B., and Shiloach, J. (2005) Large-scale expression and purification of a G protein-coupled receptor for structure determination – an overview. *J. Struct. Funct. Genomics* **6**, 159–163.

66. Winter-Vann, A.M., Martinez, L., Bartus, C., Levay, A., and Turner, G.J. (2001) G protein-coupled expression in *Halobacterium salinarum*. In *Perspectives on Solid State NMR in Biology*. Kuehne, S.R. and de Groot, H. (eds.), Doordrecht, Kluwer, The Netherlands, pp. 141–159.

67. Kunji, E.R., Slotboom, D.J. and Poolman, B. (2003) *Lactococcus lactis* as host for overproduction of functional membrane proteins. *Biochim. Biophys. Acta* **1610**, 97–108.

68. David, N.E., Gee, M., Andersen, B., Naider, F., Thorner, J., and Stevens, R.C. (1997) Expression and purification of the *Saccharomyces cerevisiae* alpha-factor receptor (Ste2p), a 7-transmembrane-segment G protein-coupled receptor. *J. Biol. Chem.* **272**, 15553–15561.

69. Andersen, B., and Stevens, R.C. (1998) The human D1A dopamine receptor: heterologous expression in *Saccharomyces cerevisiae* and purification of the functional receptor. *Protein Expr. Purif.* **13**, 111–119.

70. Weiss, H.M., Haase, W., Michel, H., and Reilander, H. (1998) Comparative biochemical and pharmacological characterization of the mouse 5HT5A 5-hydroxytryptamine receptor and the human beta2-adrenergic receptor produced in the methylotrophic yeast *Pichia pastoris*. *Biochem. J.* **330**, 1137–1147.

71. André, N., Cherouati, N., Prual, C., Steffan, T., Zeder-Lutz, G., Magnin, T., Pattus, F., Michel, H., Wagner, R., and Reinhart, C. (2006) Enhancing functional production of G protein-coupled receptors in *Pichia pastoris* to levels required for structural studies via a single expression screen. *Protein Sci.* **15**, 1115–1126.

72. Massotte, D. (2003) G protein-coupled receptor overexpression with the baculovirus-insect cell system: a tool for structural and functional studies. *Biochim. Biophys. Acta* **1610**, 77–89.

73. Akermoun, M., Koglin, M., Zvalova-Iooss, D., Folschweiller, N., Dowell, S.J., and Gearing, K.L. (2005) Characterization of 16 human G protein-coupled receptors expressed in baculovirus-infected insect cells. *Protein Expr. Purif.* **44**, 65–74.

74. Reeves, P.J., Callewaert, N., Contreras, R., and Khorana, H.G. (2002) Rhodopsin-HEK structure and function in rhodopsin:

high-level expression of rhodopsin with restricted and homogeneous N-glycosylation by a tetracycline-inducible *N*-acetylglucosaminyltransferase I-negative HEK293S stable mammalian cell line. *Proc. Natl. Acad. Sci. USA* **99**, 13419–13424.

75. Lundstrom, K. (2003) Semliki Forest virus vectors for rapid and high-level expression of integral membrane proteins. *Biochim. Biophys. Acta* **1610**, 90–96.
76. Hassaine, G., Wagner, R., Kempf, J., Cherouati, N., Hassaine, N., Prual, C., André, N., Reinhart, C., Pattus, F., and Lundstrom, K. (2006) Semliki Forest virus vectors for overexpression of 101 G protein-coupled receptors in mammalian host cells. *Protein Expr. Purif.* **45**, 343–351.
77. Henderson, R., Baldwin, J.M., Ceska, T.A., Zemlin, F., Beckmann, E., and Downing, K.H. (1990) Model for the structure of bacteriorhodopsin based on high-resolution electron cryo-microscopy. *J. Mol. Biol.* **213**, 899–929.
78. Palczewski, K., Kumasaka, T., Hori, T., Behnke, C.A., Motoshima, H., Fox, B.A., Le Trong, I., Teller, D.C., Okada, T., Stenkamp, R.E., Yamamoto, M., and Miyano, M. (2000) Crystal structure of rhodopsin: a G protein-coupled receptor. *Science* **289**, 739–745.
79. Cherezov, V., Rosenbaum, D.M., Hanson, M.A., Rasmussen, S.G., Thian, F.S., Kobilka, T.S., Choi, H.J., Kuhn, P., Weis, W.I., Kobilka, B.K., and Stevens, R.C. (2007) High-resolution crystal structure of an engineered human beta2-adrenergic G protein-coupled receptor. *Science* **318**, 1258–1265.
80. Rosenbaum, D.M., Cherezov, V., Hanson, M.A., Rasmussen, S.G., Thian, F.S., Kobilka, T.S., Choi, H.J., Yao, X.J., Weis, W.I., Stevens, R.C., and Kobilka, B.K. (2007) GPCR engineering yields high-resolution structural insights into beta2-adrenergic receptor function. *Science* **318**, 1266–1273.
81. Zhou, W., Flanagan, C., Ballesteros, J.A., Konvicka, K., Davidson, J.S., Weinstein, H., Millar, R.P., and Sealfon, S.C. (1994) A reciprocal mutation supports helix 2 and helix 7 proximity in the gonadotropin-releasing hormone receptor. *Mol. Pharmacol.* **45**, 165–170.
82. Fong, T.M., Yu, H., Huang, R.R., and Strader, C.D. (1992) The extracellular domain of the neurokinin-1 receptor is required for high-affinity binding of peptides. *Biochemistry* **31**, 11806–11811.
83. Huang, R.R., Yu, H., Strader, C.D., and Fong, T.M. (1994) Interaction of substance P with the second and seventh transmembrane domains of the neurokinin-1 receptor. *Biochemistry* **33**, 3007–3013.
84. Gether, U., Johansen, T.E., Snider, R.M., Lowe, J.A. 3rd., Nakanishi, S., and Schwartz, T.W. (1993) Different binding epitopes on the NK1 receptor for substance P and non-peptide antagonist. *Nature* **362**, 345–348.
85. Sachais, B.S., Snider, R.M., Lowe, J.A. 3rd., and Krause, J.E. (1993) Molecular basis for the species selectivity of the substance P antagonist CP-96,345. *J. Biol. Chem.* **268**, 2319–2323.
86. Lundstrom, K., Hawcock, A.B., Vargas, A., Ward, P., Thomas, P., and Naylor, A. (1997) Effect of single point mutations of the human tachykinin NK1 receptor on antagonist affinity. *Eur. J. Pharmacol.* **337**, 73–81.
87. Tota, M.R., Candelore, M.R., Dixon, R.A. and Strader, C.D. (1991) Biophysical and genetic analysis of the ligand-binding site of the beta-adrenoceptor. *Trends Pharmacol. Sci.* **12**, 4–6.
88. Spedding, M., Newman-Tancredi, A., Millan, M.J., Dacquet, C., Michel, A.N., Jacoby, E., Vickery, B., and Tallentire, D. (1998) Interaction of the anxiogenic agent, RS-30199, with 5-HT1A receptors: modulation of sexual activity in the male rat. *Neuropharmacology* **37**, 769–780.
89. Trumpp-Kallmeyer, S., Joflack, J., Bruinvels, A., and Hibert, M. (1992) Modeling of G protein-coupled receptors: application to dopamine, adrenaline, serotonin, acetylcholine, and mammalian opsin receptors. *J. Med. Chem.* **35**, 3448–3462.
90. Schwartz, T.W., and Rosenkilde, M.M. (1996) Is there a "lock" for all agonist "keys" in 7TM receptors? *Trends Pharmacol. Sci.* **17**, 213–216.
91. Soudijn, W., Van Wijngaarden, I., and Ijzerman, A.P. (2004) Allosteric modulation of G protein-coupled receptors: perspectives and recent developments. *Drug Discov. Today* **9**, 752–758.
92. Christopoulos, A. (2002) Allosteric binding sites on cell-surface receptors: novel targets for drug discovery. *Nat. Rev. Drug Discov.* **1**, 198–210.
93. Elling, C.E., and Schwartz, T.W. (1996) Connectivity and orientation of the seven helical bundle in the tachykinin NK-1 receptor probed by zinc site engineering. *EMBO J.* **15**, 6213–6219.

94. Thirstrup, K., Elling, C.E., Hjorth, S.A., and Schwartz, T.W. (1996) Construction of a high affinity zinc switch in the kappa-opioid receptor. *J. Biol. Chem.* **271**, 7875–7878.
95. Zeng, F.Y., Hopp, A., Soldner, A., and Wess, J. (1999) Use of a disulfide cross-linking strategy to study muscarinic receptor structure and mechanisms of activation. *J. Biol. Chem.* **274**, 16629–16640.
96. Turcatti, G., Nemeth, K., Edgerton, M.D., Meseth, U., Talabot, F., Peitsch, M., Knowles, J., Vogel, H., and Chollet, A. (1996) Probing the structure and function of the tachykinin neurokinin-2 receptor through biosynthetic incorporation of fluorescent amino acids at specific sites. *J. Biol. Chem.* **271**, 19991–19998.
97. Altenbach, C., Cai, K., Khorana, H.G., and Hubbell, W.L. (1999) Structural features and light-dependent changes in the sequence 306-322 extending from helix VII to the palmitoylation sites in rhodopsin: a site-directed spin-labeling study. *Biochemistry* **38**, 7931–7937.

Chapter 5

Understanding the Ligand–Receptor–G Protein Ternary Complex for GPCR Drug Discovery

Venkata R.P. Ratnala and Brian Kobilka

Summary

Understanding the ternary complex between G protein-coupled receptors (GPCRs), cognate G proteins, and their ligands is an important landmark for drug discovery. Yet, little is known about the specific interactions between GPCRs and G proteins. For a better perspective on the ternary complex dynamics, we adapted a β_2-adrenergic receptor(β_2AR)–tetGs$_\alpha$ reconstitution system and found evidence that for efficient coupling of the β_2AR to Gs does not require specific interactions between the $\beta\gamma$-subunits and the β_2AR. Our results demonstrate that specific interactions between $\beta\gamma$ and the β_2AR are not required for G protein activation but likely serve to anchor Gs$_\alpha$ to the plasma membrane. Our results also suggests that the advantages of analysis of G protein activation by using β_2AR receptor–tetGs$_\alpha$ system *in vitro* at the close proximity of the receptor may constitute a simple screening system that avoids false positives and potentially adapted to screen drugs for other GPCRs.

Key words: GPCRs, G protein, β_2-adrenoceptor, Ternary complex, Assay development.

1. Introduction

G protein-coupled receptors (GPCRs) constitute the largest family of membrane proteins in the human genome and are responsible for the majority of transmembrane signal transduction in response to hormones and neurotransmitters. GPCRs receive extracellular signals and interact with and activate G proteins. Heterotrimeric G proteins are essential components in transmission of the majority of signals from activated GPCRs to effector molecules. The interaction between G protein and GPCRs represent a fundamental mechanism in cell signaling. Binding of an agonist to the receptor induces the formation of a ternary complex consisting of a ligand,

Wayne R. Leifert (ed.), *G Protein-Coupled Receptors in Drug Discovery, vol. 552*

Book doi: 10.1007/978-1-60327-317-6_5

the receptor, and a G protein, followed by the exchange of GDP for GTP on the G protein α-subunit. The complex then dissociates to the GTP-bound α-subunit (G_{α}GTP), $G_{\beta\gamma}$-complex, and receptor. The G_{α}GTP- and $G_{\beta\gamma}$-subunits can both interact with and regulate downstream effector enzymes and/or ion channels *(1–3)*. Early experiments with G proteins indicated that the βγ complex is a requirement for interaction of the G protein with receptors. The α-subunit alone did not effectively interact with the receptor in different assays *(4, 5)*. Although the identification of domains on the α-subunit that interacted with the receptor indicated that the α-subunit contacted the receptor directly *(6)*, it was unclear why the βγ-complex was required for G protein coupling to the receptor. The βγ-subunits form a stable dimer and, like the α subunit, can modulate the activity of a variety of enzymes and ion channels following dissociation from the α-subunit. The βγ-subunit is modified with fatty acyl groups and plays a role in anchoring the heterotrimeric complex to the plasma membrane, but little is known about the role of the βγ-subunit in GPCR–G protein interactions. The ability of the βγ-complex to interact with receptors under certain conditions and the finding that a peptide from the C-terminal tail of one of these receptors, rhodopsin, could inhibit this interaction hinted at direct contact between βγ and the receptor *(7, 8)*. G protein βγ-dimers play a crucial role in cellular signaling *(9, 10)*. The βγ-dimers are required for efficient modulation of the activities of various cellular effectors *(11)*. $G_{\beta\gamma}$ heterodimers bind to G protein-coupled receptor kinases (GRKs) and recruit them to nearby GPCRs, thus enabling phosphorylation of the intracellular C-terminal loop of the GPCR. In turn, the newly phosphorylated motif of the receptor recruits and interacts with β-arrestins. This leads to a cascade of interactions with the clathrin-based endocytic machinery, resulting in the endocytic internalization of the receptor and the desensitization of the cell to further stimulation by extracellular receptor ligand. The structure of the βγ-dimer as well as the heterotrimer has been clarified by crystallography, and contact sites with the effectors adenylyl cyclase (AC) and phospholipase C_{β}(PLC-β) have been mapped *(12–15)*. The $G_{\beta\gamma}$ contact site with the receptor remains ill defined. Biochemical evidence for a direct physical contact of the β-subunit and the third intracellular loops of the α_2-adrenergic receptor *(16)* or of the M_2- and M_3-muscarinic acetylcholine receptors was derived from interaction studies of peptides with βγ-complexes *(17)*. Deletion of the $G_{\beta\gamma}$-interacting site from the third intracellular loop of the M_3-muscarinic receptor profoundly affects agonist-induced phosphorylation by GRK2 and receptor sequestration *(17)*. Besides the third intracellular loop, other receptor regions like the intracellular C terminus have been shown to participate in receptor–$G_{\beta\gamma}$ contacts as well *(18)*. Yet, in spite of all these advances, the answer to one fundamental question, that of the molecular mechanism by which a G protein-coupled receptor promotes the GDP–GTP exchange on G_{α}, and the role that $G_{\beta\gamma}$ plays in this process, if any, is still unknown.

In order to characterize this interaction at a structural and functional level, the availability of purified recombinant G proteins are critically important. Gs_{α}, the stimulatory G protein for AC, is one of the first heterotrimeric G proteins to be identified, purified, and cloned *(1, 19, 20)*. More recently, the three-dimensional structure of this protein has been elucidated by X-ray crystallography. However, in spite of the remarkable success in characterizing the protein, it remains one of the most difficult G proteins to purify in a fully functional form. Expression and purification of this protein from *Escherichia coli (21)* was used for crystallography *(22)*; however, Gs_{α} purified from *E. coli* is not palmitoylated and therefore not capable of functionally interacting with GPCRs such as the β_2-adrenergic receptor (β_2AR). Gs_{α} has been shown to be purified from *Sf*9 insect cells, yet this process is technically challenging. We previously reported the generation of a modified, membrane-tethered Gs_{α} (tetGs_{α}) that coupled more efficiently than wild-type Gs_{α} when expressed in insect cells *(23, 24)*. Using *Sf*9–Baculovirus expression system, a general and simplified method to purify tetGs_{α} protein subunits has been developed (Ratnala et al.; data not shown). This method can be useful for purification of most of G protein subunits. We have been able to purify sufficient quantities of tetGs_{α} using this method to enable biopharmacological assays. The membrane tether facilitates large-scale production and purification of functional tetGs_{α} from insect cells. The tethering also demonstrates that reconstituting tetGs_{α} with β_2AR can yield an efficient coupling system to understand the ligand–receptor–G protein ternary complex and in turn it can be used for screening efficacies of diverse ligands. This could be further extended to other GPCR systems to examine whether the receptor–tetGs_{α} reconstitution systems can be used for high-efficacy assays and used for screening of ligands for other classes of GPCRs. We have noticed that that efficient coupling of the β_2AR to Gs_{α} does not require specific interactions between the $\beta\gamma$ subunits and the β_2AR and observed that tetGs_{α} forms a ternary complex with the β_2AR in the absence of $\beta\gamma$ subunits. The β_2AR can efficiently stimulate GTPγS binding to tetGs_{α} and also the reconstitution complex enhances the formation of the high-affinity state for agonists. The addition of purified $\beta_1\gamma_2$ has little effect on the function of β_2AR–tetGs_{α} reconstitution complex. We also noticed that specific interactions between $\beta_1\gamma_2$ and the β_2AR does not require the G protein activation, but $\beta_1\gamma_2$ is more likely involved in anchoring of Gs_{α} to the plasma membrane.

2. Reconstitution of β_2AR Receptor with Gs as a Model System for GPCR Drug Discovery

Considering the reconstituted β_2AR–tetGs$_\alpha$ as a model system, we examined the influence of different $\beta\gamma$-complexes on β_2AR coupling to Gs$_\alpha$ and to facilitate β_2AR-induced guanosine 5′-*O*-(3-thiotriphosphate) (GTPγS) binding to Gs$_\alpha$. Our results indicate that the addition of $\beta\gamma$ in the reconstitution complex does not play a major role in the nucleotide exchange of Gs$_\alpha$. The comparative studies with and without the $G_{\beta\gamma}$-dependent coupling of β_2ARsto Gs provided first experimental evidence that the $G_{\beta\gamma}$-dimer does not contribute much for the specificity of signaling by Gs-coupled receptors. Our results supports the notion that the molecular composition of the $\beta\gamma$-complex does not play a pivotal role in Gs activation via the β_2AR. Our results predicts that, by remaining closely associated with their activated receptors, the G protein $\alpha\beta\gamma$ subunits may serve as scaffolds for recruitment of other signaling molecules to the plasma membrane. For instance, kinetic evidence *(25)* favors a model in which the receptor, Gq, and phospholipase C remain associated throughout multiple GTPase cycles. In addition to effectors, numerous studies now indicate that G proteins also recruit soluble proteins *(26)*, such as receptor kinases that regulate desensitization and internalization of G protein-coupled receptors, and scaffold proteins that organize various kinase cascades. Association with such signaling complexes may contribute to receptor–G protein specificity. G proteins function as heterotrimers whose roles in a broad array of receptor signaling pathways are determined by their specific complements of the α-subunits and $G_{\beta\gamma}$ may serve as an adaptor protein.

The efficiency of receptor–tetGs$_\alpha$ protein coupling was assessed in several ways. GTP-sensitive, high-affinity agonist binding reflects the formation of the ternary complex between agonist, receptor, and guanine nucleotide-free G protein. GTPγS binding assay measures the uptake of the non-hydrolyzable GTP analogue GTPγS to the α-subunit and is therefore not a steady-state assay. However, this assay provides information about the number of G proteins accessible to receptors during a given period of time. Purified and reconstituted β_2AR–tetGs$_\alpha$complex derived from *Sf*9 cells were examined for binding with [^{3}H]DHA or [^{35}S]GTPγS. **Figure 1** shows the displacement curve of [^{3}H]DHA binding in the absence or presence of 0.1 m*M* GTPγS for the purified and reconstituted β_2AR–tetGs$_\alpha$ complex. The displacement curve with a full agonist, isoproterenol, shifted to the right in presence of GTPγS for reconstituted β_2AR–tetGs$_\alpha$complex. The displacement curve with a full agonist, isoproterenol, shifted to the left in the absence of GTPγS for reconstituted β_2AR–tetGs$_\alpha$ complex. Approximately

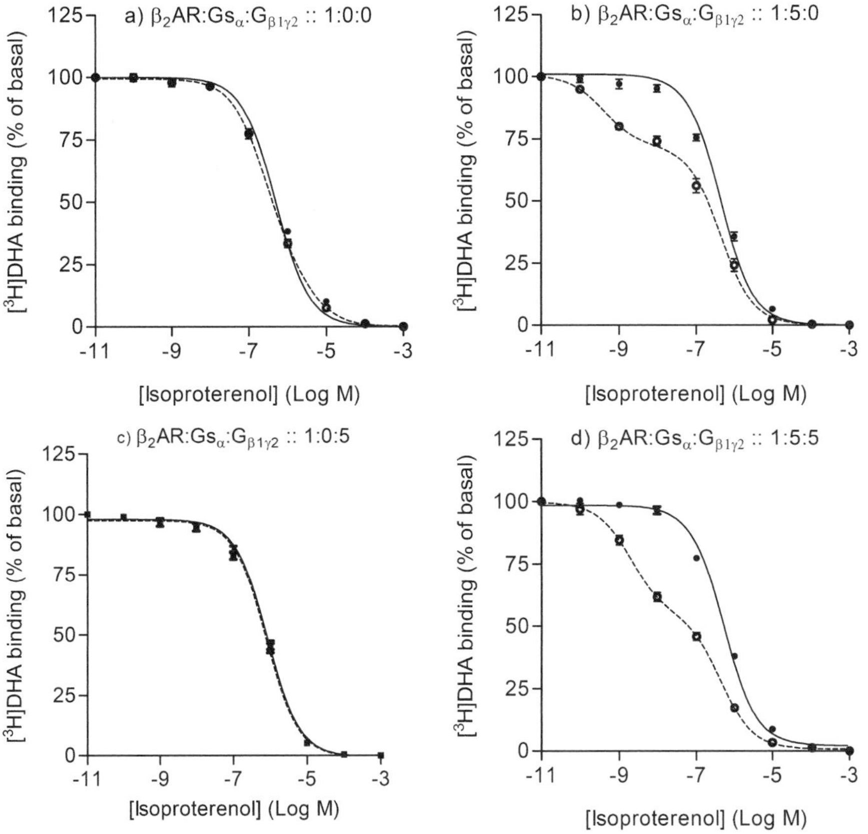

Fig. 1. Competition by isoproterenol of [^{3}H]dihydroalperenol ([^{3}H]DHA) binding in various reconstitution conditions of β_2-AR and G protein subunits with or without GTPγ[S]. [^{3}H]DHA binding in reconstitution complex was performed as described in **Section 2**. Reconstitution complexes containing different G protein subunits, [^{3}H]DHA and isoproterenol of the concentrations indicated on the abscissa. Reaction mixtures additionally contained binding buffer (control) (○) or GTPγS (10μ*M*) (•). Data points are expressed as percent of basal bound [^{3}H]DHA. Data shown are the mean±S.D. of three independent experiments performed in triplicate. (**A**) β_2-AR reconstituted with lipids alone. (**B**) β_2-AR reconstituted with tetGs$_\alpha$ in the molar ratio of 1:5. (**C**) β_2-AR reconstituted with tetGs$_\alpha$ and $\beta_1\gamma_2$ in the molar ratio of 1:0:5. (**D**) β_2-AR reconstituted with tetGs$_\alpha$ and $\beta_1\gamma_2$ in the molar ratio of 1:5:5.

50% GTPγS-sensitive high-affinity agonist binding sites were observed for the reconstituted β_2AR–tetGs$_\alpha$ complex in the molar ratio of 1:5. We then examined the effect of $\beta_1\gamma_2$ on the above reconstitution complex. We reconstituted β_2AR/tetGs$_\alpha$/$\beta_1\gamma_2$ in the ratio of 1:5:5, respectively, and performed the above experiments and noticed a similar GTPγS-sensitive high-affinity agonist binding sites, indicating the lack of a major influence of $\beta\gamma$ proteins in the formation of the high-affinity sites.

2.1. Effects of β_2 AR Ligands on [^{35}S]GTPγS Binding

Figure 2 shows the time course of [^{35}S]GTPγS binding to reconstitution complex in presence of 10 μM isoproterenol and 10 μM ICI. **Figure 3** shows the effect of isoproterenol and other ligands

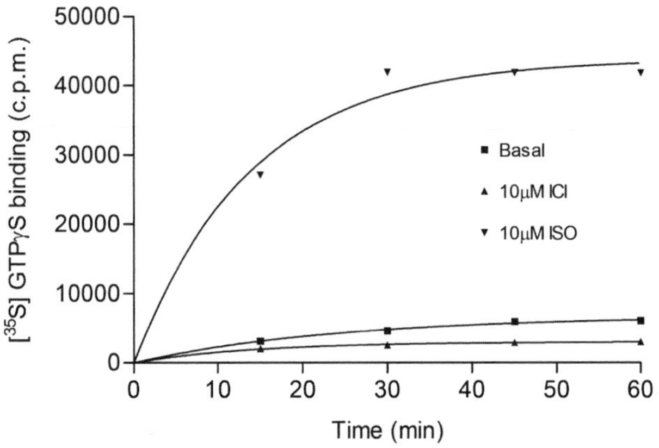

Fig. 2. Time course of [^{35}S]GTPγS binding in reconstitution complex containing β2-AR and tetGs$_{\alpha}$. The reconstitution complexes were incubated with 1 n*M* [^{35}S]GTPγS and 1 μ*M* GDP in the absence (basal;■) or in presence of 10 μ*M* isoproterenol (ISO;▼) or in presence of 10 μ*M* ICI118551 (ICI;▲). Data shown are the mean±S.D. of three independent experiments performed in triplicate.

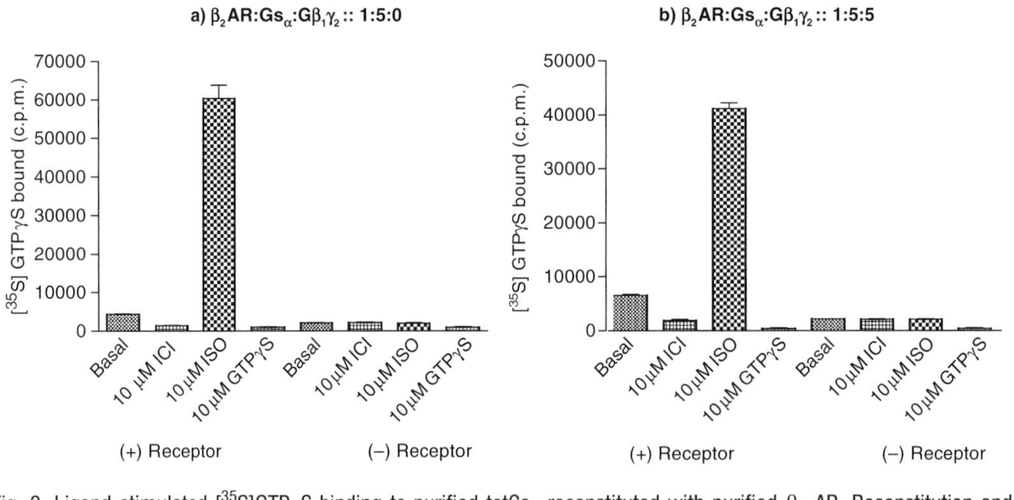

Fig. 3. Ligand-stimulated [^{35}S]GTPγS binding to purified tetGs$_{\alpha}$ reconstituted with purified β_2-AR. Reconstitution and [^{35}S]GTPγS binding were performed as described above. The effects of agonist isoproterenol and the inverse agonist ICI118551 on basal [^{35}S]GTPγS binding in the presence and absence of β_2-AR are shown in the histograms. (**A**) β_2-AR reconstituted with tetGs$_{\alpha}$ and $\beta_1\gamma_2$ in the molar ratio of 1:5:0. (**B**) β_2-AR reconstituted with tetGs$_{\alpha}$ and $\beta_1\gamma_2$ in the molar ratio of 1:5:5. The data for each panel represent the average ±S.E. of three determinations and representative of three independent experiments.

on the binding of [^{35}S]GTPγS to the reconstitution complex in the presence of 1 μ*M* GDP. The extent of [^{35}S]GTPγS binding was approximately 13 times greater in the presence of isoproterenol than in its absence.

2.2. Effects of β_2 AR Ligands on the Affinities of β_2 AR–tetGs$_\alpha$ for Guanine Nucleotides

We also examined effects of ligands on displacement of [^{35}S]GTPγS binding by guanine nucleotides. The displacement curves by GDP shifted to right in the presence of agonist, indicating that the affinity for GDP of β_2AR–tetGs$_\alpha$ reconstitution system decreased by agonist binding (**Fig. 4**). The full agonist, partial agonist, and antagonist differed in their effects on the apparent affinity of the reconstitution system for GDP. These results indicated that the agonist-bound β_2AR–tetGs$_\alpha$ reconstitution system had a lower affinity for GDP than the ligand-free or antagonist-bound β_2AR–tetGs$_\alpha$ reconstitution system, and that the affinity for GDP of salbutamol-bound β_2AR–tetGs$_\alpha$ reconstitution system was intermediate. A similar shift was also observed in the displacement curves by GTP in the presence of full and partial agonists, although the extent of the shift was smaller than in the displacement by GDP. No shifts were observed for displacement by GTPγS with and without ligands (Ratnala et al.; data not shown). These results indicate that the β_2AR–tetGs$_\alpha$ reconstitution system provides a useful means to characterize ligand–receptor–G$_\alpha$–guanine–nucleotide interactions.

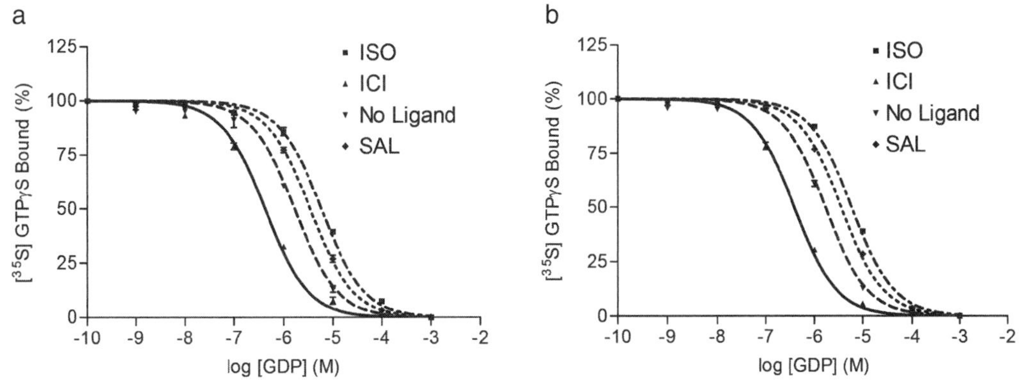

Fig. 4. Displacement of [^{35}S]GTPγS binding by GDP in the presence of various β_2-AR ligands. The purified β_2-AR reconstituted with purified tetGs$_\alpha$±βγ in the molar ratio of 1:5 or 1:5:5 were incubated with 1 m*M* isoproterenol (ISO;■), ICI118551(ICI;▲), salbutamol (SAL;◆), and in absence of ligand (▼) and with indicated concentrations of GDP at 30°C for 30 min in binding buffer with 100p*M* [^{35}S]GTPγS, and 10m*M* $MgCl_2$. The membranes were trapped on GF/B glass filters, which were washed three times with ice-cold binding buffer. Radioactivity was then counted with liquid scintillation counter. Data points are expressed as percentage of basal bound [^{35}S]GTPγS. Data shown are the mean±S.E. of three independent experiments performed in triplicate. (**A**) β_2-AR reconstituted with tetGs$_\alpha$ in the molar ratio of 1:5. (**B**) β_2-AR reconstituted with tetGs$_\alpha$ and $\beta_1\gamma_2$ in the molar ratio of 1:5:5.

3. Conclusions

Development and improvement of novel subtype-specific ligands for known GPCRs is a key step in elucidating receptor functions and developing new drugs. Thus, screening many thousands of samples for each target GPCR is a regular practice to identify novel ligands or drugs in pharmacological research. Current conditions of ligand screening procedures promoted the development of a functional assay system with precise efficacies that could be extended for high-throughput screening. The high-throughput screening of GPCR ligands has generally been based on cell-based assay systems that monitor downstream events of signaling cascades. The representative downstream events for G_s- and G_q-coupled receptors are usually an increase in intracellular cAMP concentrations and Ca^{2+} concentration, respectively. Thus, measurements of cAMP and Ca^{2+} are now the most popular assay systems that are available for GPCRs. The cell-based assay systems have been applied to several receptors and contributed to the finding of novel ligands like AC-90179 *(27)* and ghrelin *(28)*. However, these cell-based assays have the disadvantage that endogenous receptors on host cells respond to their ligands resulting in false-positive signals and also since the signal being collected at the very distal end of the activation processes, which does not give the clear picture of the proximal events that take place near the receptor and seldom give false positives. Assay protocols that directly estimate G protein activation by a target receptor *in vitro* may constitute a simple screening system that avoids such false-positive reactions in high-throughput screening. Since the GTPγS binding studies reflect the efficiency of G protein activation, we see much more efficient basal and agonist-stimulated GTPγS binding activation in tetGs_α membranes without the $\beta_1\gamma_2$ proteins compared to the presence of $\beta_1\gamma_2$ proteins. The most important advantage of [^{35}S]GTPγS binding assay using the β_2AR–tetGs_α reconstitution system over cell-based assays is that false-positive reactions are negligible. The cell-based assay systems are affected by different circumstances causing false-positive responses by endogenous receptors.

We planned to construct a new ligand screening system and apply it to β_2AR. The reconstitution system between a GPCR and its partner G protein α-subunit has been shown to be useful for studies of receptor–G protein interactions because of their efficient coupling *(23)*. Purification of G proteins from natural tissue requires lengthy procedures with limited yields and it is also difficult to resolve closely related members of Gs_α subunits. The *Sf*9-Baculovirus expression system has many advantages to overcome these problems. First, a variety of posttranslational modification mechanisms, especially lipid modifications, such as palmitoylation, myristoylation, and prenylation, are present in *Sf*9 cells. These lipid modifications are critically important for the interactions of G protein subunits with receptors, RGS proteins, or effectors. With these modifications present, the recombinant G protein subunits from *Sf*9 expression system are almost as active as native proteins *(29, 30)*. Thus, the receptor–tetGsα reconstitution complex could be a useful candidate for a new screening system. Using a β_2AR–tetGs$_\alpha$ reconstitution system (β_2AR–Gs$_\alpha$) as a model system, we have examined this system's sensitivity and efficacies on various drugs. As shown in **Fig. 4**, β_2AR–tetGs$_\alpha$ reconstitution complex shows low, intermediate, and high affinity for GDP when it is bound with full agonist, partial agonist, and antagonist, respectively. It is reasonable to assume that the agonist-bound receptor in the reconstitution system accelerates the dissociation of GDP from tetGs$_\alpha$, and that the partial agonist does so to a lesser extent.

In summary, we have observed that a membrane tether facilitates the expression and purification of functional tetGs$_\alpha$ from *Sf*9 insect cells.The purified protein can be efficiently reconstituted with purified β_2AR and functional coupling was observed. This preparation should facilitate biophysical studies to characterize interactions between the β_2AR and tetGs$_\alpha$. Our results also indicate that the receptor–tetGs$_\alpha$ reconstitution system is a good model system for studies on the interaction of receptors and G proteins and also provides evidence that the G$_{\beta\gamma}$-subunit is not required for the formation of the ternary complex between Gs$_\alpha$ and the β_2AR. These results indicate that the β_2AR–tetGs$_\alpha$ reconstitution system is useful for ligand screening because of its high specificity and efficacy. Another benefit of the β_2AR–tetGs$_\alpha$ reconstitution system is the high signal-to-noise ratio of roughly 10-fold to basal in the presence and absence of agonist (**Fig. 3**). These results also suggest the potential usefulness and advantages of β_2AR–Gs$_\alpha$ reconstitution system for screening of ligands, ligand efficacies for β_2AR, and which could be possibly extended to other classes of GPCRs for the drug discovery efforts.

Acknowledgment

We thank Roger Sunahara for providing us with purified $\beta_1\gamma_2$-subunits of G proteins.

References

1. Gilman, A.G. (1987) G proteins – transducers of receptor-generated signals. *Annu. Rev. Biochem.* **56**, 615–649.
2. Neer, E.J. (1995) Heterotrimeric G proteins – organizers of transmembrane signals. *Cell* **80**, 249–257.
3. Bourne, H. R. (1997) How receptors talk to trimeric G proteins. *Curr. Opin. Cell Biol.* **9**, 134–142.
4. Hekman, M., Holzhofer, A., Gierschik, P., Im, M.J., Jakobs, K.H., Pfeuffer, T., and Helmreich, E.J.M. (1987) Regulation of signal transfer from beta-1-adrenoceptor to adenylate-cyclase by beta-gamma-subunits in a reconstituted system. *Eur. J. Biochem.* **169**, 431–439.
5. Florio, V.A., and Sternweis, P.C. (1989) Mechanisms of muscarinic receptor action

on G0 in reconstituted phospholipid-vesicles. *J. Biol. Chem.* **264**, 3909–3915.

6. Hamm, H.E., Deretic, D., Arendt, A., Hargrave, P. A., Koenig, B., and Hofmann, K.P. (1988) Site of G protein binding to rhodopsin mapped with synthetic peptides from the alpha-subunit. *Science* **241**, 832–835.
7. Im, M.J., Holzhofer, A., Bottinger, H., Pfeuffer, T., and Helmreich, E.J.M. (1988) Interactions of pure beta-gamma-subunits of G proteins with purified beta-1-adrenoceptor. *FEBS Lett.* **227**, 225–229.
8. Phillips, W.J., and Cerione, R.A. (1992) Rhodopsin transducin interactions. I. Characterization of the binding of the transducin-beta-gamma subunit complex to rhodopsin using fluorescence spectroscopy. *J. Biol. Chem.* **267**, 17032–17039.
9. Gautam, N., Downes, G. B., Yan, K., and Kisselev, O. (1998) The G protein beta gamma complex. *Cell. Signal.* **10**, 447–455.
10. Schwindinger, W.F., and Robishaw, J.D. (2001) Heterotrimeric G protein beta gamma-dimers in growth and differentiation. *Oncogene* **20**, 1653–1660.
11. Gutkind, J. S. (1998) The pathways connecting G protein-coupled receptors to the nucleus through divergent mitogen-activated protein kinase cascades. *J. Biol. Chem.* **273**, 1839–1842.
12. Chen, Y.B., Weng, G.Z., Li, J.R., Harry, A., Pieroni, J., Dingus, J., Hildebrandt, J.D., Guarnieri, F., Weinstein, H., and Iyengar, R. (1997) A surface on the G protein beta-subunit involved in interactions with adenylyl cyclases. *Proc. Natl. Acad. Sci. USA* **94**, 2711–2714.
13. Ford, C. E., Skiba, N. P., Bae, H. S., Daaka, Y. H., Reuveny, E., Shekter, L. R., Rosal, R., Weng, G. Z., Yang, C. S., Iyengar, R., Miller, R. J., Jan, L. Y., Lefkowitz, R. J., and Hamm, H. E. (1998) Molecular basis for interactions of G protein beta gamma subunits with effectors. *Science* **280**, 1271–1274.
14. Li, Y., Sternweis, P.M., Charnecki, S., Smith, T.F., Gilman, A.G., Neer, E.J., and Kozasa, T. (1998) Sites for G alpha binding on the G protein beta subunit overlap with sites for regulation of phospholipase C beta and adenylyl cyclase. *J. Biol. Chem.* **273**, 16265–16272.
15. Panchenko, M.P., Saxena, K., Li, Y., Charnecki, S., Sternweis, P.M., Smith, T.F., Gilman, A.G., Kozasa, T., and Neer, E.J. (1998) Sites important for PLC beta(2) activation by the G protein beta gamma subunit map to the sides of the beta propeller structure. *J. Biol. Chem.* **273**, 28298–28304.
16. Taylor, J.M., JacobMosier, G.G., Lawton, R.G., VanDort, M., and Neubig, R.R. (1996) Receptor and membrane interaction sites on G beta – a receptor-derived peptide binds to the carboxyl terminus. *J. Biol. Chem.* **271**, 3336–3339.
17. Wu, G.Y., Bogatkevich, G.S., Mukhin, Y.V., Benovic, J.L., Hildebrandt, J.D., and Lanier, S.M. (2000) Identification of G beta gamma binding sites in the third intracellular loop of the M-3-muscarinic receptor and their role in receptor regulation. *J. Biol. Chem.* **275**, 9026–9034.
18. El Far, O., Bofill-Cardona, E., Airas, J. M., O'Connor, V., Boehm, S., Freissmuth, M., Nanoff, C., and Betz, H. (2001) Mapping of calmodulin and G beta gamma binding domains within the C-terminal region of the metabotropic glutamate receptor 7A. *J. Biol. Chem.* **276**, 30662–30669.
19. Harris, B.A., Robishaw, J.D., Mumby, S.M., and Gilman, A.G. (1985) Molecular-cloning of complementary-DNA for the alpha-subunit of the G protein that stimulates adenylate-cyclase. *Science* **229**, 1274–1277.
20. Neer, E.J., and Clapham, D.E. (1988) Roles of G protein subunits in transmembrane signaling. *Nature* **333**, 129–134.
21. Lee, E., Linder, M.E., and Gilman, A.G. (1994) Expression of G protein alpha-subunits in *Escherichia coli*. In: "Heterotrimeric G proteins," Vol. 237, pp. 146–164.
22. Sunahara, R.K., Tesmer, J.J.G., Gilman, A.G., and Sprang, S.R. (1997) Crystal structure of the adenylyl cyclase activator G(S alpha). *Science* **278**, 1943–1947.
23. Lee, T.W., Seifert, R., Guan, X.M., and Kobilka, B.K. (1999) Restricting the mobility of G(s)alpha: impact on receptor and effector coupling. *Biochemistry* **38**, 13801–13809.
24. Seifert, R., Lee, T.W., Lam, V.T., and Kobilka, B.K. (1998) Reconstitution of beta(2)-adrenoceptor-GTP-binding-protein interaction in *Sf9* cells – high coupling efficiency in a beta(2)-adrenoceptor-G(s alpha) fusion protein. *Eur. J. Biochem.* **255**, 369–382.
25. Mukhopadhyay, S., and Ross, E.M. (1999) Rapid GTP binding and hydrolysis by G(q) promoted by receptor and GTPase-activating proteins. *Proc. Natl. Acad. Sci. USA* **96**, 9539–9544.
26. Li, Z., Hannigan, M., Mo, Z.C., Liu, B., Lu, W., Wu, Y., Smrcka, A.V., Wu, G.Q., Li, L.,

Liu, M.Y., Huang, C.K., and Wu, D.Q. (2003) Directional sensing requires G beta gamma-mediated PAK1 and PIX alpha-dependent activation of cdc42. *Cell* **114**, 215–227.

27. Weiner, D.M., Burstein, E.S., Nash, N., Croston, G.E., Currier, E.A., Vanover, K.E., Harvey, S.C., Donohue, E., Hansen, H.C., Andersson, C.M., Spalding, T.A., Gibson, D.F.C., Krebs-Thomson, K., Powell, S.B., Geyer, M.A., Hacksell, U., and Brann, M.R. (2001) 5-hydroxytryptamine(2A) receptor inverse agonists as antipsychotics. *J Pharmacol. Exp. Ther.* **299**, 268–276.

28. Kojima, M., Hosoda, H., Date, Y., Nakazato, M., Matsuo, H., and Kangawa, K. (1999) Ghrelin is a growth-hormone-releasing acylated peptide from stomach. *Nature* **402**, 656–660.

29. Iniguezlluhi, J.A., Simon, M.I., Robishaw, J.D., and Gilman, A.G. (1992) G protein beta-gamma subunits synthesized in *Sf9* cells – functional-characterization and the significance of prenylation of gamma. *J. Biol. Chem.* **267**, 23409–23417.

30. Hepler, J.R., Kozasa, T., Smrcka, A.V., Simon, M.I., Rhee, S.G., Sternweis, P.C., and Gilman, A.G. (1993) Purification from *Sf9* cells and characterization of recombinant Gq-alpha and G11-alpha – activation of purified phospholipase-C isozymes by G-alpha subunits. *J. Biol. Chem.* **268**, 14367–14375.

Chapter 6

Assay Data Quality Assessment

Hanspeter Gubler

Summary

An overview of the characteristics of classical and outlier-resistant data summaries is provided. The latter are important because outlier data can skew results and decisions based on them. The simple data summaries are the basis for all composite assay and screening data quality measures, for example, the signal-to-noise ratio, signal-to-background ratio, assay and screening window coefficients Z' and Z, or strictly standardized mean difference (*SSMD*). In addition to the measures of assay reliability which are based on assessing the size of the "signal windows," some measures for the characterization of the degree of agreement of repeated measurements are also outlined.

Key words: Assay data analysis, Screening data analysis, Data quality indicators, Assay performance indicators, Robust statistics, Outlier-resistant methods, Reproducibility.

1. Introduction

Microtiter plate-based assay and screening technologies have become essential tools in the field of drug discovery. They are widely used in the pharmaceutical and biotech industries *(1–3)*, as well as in academic laboratories *(4, 5)*. Progress in assay miniaturization and the application of robotic technologies in compound management and screening have increased the throughput in a dramatic way *(6)*. Appropriate data management and statistical data analysis tools are essential to cope with the large amounts of primary screening data ($n = 1$, single well at one concentration per compound), confirmation data (usually run in replicates or as small titration series, e.g., $n = 2$ or 4) and increasingly larger numbers of full concentration–response curve (CRC) or dose–response curve (DRC) experiments

Wayne R. Leifert (ed.), *G Protein-Coupled Receptors in Drug Discovery, vol. 552*

Book doi: 10.1007/978-1-60327-317-6_6

(7, 8). Several statistical quantities and procedures described in more detail later in this article are available to assess the assay quality and reproducibility of a particular assay and screening setup.

Particular emphasis is put on the description and application of outlier-resistant methods because the latter, if present in the data set, can have an unduly large influence on the classical statistical measures. Even when assuming that the initial assay development process has resulted in a stable and sensitive readout, a series of systematic – but locally and temporally variable – errors of different origins and sizes can occur over the course of a screening campaign (**Fig. 1**). It is a great advantage for the routine analysis of the screening data if automated software for quality control, as well as detection and correction of systematic errors in the data sets, is available *(9–16)*.

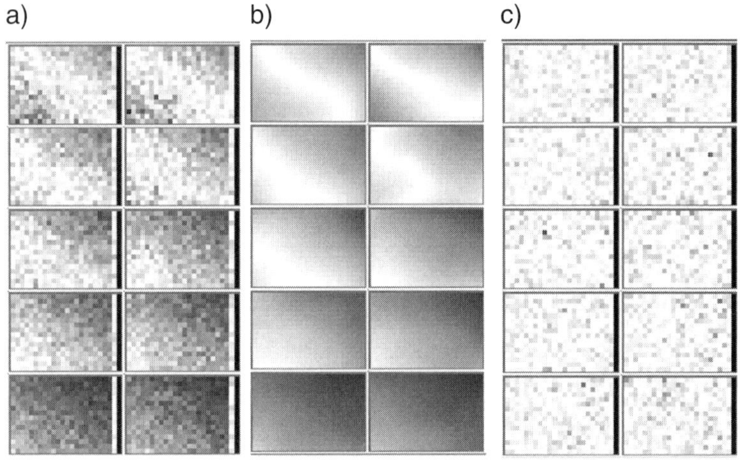

Fig. 1. Plate image representation of measured or calculated activity values. Usually a color scale (e.g., *blue–white–red*, "heat map") is used to represent the % activity values instead of the gray scale employed in this figure. (**a**) Normalized data are strongly affected by systematic response background trends, (**b**) 2D robust local regression surface representation of the systematic effect, and (**c**) corrected response data, *see (12)*.

2. Data Summaries

All of our measures of assay quality, stability, and reproducibility as well as the calculations determining the biological effect are finally based on simple summary statistical quantities for the *location* and the degree of variability, that is, the spread, or *scale* of the data. The term sample in the context of this section means "statistical sample," that is, a set of n measurements which are taken under the same experimental conditions. For a set of n data points $x_1, \ldots, x_n$ the usual *sample mean* is given by

$$mean_n = mean_n(x) = \bar{x} = \frac{1}{n}\sum_{i=1}^{n} x_i \qquad [1]$$

and is an estimator of the mean of the underlying population. The *sample variance*

$$sd_n^2 = sd_n^2(x) = \frac{1}{n-1}\sum_{i=1}^{n}(x_i - \bar{x})^2 \qquad [2]$$

and its square root value, the *sample standard deviation*

$$sd_n = \sqrt{sd_n^2} \qquad [3]$$

are the usual measures of data variability or spread of data. The standard deviation is a measure for the "typical (average) distance" between the mean and the data points. For a large number of identically and independently distributed data values x_i from a normal distribution with center μ and variance σ^2 the values of [1] and [2] will asymptotically tend toward these two respective population parameters *(17)*. The sample mean and standard deviation as defined above can be calculated for *any* data set, one just needs to be aware that they do not necessarily correspond to the defining parameters of the underlying distribution if it is not normal. The "uncertainty" of the sample mean, the *standard error of the mean*, or simply, the *standard error* is given by

$$se_n = \frac{sd_n}{\sqrt{n}} \qquad [4]$$

and indicates how "precise" our sample mean is determined by our n data values. It is a measure of the "typical variability" of the mean if the experiments are repeated many times.

Unfortunately, all the quantities described above are vulnerable even to single outlier values and are thus prone to be "thrown off" by data points which are unusual in a sense that they deviate from the pattern given by the majority of the data. The data analyst should refrain from simply deleting such data points because they look "odd," unless there is other evidence from the assay execution phase suggesting a malfunction of one or more experimental steps. A whole series of estimation methods which are resistant to the presence of outliers make the decision whether "to delete or not to delete" unnecessary. It can be shown that both the *sample median* $med_n = median_n(x)$ of the sorted data set $x_1, \ldots, x_n$ which is determined as

$$med_n = x_{(n+1)/2} \text{ if } n \text{ is odd, and } med_n = \frac{1}{2}(x_{n/2} + x_{(n/2)+1}) \text{ if } n \text{ is even} \quad [5]$$

and the *sample median absolute deviation* (which is "unfortunately" abbreviated as *mad*)

$$mad_n = 1.4826 \cdot med_n(|x_i - med_n|) \quad [6]$$

provide a high degree of resistance against outliers *(18)*. The factor 1.4826 guarantees the asymptotic equivalence of [6] with [3] for normally distributed data, so that mad_n can be interpreted as an *outlier-resistant version of the sample standard deviation* sd_n.

Other data summaries are based on the quantiles of the sample distribution. Empirical quantile values *quantile* (x, p) can be calculated from the sorted data set $x_1, \ldots, x_n$, as an interpolated value for each probability $0 \le p \le 1$ *(18)*. Note also that $med_n = quantile(x, 0.5)$. An alternative robust measure of variability is based on the interquartile range (*IQR*), that is, the span between the 75 and 25% sample distribution quantiles. It is obviously a measure of data spread which eliminates a considerable part of tail region at both ends and is thus highly resistant to the presence of outliers. The *iqr* variability scale estimator *(18)*, which is again designed to be equivalent to the normal distribution standard deviation in its asymptotic limit, is

$$iqr_n = 0.7413 \cdot IQR = 0.7413 \cdot (quantile(x, 0.75) - quantile(x, 0.25)) \quad [7]$$

It was found *(19)* that less than 0.2% contamination of a normal distribution with a component three times as broad was enough to make *mad* a more reliable estimator of the distribution "width" than the classical *sd* value. The reason is simply that large deviations contribute according to their squared magnitudes to *sd*, which gives an overly large influence on the results. Another outlier-resistant measure of location is the *trimmed mean (20)*. It is calculated in the same way as the mean after discarding a certain percentage of the samples at the high and low ends. Typically between $\alpha = 5\%$ and $\alpha = 25\%$ of the data are eliminated from the lower and upper ends, respectively, when calculating the *α-trimmed means.* The special case of the *interquartile mean* (*iqm*) corresponds to $\alpha = 25\%$. Interestingly the *mean* and the *median* can be considered to be the extreme cases of trimmed means with $\alpha = 0\%$ and $\alpha = 50\%$, that is, minimal and maximal trimming, respectively.

Making summary plots of the data is another important "robust" technique and can quickly reveal irregularities in the data set. Dot plots, box plots, histograms, density estimates, and quantile plots, many of which are based on the presented summary statistics values, can be used for the purpose of checking the homogeneity of the data set and look for the presence of outliers *(21)*. A simple graphical method to look for asymmetries in the data distribution and for potential outliers is the box plot, also called box-and-whisker plot *(20, 21)*. It is based on the determination of the sample median and other distribution quantiles. Visual limits (box) are drawn at the 1st and 3rd quartile and at the most extreme data values which are still within the $Q_{1,3} \pm 1.5IQR$ range on both sides of the median (whiskers). Data points outside this limit are plotted individually.

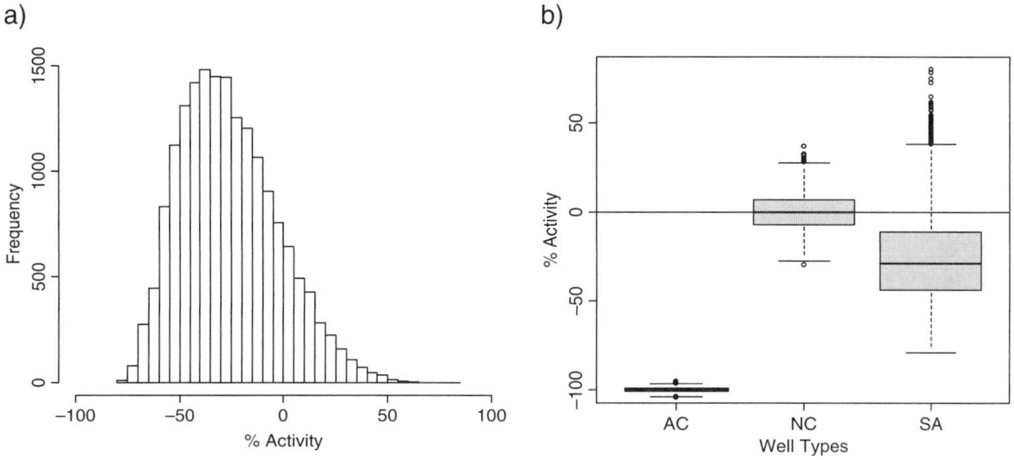

Fig. 2. (**a**) Histogram of compound sample activity values and (**b**) box plot categorized by well types (AC, active control; NC, neutral control; SA, compound sample). This data set is obviously strongly affected by systematic response distortions and average response shifts between the neutral (zero-effect) controls and the sample wells. The plots are based on the normalized screening data, as depicted in **Fig. 1a**. The *Z* value (*see* **Section 3.5**) for the normalized sample data is –0.01.

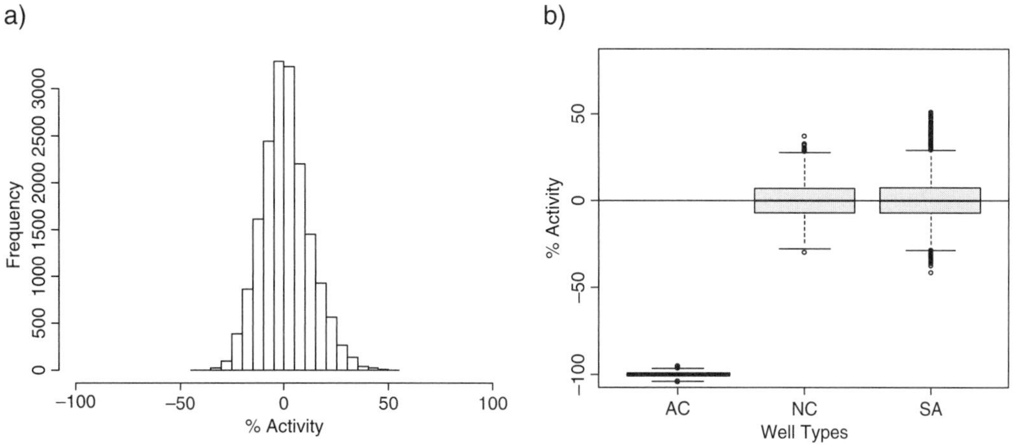

Fig. 3. (**a**) Histogram of compound sample activity values and (**b**) box plot categorized by well types (AC, active control; NC, neutral control; SA, compound sample) based on the corrected screening data depicted in **Fig. 1**. The corrected sample data corresponding to **Fig. 1c** is now centered on the zero activity level as given by the neutral control group and exhibits a much smaller spread. The *Z* value for the corrected sample data is 0.61. Compare this situation to **Fig. 2**.

The box and whisker limits correspond to approximately $\pm 0.6745\sigma$ (50% probability) and $\pm 2.678\sigma$ (99.3% probability) values of a normal distribution, respectively. Box plots are especially useful because they can at the same time represent location, spread, skewness, tail length, and outlying data points. Example histograms and box plots based on the plate data set shown in **Fig. 1** are displayed in **Fig. 2** for the corresponding normalized data and in **Fig. 3** for the results after a correction step to eliminate the systematic errors *(12)*. Selected assay performance indicators, which are explained in the next section, show a clear improvement of the assay data quality after the data correction step.

3. Indicators of Assay Performance

In the following sections the indices *min* and *max* are used to indicate the respective magnitude of the signals, that is, the "low" and "high" control values. For inhibition assays the *max* signal usually corresponds to the neutral control (*NC*; zero compound effect) and the *min* signal to the maximal inhibition level. In stimulatory assays the *min* signal usually corresponds to the baseline, that is, *NC* and an increased signal level (*max*) to the positive control. Some assay designs can lead to an inverted signal direction. All quantities outlined below are based on the basic summary statistics for location and variability scale defined in **Section 2**. Not all of the mentioned assay quality indicators provide a completely independent assessment of assay performance because they are directly or indirectly related to each other. An example is shown in **Section 3.6**. The Z' and Z factors, as well as strictly standardized mean difference (*SSMD*; *see* **Sections 3.5** and **3.7**, respectively), provide a data quality assessment which combines signal range and variability measures in a concise summary number.

It is worth noting that assay quality indicators should not be "blindly" optimized without consideration of the necessary assay sensitivity, that is, the capability to actually detect and rank compounds with the desired mode of action.

3.1. Classical and Outlier-Resistant Versions of Data Quality Indicators

In the following chapters, the population means μ and standard deviations σ are always used to indicate the use of the measures of location and spread in the corresponding expressions. In actual practice the sample mean and sample standard deviation *mean* and *sd*, or better, one of the robust (outlier-resistant) equivalents listed in **Table 1** are used in their respective place.

So for example a robust Z' factor, denoted RZ', is obtained as

$$RZ' = 1 - 3(mad_{max} + mad_{min})/|median_{max} - median_{min}| \quad [8]$$

Table 1
Equivalence between normal distribution population parameters and various classical and robust sample summary statistics

Population parameters of the normal distribution	Classical estimators	Robust estimators
μ	*mean*	*median, trimmed mean, biweight-location*
σ	*sd*	*mad, iqr, biweight scale*

Robust estimators can be used as plug-in values in place of the classical quantities.

given the basic expression [16] for the assay window coefficient Z' (*see* **Section 3.5**) and the corresponding entries in **Table 1**.

3.2. Coefficient of Variation

The coefficient of variation *(22)* is a measure of the readout precision relative to the average value. The coefficient of variation (sometimes also called the "relative error") is defined as

$$CV = \sigma/\mu \qquad [9]$$

and the coefficient variation in percent simply as

$$\%CV = 100CV = 100\,\sigma/\mu \qquad [10]$$

As mentioned in the introduction to this section, the various assay performance indicators are determined at *min*, *max*, and possibly midpoint level. In typical assays the $\%CV$ value at the max and mid level should be below ~15%, *see also* **Section 3.6**. The $\%\,CV$ value for the minimal readout signal could well surpass this limit if the absolute signal size is very small. The relation between CV and other assay data quality indicators (Z', S/B) is explained and illustrated in **Section 3.6**.

3.3. Signal-to-Background Ratio

The signal-to-background ratio S/B or SBR is simply defined as the ratio of the two extreme signal levels in the assay

$$S/B = SBR = \mu_{max}/\mu_{min} \qquad [11]$$

The signal-to-background ratio has essentially no significance in terms of being a direct indicator of statistical assay quality, because the relationship of the signal to the level of its precision is not at all reflected in this particular parameter. It is sometimes used as a "surrogate" indicator in a particular context, because for a stable assay system and the given experimental variability (σ or CV) there is of course a direct empirical relationship between S/B

and, for example, the Z' factor, *see* **Section 3.6**. In terms of defining a biologically meaningful change of the signal level it clearly needs to be considered in the assay design phase. So *SBR* is not directly concerned with statistical significance or quality of an assay, but simply with biological or pharmacological significance and sensitivity of the readout change. The *SBR* is "adequate" if the assay system is tuned to allow the unequivocal identification of potent and efficacious compounds. The mentioned fact that *SBR* and a related *CV* value "determine" the corresponding Z' factor values is only an indirect effect from this point of view.

3.4. Signal-to-Noise Ratio

The signal-to-noise ratio *S/N* or *SNR* is a measure of the size of the signal change (i.e., the dynamic range of the assay signal) in relation to the variability of the baseline signal or the signal difference, so it is a measure of the statistical "significance" of the useable signal change. The original concept originates from field of electrical engineering *(23)*. In contrast to *SBR* the signal-to-noise ratio can be used as a statistical indicator on how well the maximal signal can be determined as being "different" from the background signal. It is defined as

$$S/N = SNR = (\mu_{max} - \mu_{min})/\sigma_{min} \qquad [12]$$

or *alternatively* – and in the assay development and screening field sometimes more adequately – as

$$S/N = SNR = (\mu_{max} - \mu_{min})/\sqrt{\sigma^2_{max} + \sigma^2_{min}} \qquad [13]$$

where the *overall* standard deviation of the difference $(\mu_{max} - \mu_{min})$ instead of simply the standard deviation at the *min* (i.e., background) level appears in the denominator. For some assay technologies and assay conditions the *SNR* may well behave differently than the *SBR* and even show an "inverse" relationship when assay and process parameters (reagent composition, reaction parameters, etc.) are varied. Equation [13] is also used in the context of the *SSMD* data quality indicator (*see* **Section 3.7**).

3.5. Assay and Screening Window Coefficients: Z and Z′ Factors

The assay and screening window coefficients Z' and Z (also called Z' and Z factors) as defined in *(24)* has become ubiquitously used in the screening community. The Z' factor is a dimensionless quantity which is calculated as the ratio of the signal window *SW* between the two control signal levels *(25)* to the signal range $SR = |\mu_{max} - \mu_{min}|$ of the assay (**Fig. 4**). It is a normalized quantity measuring data variation and dynamic range in a combined score. The signal window *SW* is defined as

$$\begin{aligned} SW = SW_{max,min} &= (\mu_{max} - 3\sigma_{max}) - (\mu_{min} + 3\sigma_{min}) \\ &= (\mu_{max} - \mu_{min}) - 3(\sigma_{max} + \sigma_{min}) \end{aligned} \qquad [14]$$

and Z' is simply the above-mentioned ratio

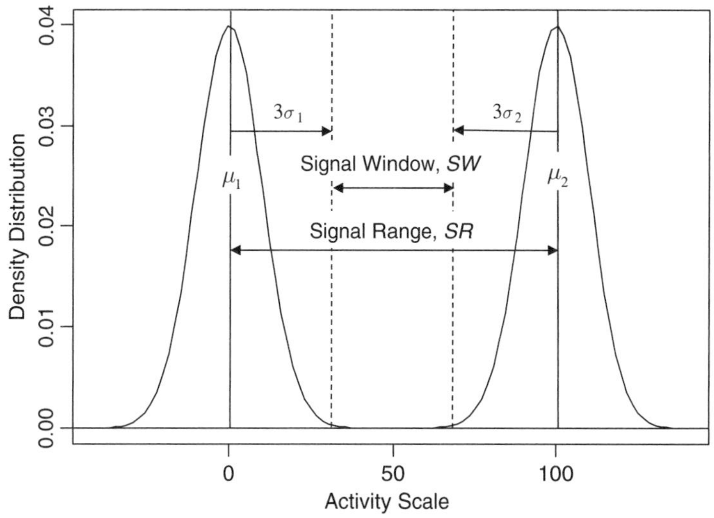

Fig. 4. Illustration of the signal window *SW* and the signal range *SR* between the two types of control sample populations in a typical assay. The ratio of *SW* to *SR* is the Z' factor.

$$Z' = SW/SR = 1 - 3(\sigma_{max} + \sigma_{\min})/|\mu_{max} - \mu_{min}| \quad [15]$$

The Z' factor quantifies the relative size of the "usable window" between the control signals used in the assay, for example, the neutral controls (*NC*) and inhibition controls (*IC*) for *max* and *min*, respectively. In terms of these mentioned control indices [15] is then simply

$$Z' = 1 - 3(\sigma_{NC} + \sigma_{IC})/|\mu_{NC} - \mu_{IC}| \quad [16]$$

The Z factor is defined in an equivalent way and measures the relative signal window between the compound samples (*SA*) and the *IC*:

$$Z = 1 - 3(\sigma_{SA} + \sigma_{IC})/|\mu_{SA} - \mu_{IC}| \quad [17]$$

Limits for both the Z' and Z parameters are $-infinity \leq Z', Z \leq 1$. The limit case $Z = 1$ corresponds to the situation where $\sigma = 0$, or the signal range becomes very large (infinity), or both.

Good values for Z' and Z are > 0.5, but some assay types, especially the ones using ratiometric readouts, can still give useful results for smaller values with $Z' > 0$. Also, if one is only interested in strongly active compounds, then the false-negative rates for assays with $Z' < 0.5$ (which usually means that hit thresholds needs to be set at a higher level) can be still very small and the results of the assay can be very reliable. For $Z', Z < 0$ the data variability bands start overlap and the assignment of a sample as an active "hit" becomes more and more uncertain.

The Z and Z' factors are useful quantities to directly compare the quality of different assays or the behavior of a given assay over time on the same normalized and "universal" relative scale, but they need to be interpreted with caution when data are highly nonnormal and exhibit asymmetric distributions. It is also obvious from [16] or [17] that the same Z' or Z values can be obtained for different combinations of the two σ terms and the signal range. *See* **Section 3.7** for view of these quantities in a probabilistic context.

3.6. Relationship between SBR, CV, and Z′

It is illustrative to rewrite the expression for Z' in terms of other assay performance indicators *(26)*. Using previously defined relationships one obtains

$$Z' = 1 - 3(1 + k)CV_{max}/(1 - 1/SBR) \qquad [18]$$

Where $k = \sigma_{min}/\sigma_{max}$.

In practice the factor k is between 0 (if σ_{min} becomes negligibly small compared to σ_{max}) and 1 (if the respective standard deviations at the two comparison levels are equal in size). When requiring $0 \leq Z'$ then the largest CV_{max} values, which are tolerated for large *SBR*s, are 0.33 or 0.167 for $k = 0$ or $k = 1$. For $0.5 \leq Z'$ the corresponding CV_{max} limits are 0.167 and 0.083. Correspondingly smaller values are tolerated if the *SBR* is getting smaller (e.g., only half of these values for $SBR = 2$). In an assumed "worst case" scenario with $SBR=2$ and $k = 1$ the largest CV_{max} value for $Z' > 0$ is only 0.083 or 0.042 for $Z' > 0.5$. It is obvious from [18], and also intuitively clear, that small CV_{max} values, large *SBR* values, and small values of k (which often go together with a large *SBR*) lead to larger (better) Z' factors.

3.7. Strictly Standardized Mean Difference (SSMD)

In **Section 3.4**, Equation [13], the "alternative" formulation of the *S/N* ratio was defined as $S/N = (\mu_{max} - \mu_{min})/\sqrt{\sigma_{max}^2 + \sigma_{min}^2}$, where the asymptotic *standard deviation of the difference of the means*, that is, $\sqrt{\sigma_{max}^2 + \sigma_{min}^2}$, is used as a measure of variability. This alternative formulation of *S/N* was also termed "strictly standardized mean difference" (*SSMD*) and was investigated as an assay quality indicator in *(27, 28)*. *SSMD* has similar properties as Z' or Z, but allows a meaningful interpretation of decision error rates which are based on (normal) probability theory. Such an interpretation is difficult to obtain for the Z' and Z factors. In **Section 3.5** it was already mentioned that the same *Z or* Z' factors can result from a combination of different values of σ_{max} and σ_{min}. Related to this fact one can also find different false negative rates (FNR) and statistical power values *(29–31)* with respect to the standard 3σ threshold setting and %-activity values of interest (see examples in **Table 2**). This fact reflects the difficulty of direct interpretation of the Z factors in terms of probability values because they cannot be determined in a unique way from the Z factor alone. In a related approach to assess data quality in probabilistic terms, Sui and Wu *(32)* have proposed to use directly the power value as alternative data quality indicator.

Table 2
Illustration of the influence of differences in the $k = sd_{min}/sd_{max}$ ratio on Z', *SSMD*, as well as FN and power values for samples with 50% activity ($\mu_{sample} = 30$)

μ_{min}	μ_{max}	*SBR*	σ_{min}	σ_{max}	*k*	CV_{max}(%)	Z'	*SSMD*	T $\mu_{max}-3\sigma_{max}$	μ_{sample}	FNR (%)	Power (%)
10	50	5	0.0	6.7	0	13.3	0.5	6.0	30.0	30.0	50	50
10	50	5	3.3	3.3	1	6.7	0.5	8.5	40.0	30.0	0	100
10	50	5	0.0	10.0	0	20.0	0.25	4.0	20.0	30.0	98	2
10	50	5	5.0	5.0	1	10.0	0.25	5.7	35.0	30.0	16	84
10	50	5	0.0	13.3	0	26.7	0	3.0	30.0	30.0	100	0
10	50	5	6.7	6.7	1	13.3	0	4.2	10.0	30.0	50	50
10	50	5	0.0	20.0	0	40.0	–0.5	2.0	–10.0	30.0	100	0
10	50	5	10.0	10.0	1	20.0	–0.5	2.8	20.0	30.0	84	16

The two "extreme" cases $k = 0$ and $k = 1$ are always constructed such that the identical Z' values (0.5, 0.25, 0, and –0.5) result from the example data. The hit detection threshold is chosen as $T = \mu_{max} - 3\sigma_{max}$. Samples with expected mean value of $\mu_{sample} = 30$ and a given threshold *T* lead to expected false-negative rates FNR and detection power (1-FNR). It is obvious that different data variability situations can result in equal Z' but different expected FNR and power values. *SSMD* correlates more closely with the hit detection power.

The finite sample expression for the expected population *SSMD* is

$$SSMD = mean_{SSMD}$$
$$= (mean_{max} - mean_{min}) / \sqrt{\frac{n_{max}-1}{n_{max}} sd^2_{max} + \frac{n_{min}-1}{n_{min}} sd^2_{min}} \quad [19]$$

which tends toward [13] for normal distributions in the limit of large $n_{\max}$ and $n_{\min}$. From the *SSMD* value one can derive the probability that a value from the positive control population is actually greater than a value from the negative control population. This is meaningful and easily interpreted information on the difference between the two types of controls in an assay. Using the 3σ limit on *SSMD* is conceptually equivalent to performing a statistical test and rejecting the null hypothesis (i.e., that no difference exists between the two means) at the 0.27% (two-tailed test) or 0.13% (one-tailed test) level *(28, 33)*.

Because of the general relationship $\sqrt{\sigma^2_{max} + \sigma^2_{min}} < \sigma_{max} + \sigma_{min}$ and by using Equations [13] and [15], one obtains the following inequality for large n

$$|SSMD| > 3/(1 - Z') \quad [20]$$

as also demonstrated in *(27)*. It is shown that if $1 > Z' > 0$, then $|SSMD|$ is > 3, but that the inverse is not true, because of the inequality in [20]. This can be illustrated as follows: with $sd_{min} = k\ sd_{max}$, as

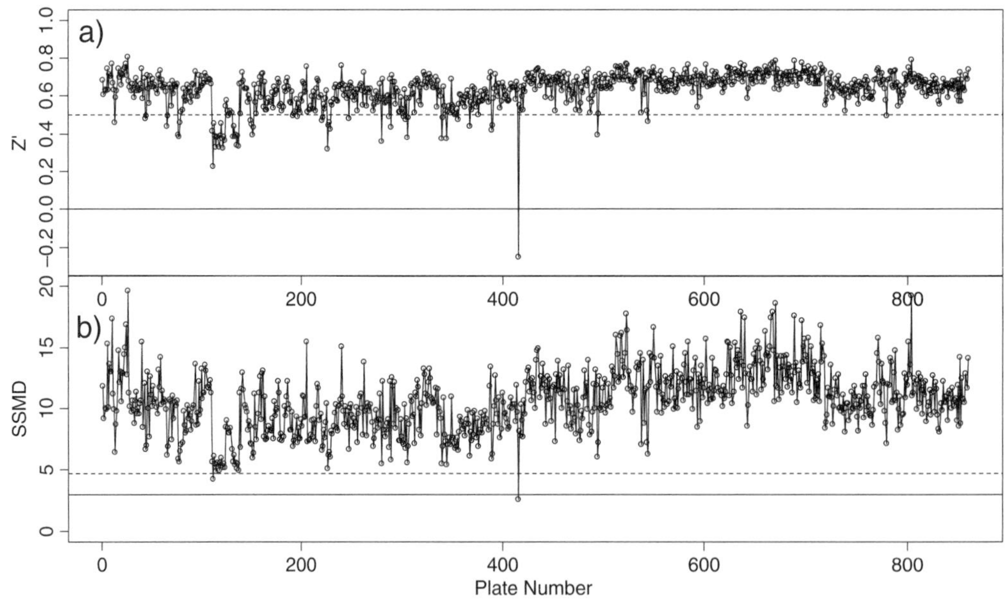

Fig. 5. (**a**) Z' factor and (**b**) corresponding *SSMD* values for the same 900 set of 1536-well plates. Typical decision levels for Z' are 0.5 ("excellent assay" if larger; dashed line) and 0 ("screening essentially impossible" if smaller; solid line). The corresponding *SSMD* limits are 4.7 (dashed line) and 3 (solid line). It can be easily seen that the Z' limit is more conservative, that is, more points are found below the dashed lines in (a) than in (b).

defined previously in **Section 3.6**, it is easily shown that $SSMD = 3f/(1 - Z')$, where $f = (1 + k)/\sqrt{1 + k^2}$. The factor f lies between 1 for k=0 and $\sqrt{2}$ for k=1, that is, $f \geq 1$ for the defined range of k. As long as the value of Z' fulfills the condition $Z' > 1 - f$ (i.e., $Z' > 0$ for $k = 0$ and $Z' > -0.414$ for $k = 1$), then *SSMD* is > 3. The $Z' > 0$ criterion is thus in general more conservative than the $|SSMD| > 3$ limit. In the same way as Z' and Z can be calculated as separate quantities based on the *NC* and *SA* data subsets, respectively, two variants of the *SSMD* measure can of course also be calculated based on the same data alternatives. *SSMD* can clearly be used as plate QC indicator instead of or in parallel to Z' or Z. When requiring $Z' > 0.5$ (indicating an "excellent" assay according to *(24)*, then the "equivalent" *SSMD* limit needs to be chosen as $|SSMD| > 4.7$, *see (34)*. In (**Fig. 5**) a comparison of the Z' and the *SSMD* data quality indicators for a series of screening plates is shown.

4. Reproducibility, Reliability

Tests of assay reproducibility and agreement between repeat runs of the same assay are further important steps for assessing the quality and stability of an assay. A simple comparison method for clinical measurements which is also applicable in the drug discovery field was published by Bland and Altman in *(35)*. Sun et al. *(36)* have described the corresponding applications and some extensions for potency (*AC50*) determinations.

In the case of duplicate runs the approach which comes usually first to mind is to calculate the simple Pearson or the Spearman correlation coefficients *(17)*. While both of these provide a measure for (linear) *association* of the two repeat runs, they do not provide any information about the degree of *agreement* of the replicate determinations of the test compound set. In this type of reproducibility analysis it is actually crucial to assess the size and distribution of the observed *differences* between the measurements in the two groups, that is, $(x_{i,1} - x_{i,2})$, or more generally, all pairwise differences $(x_{i,j} - x_{i,k})$ between the measurements in all groups j, $k = 1 .. n$. When comparing more than $n = 2$ groups the intraclass correlation coefficient ICC *(37, 38)* can be used to characterize the degree of reproducibility of groups of repeated measurements. In short and simplified terms the intraclass correlation is the ratio of the inter-subject variance to the total variance. In the following paragraph, the quantitative assessment of the "degree of agreement" of duplicate determinations or of comparison measurements employing different technologies is outlined.

The minimum significant ratio *MSR*, the minimum significant difference *MSD*, and the corresponding limits of agreement *LsA* are quantities of interest in this context *(39, 40)*. Potency and efficacy determinations are usually based on fitting the parameters of the four-parameter logistic (*4PL*) model – often called the Hill-slope model – to the experimental data. The inflection point (the AC50 parameter), the concentration giving 50% of a compound's maximal response in an antagonist/inhibition assay (IC_{50}) or in an agonist/activator assay (EC_{50}) is the usual measure of potency of a compound. The proper treatment of outliers is at least as important in the nonlinear regression methods used to find the best fit parameters of the *4PL* or other concentration–response models as for the simple summary statistics which were described in **Section 2**. One possible way of handling outliers in CRC fitting through iterative reweighing of the residuals is described in a number of articles *(41– 43)*. The approach is again one of "accommodation," that is, making the method insensitive to the presence of outlier points.

The ratio $AC50_{1,i}/AC50_{2,i}$ or, equivalently, the log potency differences $d_i = log10(AC50_{1,i}) - log10(AC50_{2,i})$ are used to derive the mean log potency difference $d = mean(d_i) = log10(MR)$ and their standard deviation $sd = sd(d_i)$.

The mean ratio *MR* is thus $MR = 10^d$. The asymptotic 95% confidence limits of *MR* are $[CLMR_L, CLMR_U] = 10^{d \pm 1.96\, sd/\sqrt{n}}$. The mean significant ratio (MSR) at the usual 100(1–α)%=95% confidence level is defined as

$$MSR_{\alpha=5\%} = 10^{Z_{1-\alpha/2} sd} = 10^{1.96 sd} \quad [21]$$

The corresponding "limits of agreement" *LsA* are

$$LsA_\alpha = 10^{d \pm Z_{1-\alpha/2} sd} \quad [22]$$

and the lower and upper limit values *LLsA* and *ULsA* are

$$[LLsA_\alpha, ULsA_\alpha] = [MR/MRS_\alpha, MR \times MSR_\alpha] \quad [23]$$

Confidence levels α other than 5% can, of course, also be used. Plots of the geometric mean of the potency values $GM_i = \sqrt{AC50_{1,i} AC50_{2,i}} = 10^{(\log 10(AC50_{1,i}) + \log 10(AC50_{2,i}))/2}$ vs. the difference of log potency pairs d_i and graphical indications of the *MR* and *LsA* values are very useful tools to visualize assay reproducibility or the agreement of measurements using different methods. The "ratio – geometric mean plot," which is a variant of the Bland–Altman plot, incorporates all these features. *See* **Fig. 6** for an example. A typical recommended upper limit for the minimum significant ratio is *MSR* <3, but actual "acceptance limits" in a particular context depend strongly on the intended use of the final results.

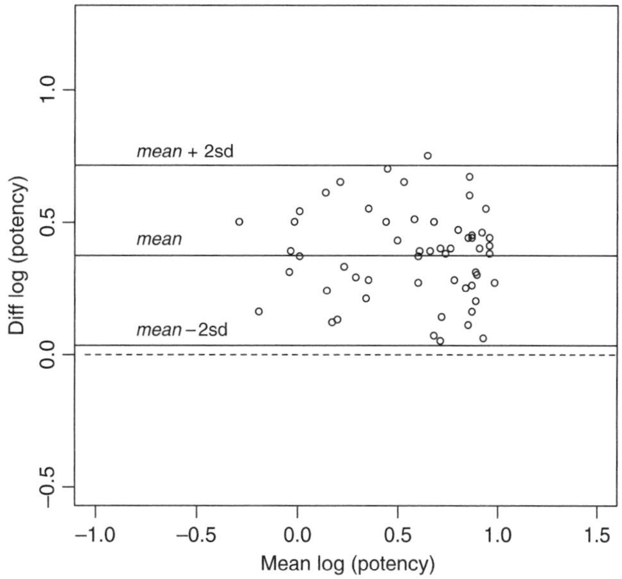

Fig. 6. Example *MR-GM* (mean ratio – geometric mean), or mean log(potency)-difference vs. mean log(potency) plot, to assess the variability and degree of agreement between repeated determinations of compound potency in an assay, or between two different assays. In this example the agreement of the IC_{50} determinations of a series of compounds between two assay technologies was investigated. The lower limit of agreement, that is, the *mean–2sd* line does not include the diff(log(potency)) = 0, that is, the *MR* = 1 line. A clear shift between the potency determinations based on the two different technologies is apparent.

Similar calculations for the mean difference *MD*, the minimum significant difference *MSD* and the corresponding limits of agreement can be defined for linear quantities (e.g., efficacy values derived from curve fits or duplicate determinations of %-activity values in primary screening). The mean $M_i = 0.5^* (E_{1,i} + E_{2,i})$ and the difference $\Delta_i = E_{1,i} - E_{2,i}$ of the duplicate determinations are used to calculate the mean difference $MD = mean(\Delta_i)$ and the respective standard deviation $sd{=}sd(\Delta_i)$. In this case plots of the mean M_i vs. Δ_i and the indication of *MD* and *LsA* is the equivalent graphical representation for observed quantities on the linear scale ("mean-difference plots").

5. Summary and Conclusion

This chapter has given an overview of classical and outlier-resistant methods for summarizing the experimental data and for characterizing their statistical quality. Outlier-resistant methods are especially important for the analysis of screening results, because outlier data can skew results and decisions based on them. Simple data summaries are the basis for all composite assay and screening data quality measures, for example, the signal-to-noise ratio, signal-to-background ratio, assay and screening window coefficients Z' and Z, or strictly standardized mean difference *SSMD*. Besides the measures of assay reliability which are based on the size of signal windows and their statistical variability, simple methods for the assessment of the degree of agreement of repeated measurements were reviewed.

Acknowledgment

The author thanks Christian N. Parker for the careful review of the manuscript.

References

1. Fox, S.J. (ed.) (2002) *High Throughput Screening 2002: New Strategies and technologies*. High Tech Business Decisions, Moraga, CA, USA.
2. Fox, S.J. (ed.) (2005) *High Throughput Screening 2005: New Users, Cell Based Assays, and a Host of New Tools*. HighTech Business Decisions, Moraga, CA, USA.
3. Downey, W.P. (ed.) (2007) *High Throughput Screening 2007: New Strategies, Success Rates, and Use of Enabling Technologies*. HighTech Business Decisions, San Jose, CA, USA.
4. Editorial (2007) The academic pursuit of screening. *Nature Chemical Biology* **3**, 433.
5. Austin, C.P., Brady, L.S., Insel, T.R., and Collins F.S. (2004) NIH molecular libraries initiative. *Science* **306**, 1138–1139.
6. Mayr, L.M., and Fuerst, P. (2008) The future of high-throughput screening. *J. Biomol. Screen.* **13**, 443–448.
7. Inglese, J., Auld, D.S., Jadhav, A., Johnson, R.L., Simeonov, A., Yasgar, A., Zheng, W., and Austin, C.P. (2006) Quantitative high-throughput screening: a titration-based approach that efficiently identifies biological activities in large chemical libraries. *Proc. Natl. Acad. Sci. USA* **31**, 11473–11478.
8. Auld, D.S., Inglese, J., Jadhav, A., Austin, C.P., Sittampalam, G.S., Montrose-Rafizadeh, C., Mcgee, J.E., and Iversen, P.W. (2007) HTS technologies to facilitate chemical genomics. *Eur. Pharm. Rev.* **2**, 53–63.
9. Gunter, B., Brideau, C., Pikounis, B., and Liaw, A. (2003) Statistical and graphical methods for quality control determination of high-throughput screening data. *J. Biomol. Screen.* **8**, 624–633.
10. Brideau, C., Gunter, B., Pikounis, B., and Liaw, A. (2003) Improved statistical methods for hit selection in high-throughput screening. *J. Biomol. Screen.* **8**, 634–647.
11. Malo, N., Hanley, J.A., Cerquozzi, S., Pelletier, J., and Nadon, R. (2006) Statistical practice in high-throughput screening data analysis. *Nat. Biotechnol.* **24**, 167–175.
12. Gubler H. (2006) Methods for statistical analysis, quality assurance and management of primary HTS data. In: Hüser, J. (ed.), *High-Throughput Screening in Drug Discovery*, Vol. 28 of Methods and Principles in Medicinal Chemistry, Series Editors Mannhold, R., Kubinyi, H., Folkers, G., Wiley-VCH, Weinheim, Germany, pp. 151–205.
13. Gribbon, P., Lyons, R., Laflin, P., Bradley, J., Chambers, C., Williams, B.S., Keighley, W., and Sewing, A. (2005) Evaluating real-life high-throughput screening data. *J. Biomol. Screen.* **10**, 99–107.
14. Reimann, S., Lindemann, M., Rinn, B., Lefevre, O., and Heyse, S. (2003) Large Scale, comprehensive quality control and analysis of high-throughput screening data. *European BioPharmaceutical Review, Applied R&D*, Spring 2003 issue, Samedan Ltd., London.
15. Root, D.E., Kelley, B.P., and Stockwell, B.R. (2003) Detecting spatial patterns in biological array experiments. *J. Biomol. Screen.* **8**, 393–398.
16. Kevorkov, D., and Makarenkov, V. (2005) Statistical analysis of systematic errors in

high-throughput screening. *J. Biomol. Screen.***10**, 557–567.

17. Box, G.E.P., Hunter, W.G., and Hunter, J.S. (1978) *Statistics for Experimenters.* John Wiley & Sons, New York.
18. Venables, W.N., and Ripley, B.D. (1994) *Modern Applied Statistics with S-Plus*, Springer, New York.
19. Tukey, J. W. (1960) *Contributions to Probability and Statistics*, Olkin, I., (ed.). Stanford University Press, p. 448.
20. Hoaglin, D., Mosteller, F., and Tukey, J.W. (2000) *Understanding Robust and Exploratory Data Analysis.* Wiley Classic Library Series, John Wiley & Sons, New York.
21. Cleveland, W.S. (1993) *Visualizing Data.* Hobart Press, Summit, NJ.
22. Frank, H. and Althoen, S.C. (1995) *The Coefficient of Variation, in Statistics: Concepts and Applications.* Cambridge University Press, Cambridge, pp. 58–59.
23. Johnson, D.J. (2006) *Signal-to-noise Ratio.* Scholarpedia, 1(12):2088, http://www.scholarpedia.org/article/Signal-to-noise ratio.
24. Zhang, J.H., Chung, T.D., and Oldenburg, K.R. (1999) A simple statistical parameter for use in evaluation and validation of high throughput screening assays. *J. Biomol. Screen.* **4**, 67–73.
25. Sittampalam, G.S., Iversen, P.W., Boadt, J.A., Kahl, S.D., Bright, S., Zock, J.M., Janzen, W.P., and Lister, M.D. (1997) Design of signal windows in high throughput assays for drug discovery. *J. Biomol. Screen.* **2**, 159–169.
26. Iversen, P.W., Eastwood, B.J., and Sittampalam, G.S. (2006) A comparison of assay performance measures in screening assays: signal window, Z′-factor and assay variability ratio. *J. Biomol. Screen.* **11**, 247–252.
27. Zhang, X.D. (2007) A pair of new statistical parameters for quality control in RNA interference high-throughput screening assays. *Genomics* **89**, 552–561
28. Zhang, X.D. (2007) A new method with flexible and balanced control of false negatives and false positives for hit selection in RNA interference high-throughput screening assays. *J. Biomol. Screen.* **12**, 645–655.
29. Bland, M. (2000) *An Introduction to Medical Statistics.* Oxford University Press, Oxford.
30. Le, C.T. (2003) *Introductory Biostatistics.* John Wiley & Sons, New York.
31. StatSoft, Inc. (2007) *Electronic Statistics Textbook.* Tulsa, OK, StatSoft. WEB: http://www.statsoft.com/textbook/stathome.html.
32. Sui, Y., and Wu, Z. (2007) Alternative statistical parameter for high-throughput screening assay quality assessment. *J. Biomol. Screen.* **12**, 229–234.
33. Schechtman, E. (2008) A method with flexible and balanced control of false negatives and false positives for hit selection in RNA interference high-throughput screening assays: a statistical terminology. *J. Biomol. Screen.* **13**, 309–311.
34. Zhang, X.D. (2008) Novel analytic criteria and effective plate designs for quality control in genome-scale RNAi screens. *J. Biomol. Screen.* **13**, 363–377.
35. Bland, J.M., and Altman, D.G. (1986) Statistical methods for assessing agreement between two methods of clinical measurements. *Lancet* **1**, 307–310.
36. Sun, D., Whitty, A., Papadatos, J., Newman, M., Deonnelly, J., Bowes, S., and Josiah, S. (2005) Adopting a practical statistical approach for evaluating assay agreement in drug discovery. *J. Biomol. Screen.* **10**, 508–516.
37. Shrout P.E., and Fleiss, J.L. (1979) Intraclass correlations: uses in assessing rater reliability. *Psychol. Bull.* **86**, 420–428.
38. Müller, R., and Büttner, P. (1994) A critical discussion of intraclass correlation coefficients. *Stat. Med.* **13**, 2465–2476.
39. Eastwood, B.J., Farmen, M.W., Iversen, P.W., Craft, T.J., Smallwood, J.K., Garbison, K.E., Delapp, N., and Smith, G.F (2006) The minimum significant ratio: A statistical parameter to characterize the reproducibility of potency estimates from concentration-response assays and estimation by replicate-experiment studies. *J. Biomol. Screen.* **11**, 253–261.
40. Eastwood, B.J., Chesterfield, A.K., Wolff, M.C., and Felder, C.C. (2005) *Methods for the Design and Analysis of Replicate-Experiment Studies to Establish Assay Reproducibility and the Equivalence of Two Potency Assays, in Drug Discovery Handbook*, Gad, S.C. (ed.). John Wiley & Sons, New York, pp. 667–688.
41. Formenko, I., Durst, M., and Balaban, D. (2006) Robust regression for high-throughput screening. *Comput. Methods Programs Biomed.* **82**, 31–37.
42. Normolle, D.P. (1993) An algorithm for robust non-linear analysis of radioimmunoassay and other bioassays. *Stat. Med.* **12**, 2025–2042.
43. Johnson, M.L. (2000) Outliers and robust parameter estimation. *Methods Enzymol.* **321**, 417–424.

Chapter 7

Homology Modeling of GPCRs

John Simms, Nathan E. Hall, Polo H.C. Lam, Laurence J. Miller, Arthur Christopoulos, Ruben Abagyan, and Patrick M. Sexton

Summary

Over 1000 sequences likely to encode G protein-coupled receptors (GPCRs) are currently available in publicly accessible and proprietary databases and this number may grow with the refinement of a number of different genomes. However, despite recent efforts in the crystallization of these proteins, homology modeling approaches are becoming widely used as a method for obtaining quantitative and qualitative information for structure-based drug design as well as the interpretation of experimental data.

Key words: GPCR modeling, Homology modeling, β2-Adrenergic receptor, Rhodopsin, GPCR alignment, Spatial restraints, MODELLER.

1. Introduction

The functional characterization of a protein sequence is one of the most frequent problems in biology. This task is usually facilitated by a three-dimensional (3D) structure of the studied protein *(1)*. However, despite numerous efforts, only the structures for members of the rhodopsin (Rh) *(2–4)*and more recently the adrenergic receptor (βAR) *(5)* families have been solved at high resolution. Homology modeling and prediction of G protein-coupled receptors (GPCR) structure is therefore expected to be a valuable tool for understanding the function of this class of membrane proteins.

In recent years homology modeling has become increasingly common and although the number of techniques has increased, any homology modeling procedure consists of four sequential steps:

i. Template recognition.

ii. Alignment of the target sequence and template structure(s).

Wayne R. Leifert (ed.), *G Protein-Coupled Receptors in Drug Discovery, vol. 552*

Book doi: 10.1007/978-1-60327-317-6_7

iii. Model building.

iv. Model verification, which may be used iteratively with Steps i–iii.

1.1. Template Selection for Homology Modeling

The first step of any homology modeling method begins with the selection of a suitable structural template from the Protein Data Base (PDB, http://www.pdb.org *(6)*). If the target sequence (i.e., the query sequence to be modeled) shares a moderate sequence identity to the template, homology detection is reasonably straightforward and can be achieved by using software such as BLAST (http://www.ncbi.nlm.nih.gov/blast/ *(7)*).

1.2. Transmembrane (TM) Region Modeling including Interconnecting Loops

To date, the only suitable templates for the TM region of a Family A GPCR are the X-ray crystal structures for Rh *(2–4, 8–16)* and βAR *(5, 17)* families. It is important not to blindly assume that the βAR structures are better templates than Rh for modeling GPCRs a whole. Sequence alignment must be used as a guide to which sections of each structure are appropriate templates for the query sequence. This is especially important in loop regions that exhibit the greatest variability in both sequence and structure. In addition, despite the fact that a number of bovine Rh structures are available, subtleties in the crystallization procedures from different groups have resulted in slight differences between structures. This is most apparent in the region between TMs 5 and 6 of the bovine Rh structures, which show differences in the proximal and distal ends of intracellular loop 3 (1U19 *(11)* compared with 1GZM *(10)*). In addition, squid rhodopsin, which couples to G_q rather than G_t proteins, also exhibits differences in the TM5/TM6 region compared to the other GPCR structures. A recent addition to the library of GPCR crystal structures is opsin (3CAP *(4)*), which unlike other structures has no bound ligand. This structure exhibits a number of similarities to biophysical data referring to the MetaII conformation of Rh and may be a suitable template for an active state of a GPCR.

Aligning Family B and C GPCRs with Family A templates introduces a much greater degree of difficulty. There is no agreed alignment between these two families and the lack of sequence conservation makes this area very challenging. Sequence alignment methods such as Hidden Markov Methods and Profile–Profile Alignments have only very limited reliability in this instance. One approach that does not rely on the conservation of residues between GPCR families is the "Cold Spot" approach *(18)*. This asserts that patterns of conservation will be somewhat conserved between the two GPCR families, but the amino acids will not necessarily be conserved. In practice, the cold spot approach aligns two sequences based on the positions of conservation. These "cold spots" are sequence positions that are most conserved and thus where structure is most likely preserved, providing positions at which the alignment can be based. However, even with approaches such as cold spot, high-resolution models are predicted to be only available when either a crystal structure of a Family B GPCR is released or *ab initio* modeling becomes sufficiently mature to predict membrane proteins.

1.3. N-Terminal Domains

A characteristic feature of Family B and C GPCRs as well as some Family A GPCRs is the large N-terminal domain that provides an epitope for high-affinity ligand binding. However, despite this common feature, the structures of the N-terminal domains from the respective families are distinct and different templates are required for homology modeling. A number of Family A GPCRs are characterized by a large N-terminal domain containing leucine-rich repeats (LRRs) that are capped by N- and C-terminal cysteine-rich regions. To date, a number of structures have been reported containing this motif but exhibit different properties such as the total number of LRRs and position of the cysteine residues. In this case, a number of possible templates should be identified, which can be then combined when generating homology models. Examples of LRR-containing proteins that share high sequence similarity with the thyroid-stimulating hormone receptor (TSHR), for example, are 1OZN *(19)* and 2BNH *(20)*. A limited number of high-resolution X-ray models are available for the Family B N terminus, including GIPR (2QKH *(21)*), PTH1R (3C4M *(22)*, note: a fusion protein with maltose-binding protein), and GLP1R (3C59, 3C5T *(23)*), all of which have the peptide ligand bound. The exact template to be used should be determined by the sequence identity to the target model. Two NMR models of CRF-R2 (2JND, 2JNC *(24)*) differ significantly from the X-ray structures, and are less ideal as templates for homology modeling.

In addition to three conserved disulfide bonds, the Family B N-terminal domain contains several common elements (**Fig. 1**) that include an α-helix at the distal N terminus, the first two

```
Consensus        E #  #  #   C   L    P      C   #D ##CW    P
GLP1R       TVSLWETVQKWREYRRQCQRSLTEDPPPATDLFCNRTFDEYACWPDGEPGSF
GIPR        GQTAGELYQRWERYRRECQETLAAAEPP-SGLACNGSFDMYVCWDYAAPNAT
PTH1R       VMTKEEQIFLLHRAQAQCEKRLKEVRP------CLPEWDHILCWPLGAPGEV
              HHHHHHHHHHHHHHHHHHHHHHHH          ββ    ββ      ββ

Consensus   # # CP Y## #   # G###R C   G W         W  #  C
GLP1R       VNVSCPWYLPWASSVPQGHVYRFCTAEGLWLQKDNSSLPWRDLSECEESKR
GIPR        ARASCPWYLPWHHHVAAGFVLRQCGSDGQWG-------LWRDHTQCENPE-
PTH1R       VAVPCPDYIYDF--NHKGHAYRRCDRNGSWELVPGHNRTWANYSECVKFL-
            ββββ      HHHHHH  ββββββ                  HHHHH
```

Fig. 1. Structure-based alignment of X-ray Family B GPCR N-terminal domains. Consensus residues are shown above the alignment and consensus secondary structure is shown below the alignment. "#" represents conserved hydrophobic residues, helices are denoted by "Hs," and β-strands by "βs." Six cysteine residues forming the three conserved disulfide bonds are marked above in bold.

β-strands forming a hairpin, and two additional β-strands connected by a flexible loop. These conserved elements are connected by flexible loops with variable length. Note that the first helix in the PTH1R structure is in a slightly different orientation to the rest of the domain compared with the other X-ray structures. In the case of Family C GPCRs a number of structures for the large globular ("venus flytrap"-like) N-terminal domain of the metabotropic glutamate receptor have been reported (e.g., 1ISR *(25)* and 2E4U *(26)*) in a number of liganded states and may be used as templates for this region in other receptors.

1.4. Sequence and Structure Alignments for Homology Modeling

Despite recent advances in methods used to generate homology models, a critical step is still the initial alignment between the target sequence and template structure(s) (*see* **Method 3.1**). A common method to align the target and the template is by using sequence alignment software. Recent studies have shown that multiple sequence and profile alignments are the most robust methods for generating alignments *(27)*. Methods such as T-Coffee *(28)*, ClustalW *(29)*, and SALIGN (as implemented in the MODELLER package) can generate both multiple sequence and profile alignments and have been shown to be suitable for aligning the sequences of membrane proteins *(27)*. In addition, the use of multiple sequence alignments has given rise to a number of different nomenclatures for identifying residues across divergent GPCR families *(30)*. Generic numbering systems can then be used to check a sequence alignment, such that conserved residues are aligned (**Fig. 2**).

1.5. Homology Modeling of a GPCR

Once a suitable template has been found and an alignment of between the target and the template structures has been generated, a model of the target protein can be created using spatial restraints, much in the same way as NMR structures are generated (*see* **Method 3.2**). An example of a program that uses this style of homology modeling is MODELLER *(31)*. Spatial restraints can be obtained from a number of sources that include homology-derived restraints and molecular mechanics based or statistically derived preferences for bonded and non-bonded interactions. In addition, restraints may be obtained from a number of external sources such as spin labeling *(32)*, fluorescence labeling *(33)*, cysteine cross-linking *(32)*, engineered Zn-binding sites *(34)*, and double mutant constructs *(35)*. In addition to the satisfaction of spatial restraints the concept of positional tethers is a further method which has been successfully used to generate homology models. Tethering and other proprietary methods are available in ICM Pro (Molsoft LLC) that contain integrated bioinformatics, modeling, and visualization software, which is also supported by a Graphical User Interface. The integrated environment in this type of software would then enable easy transitions for a number of different modeling tasks. A number of publicly accessible

```
                                       N                       L   D                           C
bovine rhodopsin EPWQFSMLAAYMFLLIMLGFPINFLTLYVTVQHKKLRTPLNYILLNLAVADLFMVFGGF-TTTLYTSLHGYFVFGPTGCN
squid rhodopsin  PDAVYYSLGIFIGICGIIGCGGNGIVIYLFTKTKSLQTPANMFIINLAFSDFTFSLVNGFPLMTISCFLKKWIFGFAACK
human β2AR       DEVWVVGMGIVMSLIVLAIVFGNVLVITAIAKFERLQTVTNYFITSLACADLVMGLAVV-PFGAAHILMKMWTFGNFWCE
turkey β1AR      --QWEAGMSLLMALVVLLIVAGNVLVIAAIGSTQRLQTLTNLFITSLACADLVVGLLVV-PFGATLVVRGTWLWGSFLCE
                 |--------------TM1---------------|   |--------------TM2---------------|    |-----
                                                  ICL1                                 ECL1

                                 L     DR                          W
bovine rhodopsin LEGFFATLGGEIALWSLVVLAIERYVVVCKPM-SNFRFGENHAIMGVAFTWVMALACAA-PPLVGW    SRYIPEGMQC
squid rhodopsin  VYGFIGGIFGFMSIMTMAMISIDRYNVIGRPMAASKKMSHRRAFIMIIFVWLWSVLWAI-GPIFGW    GAYTLEGVLC
human β2AR       FWTSIDVLCVTASIETLCVIAVDRYFAITSPFKYQSLLTKNKARVIILMVWIVSGLTSFLPIQMHW YRATHQEAINCYA
turkey β1AR      LWTSLDVLCVTASIETLCVIAIDRYLAITSPFRYQSLMTRARAKVIICTVWAISALVSFLPIMMHW WRDEDPQALKCYQ
                 ----------TM3---------------|         |----------TM4-----------|    unaligned
                                                 ICL2

                      C                             P
bovine rhodopsin S    C GIDYYTPHEETN NESFVIYMFVVHFIIPLIVIFFCYGQLVFTVKEAAAQQQE                 KAE
squid rhodopsin  N    C SFDYISRDST   TRSNILCMFILGFFGPILIIFFCYFNIVMSVSNHEKEMAAMAKRLNAKELRKAQAGANAE
human β2AR       EETC C     DFFT     NQAYAIASSIVSFYVPLVIMVFVYSRVFQEAKRQL                   KFCLKE
turkey β1AR      DPGC C     DFVT     NRAYAIASSIISFYIPLLIMIFVALRVYREAKEQI                       RE
                         unaligned   |--------------TM5----------------|  variable length   |----
                     ECL2                                                     ICL3

                                    P                                  NP  Y      *   *   *
bovine rhodopsin KEVTRMVIIMVIAFLICWLPYAGVAFYIFTHQGSDFGPIFMTIPAFFAKTSAVYNPVIYIMMNKQFRNCMVTTLCCGK
squid rhodopsin  MRLAKISIVIVSQFLLSWSPYAVVALLAQFGPLEWVTPYAAQLPVMFAKASAIHNPMIYSVSHPKFREAISQTFPWVL
human β2AR       HKALKTLGIIMGTFTLCWLPFFIVNIVHVIQDN-LIRKEVYILLNWIGYVNSGFNPLIYC-RSPDFRIAFQELLCL--
turkey β1AR      HKALKTLGIIMGVFTLCWLPFFLVNIVNVFNRD-LVPDWLFVAFNWLGYANSAMNPIIYC-RSPDFRKAFKRLLAF--
                 ----------TM6-----------------|     |--------TM7----------|  |--Helix 8--|
                                                ECL3
```

Fig. 2. Structural sequence alignment of available GPCR 7TM regions. The structures used are 1GZM, 2Z73, 2RH1, and 2VT4 for bovine rhodopsin, squid rhodopsin, β_2-adrenergic receptor, and β_1-adrenergic receptor, respectively. TM helices are labeled TM1–7, extracellular loops are labeled ECL1–3, and intracellular loops are labeled ICL1–3. TM and loop regions boundaries are taken as a consensus from all four structures. Ballesteros residues are shown above in bold, other residues which have Family A conservation weights >70 in GPCRDB sequence profiles (www.gpcr.org/7tm) are also shown. The central cysteine of ECL2 (shown in bold italics above alignment) forms the conserved disulfide bond with the top TM3. The remaining ECL2 residues possess no structural alignment between the β-adrenergic receptor and Rh families and are labeled unaligned. Conserved hydrophobic residues in helix 8 which are partitioned into the membrane/solvent interface are labeled with and asterix (*). The ECL3 β-adrenergic residues missing from the structures are not shown in the alignment and this loop region is annotated as being of variable length.

programs are available to verify the integrity of the generated homology models and generally belong to one of two categories. The first category (e.g., PROCHECK *(36)* and WHATIF *(37)*) checks for proper protein stereochemistry, such as symmetry checks, geometry checks, and structural packing quality. The second category (e.g.,VERIFY3D *(38)* and PROSAII *(39)*) checks the fitness of sequence to structure and assigns a score for each residue fitting its current environment. Finally, of course, the best discriminator between good and bad models is human evaluation and should be employed at each stage of the modeling process. It is important to note that creation of a useful GPCR model may involve creating numerous different models utilizing different alignments (particularly in the loop regions) and/or different or multiple templates. However, for simplicity, the following examples will use one template.

Generating a homology model using MODELLER consists of the following steps:

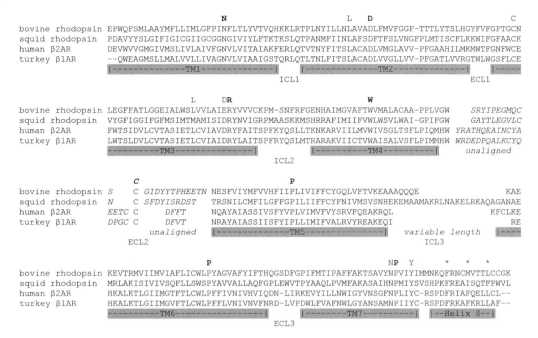

(i) Preparing an input MODELLER Python script.

(ii) Ensuring that all required files including sequences, structures and/or alignments are located the same directory.

(iii) Executing a MODELLER input to generate the homology models.

(iv) Analyzing the output model and scoring.

2. Materials

2.1. Requirements and Conventions for Methods 3.1 and 3.2

A computer running Linux/Unix, Microsoft Windows 98/NT/2000/XP, or Apple Mac OS X, 512 MB RAM or higher and approximately 100 MB of free hard disk space for the software and output files.

2.1.1. Hardware

2.1.2. Software to Obtain and Install

1. MODELLER, homology modeling software available from http://salilab.org/modeller/download_installation.html
2. DEEPVIEW *(40)*, protein structural visualization and manipulation software available from http://au.expasy.org/spdbv

2.2. Computer Skills

Although MODELLER and DEEPVIEW can run under UNIX-based, Windows, or Apple Mac operating systems, UNIX-based operating systems offer a framework and scripting system for the manipulation of files. However, while knowledge of Linux/UNIX is not necessary for modeling, some knowledge of the scripting system would be useful. In addition, MODELLER does not have a graphical user interface and is run from the command line; therefore a basic knowledge of command-line skills is necessary to follow the method described in this chapter.

2.3. Conventions Followed in the Text

The sequence for the query structure, for which a homology model is being calculated, is referred to as the "target." A "template" is an experimentally determined structure (NMR or X-ray crystallography) used for comparative modeling. Files with a ".seq" extension refer to one or more unaligned sequences in the PIR format. Files with ".ali" extensions contain the alignment of two or more sequences and/or structures. Files with ".pir" extension contain the alignment of two or more sequences and/or structures in PIR format. Files with a ".py" extension are MODELLER scripts. MODHOME is the location of the MODELLER home directory. The extensions presented here are not mandatory, and the user may adopt any systematic convention deemed necessary. The version of MODELLER is 9.4. In the methods section the symbol ">" refers to a submenu located under a main menu title in DEEPVIEW. The symbols $> refers to commands that should be applied directly to the command line and does not form part of a script. UNIX commands are represented in the main text as *italics*.Text in `Courier New font`refers to commands entered either at the command line, in a script, or the contents of a file and does not form part of the main body of text.

3. Methods

3.1. Aligning the Sequence of the Human Muscarinic M_2 Receptor with the β2AR

The following procedure uses the program SALIGN, as implemented in the MODELLER package, to align the human muscarinic M_2 receptor sequence (hum2r) and the rat muscarinic M_2 receptor (rm2r) sequence in file "hum2r.seq" with the sequence corresponding to the structure, 2RH1. The resulting file "hum2r-2RH1.pir" is then used in **Method 3.2** to generate a homology model.

1. Download the amino acid sequences for the hum2r (accession number P08172) and rm2r (accession number P10980) from http://au.expasy.org/sprot/
2. Download the structure file 2RH1 from the PBD repository (http://www.rcsb.org/pdb/home/home.do).
3. Open the file 2RH1.pdb using the File > Open PDB file function in DEEPVIEW and save the amino acid sequence using the File > Save > Sequence (FASTA) function.
4. Edit a text file such that it contains, in PIR (a) format (*see* **Note 1**; **Fig. 3**), (i) the sequence of the template (2RH1.pdb), (ii) the sequence of the protein to be modeled (hum2r), and (iii) other homologues obtained from a database search (rm2r) and save as hum2r.seq.
5. Edit a file such that it contains the following MODELLER python script and save the file as salign.py (*see* **Note 2**).

```
from modeller import *
log.verbose()
env = environ()
env.io.atom_files_directory='./'
aln = alignment(env, file='hum2r.seq',
align_codes='all')
aln.salign(rr_file='$(LIB)/as1.sim.mat',
           output='',
           max_gap_length=20,
           gap_function=True,
feature_weights=(1., 0., 0., 0., 0., 0.),
           gap_penalties_1d=(-200, 0),
            gap_penalties_2d=(3.5, 3.5,
```

```
>P1;2RH1.pdb
structure:2RH1.pdb:1:A:342:::::
DEVWVVGMGIVMSLIVLAIVFGNVLVITAIAKFERLQTVTNYFITSLACADLVMGLAVVP
FGAAHILMKMWTFGNFWCEFWTSIDVLCVTASIETLCVIAVDRYFAITSPFKYQSLLTKN
KARVIILMVWIVSGLTSFLPIQMHWYRATHQEAINCYAEETCCDFFTNQAYAIASSIVSF
YVPLVIMVFVYSRVFQEAKRQLNIFEMLRIDEGLRLKIYKDTEGYYTIGIGHLLTKSPSL
NAAKSELDKAIGRNTNGVITKDEAEKLFNQDVDAAVRGILRNAKLKPVYDSLDAVRRAAL
INMVFQMGETGVAGFTNSLRMLQQKRWDEAAVNLAKSRWYNQTPNRAKRVITTFRTGTWD
AYKFCLKEHKALKTLGIIMGTFTLCWLPFFIVNIVHVIQDNLIRKEVYILLNWIGYVNSG
FNPLIYCRSPDFRIAFQELLCL

>P1;hum2r
sequence:hum2r::::::::
MNNSTNSSNNSLALTSPYKTFEVVFIVLVAGSLSLVTIIGNILVMVSIKVNRHLQTVNNY
FLFSLACADLIIGVFSMNLYTLYTVIGYWPLGPVVCDLWLALDYVVSNASVMNLLIISFD
RYFCVTKPLTYPVKRTTKMAGMMIAAAWVLSFILWAPAILFWQFIVGVRTVEDGECYIQF
FSNAAVTFGTAIAAFYLPVIIMTVLYWHISRASKSRIKKDKKEPVANQDPVSPSLVQGRI
VKPNNNNMPSSDDGLEHNKIQNGKAPRDPVTENCVQGEEKESSNDSTSVSAVASNMRDDE
ITQDENTVSTSLGHSKDENSKQTCIRIGTKTPKSDSCTPTNTTVEVVGSSGQNGDEKQNI
VARKIVKMTKQPAKKKPPPSREKKVTRTILAILLAFIITWAPYNVMVLINTFCAPCIPNT
VWTIGYWLCYINSTINPACYALCNATFKKTFKHLLMCHYKNIGATR

>P1;rm2r
sequence:rm2r::::::::
MNNSTNSSNNGLAITSPYKTFEVVFIVLVAGSLSLVTIIGNILVMVSIKVNRHLQTVNNY
FLFSLACADLIIGVFSMNLYTLYTVIGYWPLGPVVCDLWLALDYVVSNASVMNLLIISFD
RYFCVTKPLTYPVKRTTKMAGMMIAAAWVLSFILWAPAILFWQFIVGVRTVEDGECYIQF
FSNAAVTFGTAIAAFYLPVIIMTVLYWHISRASKSRIKKEKKEPVANQDPVSPSLVQGRI
VKPNNNNMPGGDGGLEHNKIQNGKAPRDGVTENCVQGEEKESSNDSTSVSAVASNMRDDE
ITQDENTVSTSLGHSRDDNSKQTCIKIVTKAQKGDVCTPTSTTVELVGSSGQNGDEKQNI
VARKIVKMTKQPAKKKPPPSREKKVTRTILAILLAFIITWAPYNVMVLINTFCAPCIPNT
VWTIGYWLCYINSTINPACYALCNATFKKTFKHLLMCHYKNIGATR
```

Fig. 3. An example of a PIR formatted file containing the sequences of the template (β_2AR, PDB identifier 2RH1.pdb), the target (hum2r), and a homologous protein to the target (rm2r). For clarity, this example contains only three sequences whereas multiple sequence alignments for homology modeling should contain a number of homologous proteins of the target sequence.

```
3.5, 0.2, 4.0, 6.5, 2.0, 0.0, 0.0),
output_weights_file=' salign.mtx'
        similarity_flag=True)
aln.write(file=' hum2r-2RH1.pir' , align-
ment_format=' PIR' )
```

6. Execute the MODELLER python script salign.py with the command.

```
$> MODHOME/modeller9v4/bin/mod9v4 salign.py
```

```
>P1;2RH1.pdb
structure:2RH1.pdb:1:A:342:A::::
------------------DEVWVVGMGIVMSLIVLAIVFGNVLVITAIAKFERLQTVTNY
FITSLACADLVMGLAVVPFGAAHILMKMWTFGNFWCEFWTSIDVLCVTASIETLCVIAVD
RYFAITSPFKYQSLLTKNKARVIILMVWIVSGLTSFLPIQMHWYRATHQEAINCYAEETC
CDFFTN--QAYAIASSIVSFYVPLVIMVFVYSRVFQEAKRQLNIFEMLRIDEGLRLKIYK
DTEGYYTIGIGHLLTKSPSLNAAKSELDKAIG-RNTNGVITKDEAEKLFNQDVDAAVRGI
LRNAKLKPVYDSLDAVRRAALINMVFQMGETGVAGFTNSLRMLQQKRWDEAAVNLAKSRW
YNQTPNRAKRVITTFRTGTWDAYKFCLKEHKALKTLGIIMGTFTLCWLPFFIVNIVHVIQ
DNLIRKEVYILLNWIGYVNSGFNPLIYCRS-PDFRIAFQELLCL---------*
>P1;hum2r
sequence:hum2r::::::::
MNNSTNSSNNSLALTSPYKTFEVVFIVLVAGSLSLVTIIGNILVMVSIKVNRHLQTVNNY
FLFSLACADLIIGVFSMNLYTLYTVIGYWPLGPVVCDLWLALDYVVSNASVMNLLIISFD
RYFCVTKPLTYPVKRTTKMAGMMIAAAWVLSFILWAPAIL-FWQFIVGVRTVE--DGE--
CYIQFFSNAAVTFGTAIAAFYLPVIIMTVLYWHISRASKSRIKKDKKEPVANQDPVSPSL
VQGRIVKPNNNNMPSSDDGLEHNKIQNGKAPRDPVTENCVQGEEKESSNDSTSVSAVASN
MRDDEITQDENTVSTSLGHSKDENSKQTCIRIGTKTPKSDSCTPTNTTVEVVGSSGQN--
GDEKQNIVARKIVKMTKQPAKKKPPPSREKKVTRTILAILLAFIITWAPYNVMVLINTFC
APCIPNTVWTIGYWLCYINSTINPACYALCNATFKKTFKHLLMCHYKNIGATR*
>P1;rm2r
sequence:rm2r::::::::
MNNSTNSSNNGLAITSPYKTFEVVFIVLVAGSLSLVTIIGNILVMVSIKVNRHLQTVNNY
FLFSLACADLIIGVFSMNLYTLYTVIGYWPLGPVVCDLWLALDYVVSNASVMNLLIISFD
RYFCVTKPLTYPVKRTTKMAGMMIAAAWVLSFILWAPAIL-FWQFIVGVRTVE--DGE--
CYIQFFSNAAVTFGTAIAAFYLPVIIMTVLYWHISRASKSRIKKEKKEPVANQDPVSPSL
VQGRIVKPNNNNMPGGDGGLEHNKIQNGKAPRDGVTENCVQGEEKESSNDSTSVSAVASN
MRDDEITQDENTVSTSLGHSRDDNSKQTCIKIVTKAQKGDVCTPTSTTVELVGSSGQN--
GDEKQNIVARKIVKMTKQPAKKKPPPSREKKVTRTILAILLAFIITWAPYNVMVLINTFC
APCIPNTVWTIGYWLCYINSTINPACYALCNATFKKTFKHLLMCHYKNIGATR*
```

Fig. 4. The salign.py generated, PIR formatted multiple sequence alignment file (hum2r-2RH1.pir) containing the sequences for the template (β_2AR, 2RH1.pdb), the target sequence (human muscarinic M_2 receptor, hum2r), and a homologous protein to the target sequence (rat muscarinic M_2 receptor, rm2r). The experimental β_2AR structure contains an artificial t4-lysozyme insert (residues NIFE...WDAY, highlighted in gray) in the IC3 loop to facilitate crystallization and structural determination. This region must be deleted from the GPCR template. Modeling of large regions with no template structures, (e.g., N and C termini and large ICL3) requires the use of specialist techniques and should be addressed separately and as such these regions are deleted from the alignment (**Fig. 5**).

7. Manually edit the alignment file "hum2r-2RH1.pir" with a text editor such that large gaps or regions of uncertainty in the alignment and the corresponding regions in other sequences are removed (*see* **Note 3, Figs. 4** and **5**).
8. Use the program DEEPVIEW to open and edit the template file so that it corresponds to changes made in the edited sequence alignment (**Figs. 4** and **5**). This can be achieved by highlighting the relevant residues in the control panel (Window > Control Panel) and deleting them by using the Build > Remove Selected Residues function.

```
>P1;2RH1.pdb
structure:2RH1.pdb:1::283:::::
DEVWVVGMGIVMSLIVLAIVFGNVLVITAIAKFERLQTVTNYFITSLACADLVMGLAVVP
FGAAHILMKMWTFGNFWCEFWTSIDVLCVTASIETLCVIAVDRYFAITSPFKYQSLLTKN
KARVIILMVWIVSGLTSFLPIQMHWYRATHQEAINCYAEETCCDFFTN--QAYAIASSIV
SFYVPLVIMVFVYSRVFQEAKRQLXKFCLKEHKALKTLGIIMGTFTLCWLPFFIVNIVHV
IQDNLIRKEVYILLNWIGYVNSGFNPLIYCRS-PDFRIAFQELLCL*
>P1;hum2r
sequence:hum2r::::::::
KTFEVVFIVLVAGSLSLVTIIGNILVMVSIKVNRHLQTVNNYFLFSLACADLIIGVFSMN
LYTLYTVIGYWPLGPVVCDLWLALDYVVSNASVMNLLIISFDRYFCVTKPLTYPVKRTTK
MAGMMIAAAWVLSFILWAPAIL-FWQFIVGVRTVE--DGE--CYIQFFSNAAVTFGTAIA
AFYLPVIIMTVLYWHISRASKSRIXPPPSREKKVTRTILAILLAFIITWAPYNVMVLINT
FCAPCIPNTVWTIGYWLCYINSTINPACYALCNATFKKTFKHLLMC*
>P1;rm2r
sequence:rm2r::::::::
KTFEVVFIVLVAGSLSLVTIIGNILVMVSIKVNRHLQTVNNYFLFSLACADLIIGVFSMN
LYTLYTVIGYWPLGPVVCDLWLALDYVVSNASVMNLLIISFDRYFCVTKPLTYPVKRTTK
MAGMMIAAAWVLSFILWAPAIL-FWQFIVGVRTVE--DGE--CYIQFFSNAAVTFGTAIA
AFYLPVIIMTVLYWHISRASKSRIXPPPSREKKVTRTILAILLAFIITWAPYNVMVLINT
FCAPCIPNTVWTIGYWLCYINSTINPACYALCNATFKKTFKHLLMC*
```

Fig. 5. The edited multiple sequence alignment file (hum2r-2RH1.pir) containing the sequences for the template (β_2AR, 2RH1.pdb), the target sequence (hum2r), and a homologous protein to the target sequence (rm2r). Large insertions or regions of uncertainty have been deleted as specified in Fig. 4 legend. In addition the number of residues in field 5 of the structure entry (2RH1.pdb) has been changed to reflect the changes made in the alignment. See MODELLER manual for more information.

9. Use DEEPVIEW to renumber the edited template file starting from 1 using the Edit > Rename Current Layer function.
10. Save the DEEPVIEW edited file using the Save > Layer function.

3.2. Generating a Homology Model for the Human Muscarinic M_2 Receptor Based on the Structure 2RH1 Incorporating External Restraints

The following procedure uses MODELLER to generate five homology models of the hum2r using the edited alignment generated in **Method 3.1** and the β2AR structure 2RH1. In addition a number of external distance constraint will also be included that will be incorporated into the final model. For example, if an experimental technique suggests that residues 1–10 of the receptor are helical then this region can then be restrained with helical geometry. Similarly, if experimental results suggest that two residues are close in 3D space then this distance can also be restrained. For example, constrain the distance between Cα of residues 29 and 57 to 6.8 Å

1. Edit a text file such that it contains the following MODELLER python script and save the file as hum2r-model.py.

```
# Addition of restraints to the default ones
from modeller import *
from modeller.automodel import *    # Load the automodel class

log.verbose()
env = environ()

# directories for input atom files
env.io.atom_files_directory = ' ./:../atom_ files'
class mymodel(automodel):
    def special_restraints(self, aln):
        rsr = self.restraints
        at = self.atoms
#       Residues 1 through 10 should be an alpha helix:
        rsr.add(secondary_structure.alpha(self.residue_range(' 1:',
' 10:')))
#        Use a harmonic potential between residues 29 and 57.
         rsr.add(forms.gaussian(group=physical.xy_distance,
                                feature=features.distance (at[' CA:29'],

                                                           at[' CA:57']),
                                mean=6.7, stdev=0.1))
a = mymodel(env,
            alnfile  = '' hum2r-2RH1.pir ',
            knowns   = ' 2RH1.pdb',
            sequence = ' hum2r')
a.starting_model= 1
a.ending_model  = 5
a.make()
```

2. Execute the MODELLER python script with the command (*see* **Note 4**).

   ```
   $> MODHOME/modeller9v4/bin/mod9v4 hum2r-
   model.py &
   ```

3. Once the models have been generated order them on the basis of the MODELLER objective function using the following command at the UNIX prompt (*see* **Note 5**).

   ```
   $> grep' MODELLER OBJECTIVE FUNCTION:'
   hum2r.B9999*.pdb
   | sort +1
   ```

4. Visually inspect the top (lowest scoring) models using DEEP-VIEW and observe differences between the side chain packing of the models. Use web-based servers such as PROCHECK and WHATCHECK to determine the best homology model (*see* **Note 6**).

4. Notes

1. The PIR format (**Fig. 3**) for use in MODELLER is as follows: The first line contains the sequence identifier, in the format ">P1;*seqname*," where *seqname* is the name of the sequence. The identifier must be unique for all proteins and sequences in the file. The second line contains 10 fields separated by colons. However, only fields 1–6 are required for MODELLER use. Field 1 specifies whether or not the data is from a 3D structure (structure) or is sequence (sequence) data. Field 2 (2RH1.pdb, hum2r, rm2r, respectively) does not have to be unique but must correspond to the variable "sequence" in the MODELLER python script. Fields 3–6 are the residue and chain identifiers for the first (fields 3 and 4) and last residue (fields 5 and 6) of the structure file entry only, respectively. Fields 7–10 are optional, see MODELLER manual for more information. The remainder of the data contain the sequence of protein, with an asterix "*" marking the end of the entry. The standard upper case, one-letter amino acid codes are used.
2. This script will align the sequences in the file hum2r.seq and outputs the file hum2r-2RH1.pir that contains the sequence alignment in PIR format. The *salign* module accounts for structural information from the template when constructing a sequence alignment using gap penalty function that inserts gaps in loop regions that are outside regions of secondary structure see MODELLER manual for more information regarding format.
3. A further consideration in a sequence alignment for homology modeling is the length of inserted regions, denoted by gaps (–) between the target and template sequences (**Fig. 4**). Whereas, short insertions in the template alignment may be tolerated (1–4 residues), larger insertions may result in "knots" in the final structure. It is therefore a prudent step to delete any region of large insertions in the sequence alignment (shaded in gray, **Figs. 4** and **5**). It is important to maintain the overall alignment, as changes made to one sequence must also be reflected in the other sequences. Special attention should be paid to ensure that conserved residues are aligned between the sequences. Any errors introduced at this point will seriously affect the final model.
4. Once an alignment between the target and template has been generated, MODELLER can calculate a basic 3D model of the target sequence automatically using the "automodel"

routine. In this script the line "alnfile" defines the filename for the alignment between target and template in PIR format (hum2r-2RH1.pir), "knowns" defines the filename of the template structure (2RH1.pdb), and sequence defines the name of the target sequence (hum2r) in the alignment file. The two variables, starting_model and ending_model, limit the number of models that are calculated (5 in the above example). However, more models should be generated (~200) for homology modeling; only 5 models were generated with the above script for the purposes of illustration and speed. In addition to a number of housekeeping files (see MODELLER manual for more information), the files containing the coordinates of the models are defined with the suffix B9999000*.pdb, where "*" is the model number. Visual inspection of the models can then be performed using a package such as DEEPVIEW. The symbol "&" allows the program to run in the background, which allows the user to log out of the system. In addition, the nomenclature for the external restraints is described in the MODELLER manual.

5. One method of obtaining a good structure is to use the MODELLER objective function found in the model PDB file. This value is not an absolute measure of model quality and can only be used to rank models calculated from the same alignment. As with most objective functions the lower the value the better the model. Although reliable, the MODELLER objective function should be used in combination with other energy/scoring functions, thus forming a consensus approach to picking the best model. In this way, the relative strengths and weakness of the various scoring functions will not bias the results of the modeling exercise. However, it is important to note that before any external evaluation of the model, one should check the log file from the MODELLER run for runtime errors and restraint violations (see the MODELLER manual). *grep*is a command line utility that is found in most UNIX style operating systems and given a list of files (hum2r.B9999*.pdb) *grep* searches for lines of text that match a regular expressions (MODELLER OBJECTIVE FUNCTION) and outputs only the matching lines. The output of *grep*is sent, or piped, using the symbol | to a second UNIX command called *sort*. This command is able to numerically order the output of *grep*, such that it is easy to identify the best (lowest) scoring model.
6. The validity of the final model can be assessed with Ramachandran maps, such as the one implemented in the web-based server, PROCHECK. The advantage of

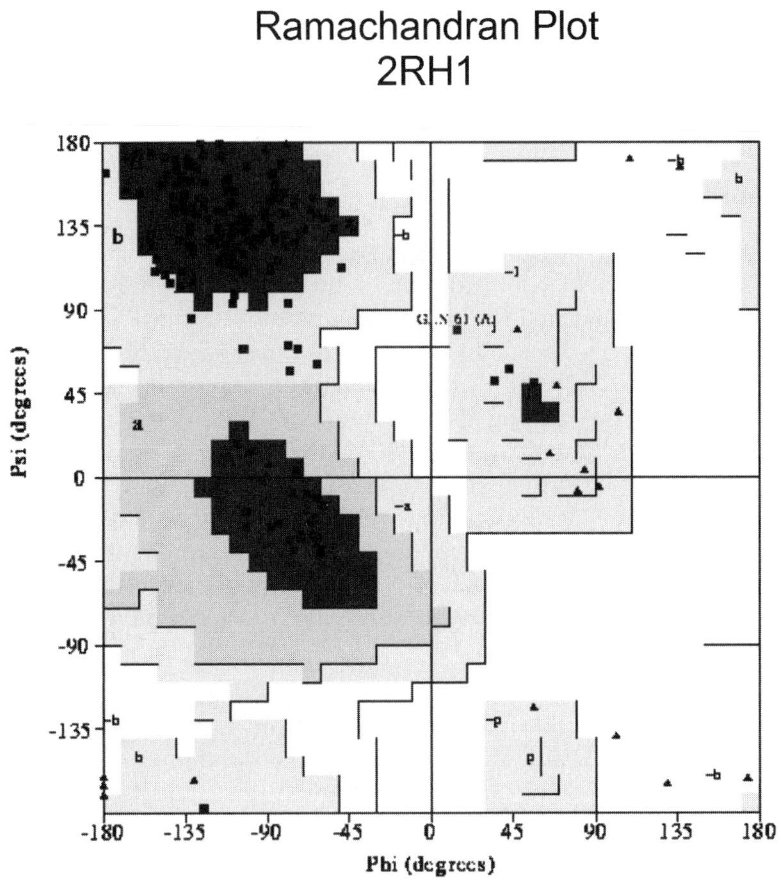

Fig. 6. Ramachandran plots calculated for the template 2RH1 using the PROCHECK server. The figure shows that all residues are within the core/allowed regions of the Ramachandran plot. This is a good measure of the quality of the structure.

PROCHECK is that a further score, referred to as the overall G-factor is also calculated and is a measure of the validity of the model. **Figure 6** and **Table 1** shows Ramachandran plot and overall scores from a homology model, respectively. The values from the template, 2RH1, have also been included in the table as a comparison. Whilst the Ramachandran plot in itself can be used as a measure of the validity of a model, the tools under WHATCHECK can be used to supplement the results from PROCHECK. The tools include packing quality of the model, deviations of bond lengths, angles, and inside/outside distribution that can also allow the user to select one model from another when the Ramachandran maps give similar results. An example of the results from WHATCHECK for a homology model of a GPCR can be found in **Table 2** and are compared to the

Table 1
Results from the PROCHECK server

Ramachandran plots (%)

Structure	Core	Allowed	Generous	Disallowed	Overall G-factor
Model	83.9	13.1	2.1	0.9	−1.39
2RH1	77.7	20.3	1.7	0.3	0.7

This figure shows the result of the PROCHECK server. The overall quality G-factor demonstrates that the models are acceptable. Precise definitions of the scoring terms can be found in the PROCHECK website.

Table 2
Results from the WHATCHECK server

Ramachandran plots (%)

Structure	Core	Allowed	Generous	Disallowed	Overall G-factor
Model	83.9	13.1	2.1	0.9	−1.39
2RH1	77.7	20.3	1.7	0.3	0.7

A further check which can be used in parallel to PROCHECK is the WHATCHECK server. The results from this server cover a number of aspects of protein structure including second-generation packing quality (PQ), Ramachandran plot appearance (RPA), rotamer normality (χNR), backbone conformation (BBC), bond lengths (BL), bond angles (BA), omega angle restraint (ΩR), side chain planarity (SCP), improper dihedral distribution (IDD), and inside/outside distribution (IOD). The precise definitions can be found in the WHATCHECK website.

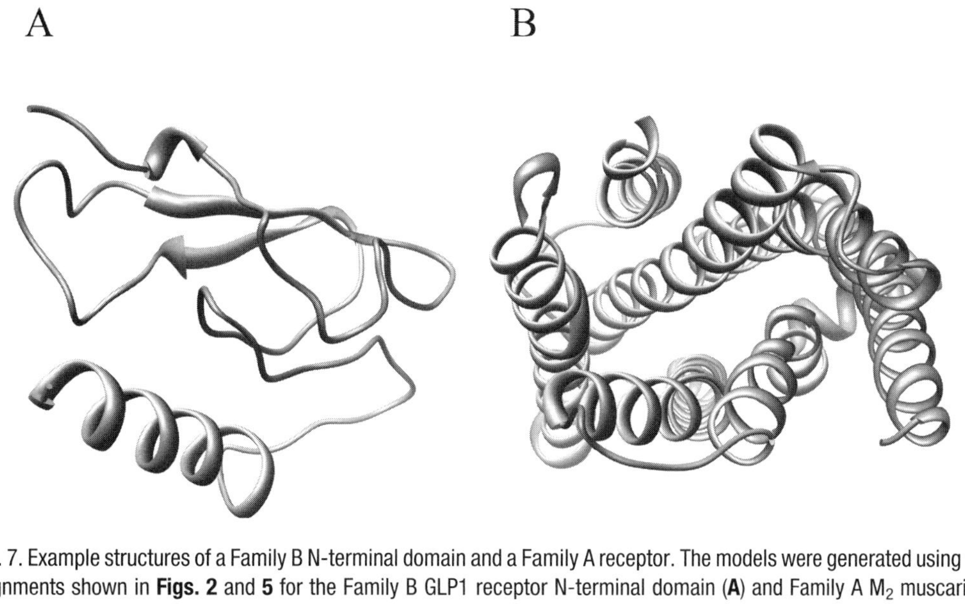

Fig. 7. Example structures of a Family B N-terminal domain and a Family A receptor. The models were generated using the alignments shown in **Figs. 2** and **5** for the Family B GLP1 receptor N-terminal domain (**A**) and Family A M_2 muscarinic receptor TM structure (**B**), respectively. ECL2 of the Family A GPCR structure (**B**) has been omitted for clarity.

template 2RH1. Examples of molecular models for the M_2 muscarinic receptor 7-TM domain core and the N-terminal domain of the GLP1 receptor are shown in **Fig. 7**

References

1. Gudermann T, Nurnberg B, Schultz G. (1995) Receptors and G proteins as primary components of transmembrane signal transduction. Part 1. G protein-coupled receptors: structure and function. *J Mol Med* **73**, 51–63.
2. Palczewski K, Kumasaka T, Hori T, et al. (2000) Crystal structure of rhodopsin: a G protein-coupled receptor. *Science* **289**, 739–745.
3. Murakami M, Kouyama T. (2008) Crystal structure of squid rhodopsin. *Nature* **453**, 363–367.
4. Park JH, Scheerer P, Hofmann KP, Choe HW, Ernst OP. (2008) Crystal structure of the ligand-free G protein-coupled receptor opsin. *Nature* **454**, 183–187.
5. Cherezov V, Rosenbaum DM, Hanson MA, et al. (2007) High-resolution crystal structure of an engineered human beta2-adrenergic G protein-coupled receptor. *Science* **318**, 1258–1265.
6. Berman HM, Westbrook J, Feng Z, et al. (2000) The protein data bank. *Nucleic Acids Res* **28**, 235–242.
7. Altschul SF, Gish W, Miller W, Myers EW, Lipman DJ. (1990) Basic local alignment search tool. *J Mol Biol* **215**, 403–410.
8. Teller DC, Okada T, Behnke CA, Palczewski K, Stenkamp RE. (2001) Advances in determination of a high-resolution three-dimensional structure of rhodopsin, a model of G protein-coupled receptors (GPCRs). *Biochemistry* **40**, 7761–7772.
9. Okada T, Fujiyoshi Y, Silow M, Navarro J, Landau EM, Shichida Y. (2002) Functional role of internal water molecules in rhodopsin revealed by X-ray crystallography. *Proc Natl Acad Sci USA* **99**, 5982–5987.
10. Li J, Edwards PC, Burghammer M, Villa C, Schertler GF. (2004) Structure of bovine rhodopsin in a trigonal crystal form. *J Mol Biol* **343**, 1409–1438.
11. Okada T, Sugihara M, Bondar AN, Elstner M, Entel P, Buss V. (2004) The retinal conformation and its environment in rhodopsin in light of a new 2.2 A crystal structure. *J Mol Biol* **342**, 571–583.
12. Nakamichi H, Okada T. (2006) Local peptide movement in the photoreaction intermediate of rhodopsin. *Proc Natl Acad Sci USA* **103**, 12729–12734.
13. Nakamichi H, Okada T. (2006) Crystallographic analysis of primary visual photochemistry. *Angew Chem Int Ed Engl* **45**, 4270–4273.
14. Salom D, Lodowski DT, Stenkamp RE, et al. (2006) Crystal structure of a photoactivated deprotonated intermediate of rhodopsin. *Proc Natl Acad Sci USA* **103**, 16123–16128.
15. Standfuss J, Xie G, Edwards PC, Burghammer M, Oprian DD, Schertler GF. (2007) Crystal structure of a thermally stable rhodopsin mutant. *J Mol Biol* **372**, 1179–1188.
16. Nakamichi H, Okada T. (2007) X-ray crystallographic analysis of 9-*cis*-rhodopsin, a model analogue visual pigment. *Photochem Photobiol* **83**, 232–235.
17. Hanson MA, Cherezov V, Griffith MT, et al. (2008) A specific cholesterol binding site is established by the 2.8 A structure of the human beta(2)-adrenergic receptor. *Structure* **16**, 897–905.
18. Frimurer TM, Bywater RP. (1999) Structure of the integral membrane domain of the GLP1 receptor. *Proteins* **35**, 375–386.
19. He XL, Bazan JF, McDermott G, et al. (2003) Structure of the Nogo receptor ectodomain: a recognition module implicated in myelin inhibition. *Neuron* **38**, 177–185.
20. Kobe B, Deisenhofer J. (1996) Mechanism of ribonuclease inhibition by ribonuclease inhibitor protein based on the crystal structure of its complex with ribonuclease A. *J Mol Biol* **264**, 1028–1043.
21. Parthier C, Kleinschmidt M, Neumann P, et al. (2007) Crystal structure of the incretin-bound extracellular domain of a G protein-coupled receptor. *Proc Natl Acad Sci USA* **104**, 13942–13947.
22. Pioszak AA, Xu HE. (2008) Molecular recognition of parathyroid hormone by its G protein-coupled receptor. *Proc Natl Acad Sci USA* **105**, 5034–5039.

23. Runge S, Thogersen H, Madsen K, Lau J, Rudolph R. (2008) Crystal structure of the ligand-bound glucagon-like peptide-1 receptor extracellular domain. *J Biol Chem* **283**, 11340–11347.
24. Grace CR, Perrin MH, Gulyas J, et al. (2007) Structure of the N-terminal domain of a type B1 G protein-coupled receptor in complex with a peptide ligand. *Proc Natl Acad Sci USA* **104**, 4858–4863.
25. Tsuchiya D, Kunishima N, Kamiya N, Jingami H, Morikawa K. (2002) Structural views of the ligand-binding cores of a metabotropic glutamate receptor complexed with an antagonist and both glutamate and Gd^{3+}. *Proc Natl Acad Sci USA* **99**, 2660–2665.
26. Muto T, Tsuchiya D, Morikawa K, Jingami H. (2007) Structures of the extracellular regions of the group II/III metabotropic glutamate receptors. *Proc Natl Acad Sci USA* **104**, 3759–3764.
27. Forrest LR, Tang CL, Honig B. (2006) On the accuracy of homology modeling and sequence alignment methods applied to membrane proteins. *Biophys J* **91**, 508–517.
28. Notredame C, Higgins DG, Heringa J. (2000) T-Coffee: A novel method for fast and accurate multiple sequence alignment. *J Mol Biol* **302**, 205–217.
29. Thompson JD, Higgins DG, Gibson TJ. (1994) CLUSTAL W: improving the sensitivity of progressive multiple sequence alignment through sequence weighting, position-specific gap penalties and weight matrix choice. *Nucleic Acids Res* **22**, 4673–4680.
30. Ballesteros JA, Shi L, Javitch JA. (2001) Structural mimicry in G protein-coupled receptors: Implications of the high-resolution structure of rhodopsin for structure-function analysis of rhodopsin-like receptors. *Mol Pharmacol* **60**, 1–19.
31. Sali A, Blundell TL. (1993) Comparative protein modelling by satisfaction of spatial restraints. *J Mol Biol* **234**, 779–815.
32. Farrens DL, Altenbach C, Yang K, Hubbell WL, Khorana HG. (1996) Requirement of rigid-body motion of transmembrane helices for light activation of rhodopsin. *Science* **274**, 768–770.
33. Gether U, Lin S, Ghanouni P, Ballesteros JA, Weinstein H, Kobilka BK. (1997) Agonists induce conformational changes in transmembrane domains III and VI of the beta2 adrenoceptor. *EMBO J* **16**, 6737–6747.
34. Elling CE, Thirstrup K, Nielsen SM, Hjorth SA, Schwartz TW. (1997) Metal-ion sites as structural and functional probes of helix-helix interactions in 7TM receptors. *Ann NY Acad Sci* **814**, 142–151.
35. Zhou W, Flanagan C, Ballesteros JA, et al. (1994) A reciprocal mutation supports helix 2 and helix 7 proximity in the gonadotropin-releasing hormone receptor. *Mol Pharmacol* **45**, 165–170.
36. Laskowski RA, Rullmannn JA, MacArthur MW, Kaptein R, Thornton JM. (1996) AQUA and PROCHECK-NMR: programs for checking the quality of protein structures solved by NMR. *J Biomol NMR* **8**, 477–86.
37. Hooft RW, Vriend G, Sander C, Abola EE. (1996) Errors in protein structures. *Nature* **381**, 272.
38. Eisenberg D, Luthy R, Bowie JU. (1997) VERIFY3D: assessment of protein models with three-dimensional profiles. *Methods Enzymol* **277**, 396–404.
39. Sippl MJ. (1993) Recognition of errors in three-dimensional structures of proteins. *Proteins* **17**, 355–362.
40. Guex N, Peitsch MC. (1997) SWISS-MODEL and the Swiss-PdbViewer: an environment for comparative protein modeling. *Electrophoresis* **18**, 2714–2723.

Chapter 8

GPCR Expression Using Baculovirus-Infected *Sf*9 Cells

Amanda L. Aloia, Richard V. Glatz, Edward J. McMurchie, and Wayne R. Leifert

Summary

Expression of proteins in insect cells using recombinant baculoviruses has gained wide use in the G protein-coupled receptor (GPCR) community. This expression system produces high yields of functional receptor, is able to perform post-translational modifications, and is readily adaptable to large-scale culture. Here, we describe the generic methods for expressing a GPCR using baculovirus-infected insect cells, including the maintenance of insect cell culture. Data are presented for *polyhedrin* promoter-driven expression of a C-terminal 6 × histidine-tagged mammalian M_2 muscarinic receptor in *Sf*9 cells. Results demonstrate that expressed receptor could be detected and quantified using radiolabeled ligand binding, that expression was maximal at approximately 72 h post-infection, and that expression levels could be altered by addition of various ligands to cultures of infected insect cells.

Key words: Baculovirus, Insect cell, GPCR expression, M_2 muscarinic receptor.

1. Introduction

Insect cell culture has proved as a valuable expression system for G protein-coupled receptors (GPCRs) owing to a combination of low maintenance requirements and the ability of insect cells to perform post-translational modifications such that vertebrate or invertebrate receptor function is not significantly altered from that *in vivo*. There are two insect cell lines in predominant use, *Sf*9 and *Sf*21, although a large range of insect cell types are used for protein expression *(1)*. The *Sf*21 cell line was originally prepared from the ovaries of *Spodoptera frugiperda* (J.E. Smith) *(2)*, the Fall armyworm, with the *Sf*9 line derived from *Sf*21 cells. In recent years, other cell lines have been developed and optimized

Wayne R. Leifert (ed.), *G Protein-Coupled Receptors in Drug Discovery, vol. 552*

Book doi: 10.1007/978-1-60327-317-6_8

to produce recombinant proteins with mammalian glycosylation profiles (e.g., Mimic™ *Sf* 9) and to increase expression of secreted proteins (e.g., High Five™ cells, which are derived from a different species, *Trichoplusia ni* (Hubner)) *(3, 4)*.

Each of these cell lines allow replication of the *Autographa californica* multiple nuclear polyhedrosis virus (a baculovirus), which will express inserted transgenes as part of the viral infection and replication process. The ease and efficiency of recombinant baculovirus production were significantly improved in 1997 by the development of an *Escherichia coli* cell line that contained modified baculovirus DNA *(5)*. This technology has subsequently been commercialized by Invitrogen (Bac-to-Bac® Baculovirus Expression System) and is now widely applied as it removes the need for homologous recombination in insect cells and the use of plaque assays for selection of cells containing pure recombinant virus. Recombination is now carried out within the specialized bacteria, which can be selected for the presence of recombinant baculovirus DNA. The DNA is then purified and used to transfect insect cells so that users can be confident that the infected cells contain pure recombinant virus.

Many GPCRs have been expressed using the baculovirus/insect cell system *(4)*. A range of baculoviral promoters that vary in strength and timing of expression are available for expression of foreign proteins. Generally, the *polyhedrin* promoter is utilized as it is an extremely strong promoter. However, this promoter is also a "very-late" baculovirus promoter which begins expression at a time point that is late in the infection cycle (within a given cell) and when cell lysis is beginning. The lytic infection process may result in degradation of recombinant proteins and limit the use of these late promoters for cellular assays. However, the strong late promoters are useful for providing maximal quantities of the receptor and so are useful, for example, if the receptor is to be purified and/or crystallized *(6, 7)*. The *p10* promoter is another example of a late promoter that could be utilized for receptor production *(8)*. This promoter has been utilized in various baculovirus vectors, including pFastBac™. Dual vector (Invitrogen) which is designed for coexpression of two genes, one driven by the *p10* promoter and the other by the *polyhedrin* promoter. If maximum protein production is required at an early stage of infection (i.e., before lysis is beginning) then early promoters can be utilized *(9)*. Alternatively, stably transformed cells can be utilized for expression using viral promoters (removing the infection process which leads to cell lysis), although vectors designed for this purpose generally utilize weaker promoters *(10, 11)*. Crude cell membrane preparations can be prepared from the infected cells providing a source of receptors for ligand binding, drug screening, or other GPCR functional assays such as interaction with purified G protein subunits.

This chapter covers the expression of a GPCR using recombinant baculovirus-infected insect cells, including the growth and maintenance of *Sf*9 cells. In addition, we discuss infection conditions and determination of optimal parameters for receptor expression.

2. Materials

2.1. Growth and Maintenance of Sf9 Cells

1. Vessels for cell culture should be thoroughly cleaned and sterilized (autoclaved).
2. Sf900-II serum-free media (Invitrogen). Store at 4°C.
3. 80% v/v ethanol in water. Caution ethanol is flammable.
4. 0.4% w/v Trypan blue prepared in phosphate-buffered saline (PBS). It can be stored at room temperature for several years.
5. 1% v/v hypochlorite solution.
6. Preservation media (for long-term storage of viable insect cells): Resuspend 15% w/v dimethyl sulfoxide (DMSO) in 10 mL of Sf900-II serum-free media. In the laminar flow hood, pass the media through a syringe filter to sterilize. The preservation media should be prepared on the day the cells are frozen and chilled to 4°C before use.
7. Hemocytometer, light microscope, sterile transfer pipettes, cryo-vials, liquid nitrogen storage facility.

2.2. Amplification of the Virus

1. Sterile syringes and 0.2 μm syringe filters.
2. Fetal bovine serum.

2.3. Infection of Sf9 Cells for Receptor Expression

1. Sterile syringes and 0.2 μm syringe filters.
2. Incubation buffer: 250 m*M* sucrose, 10 m*M* Tris-HCl (pH 8.0), and 3 m*M* $MgCl_2$ in sterile distilled H_2O. This stock can be stored at 4°C for a few months. On the day of use add the protease inhibitors: phenylmethyl sulfonyl fluoride to a final concentration of 0.02 mg/mL, benzamidine (0.03 mg/mL), bacitracin (0.025 mg/mL), and soybean trypsin inhibitor (0.03 mg/mL).

2.4. Saturation Ligand Binding

1. 4 mL (or other available size) polypropylene, round bottom tube, with cap.
2. TMN buffer: 50 m*M* Trizma®, 10 m*M* $MgCl_2$, 100 m*M* NaCl (pH 7.6).
3. 50 n*M* [^{3}H]-scopolamine prepared in TMN buffer.
4. 500 μ*M* atropine prepared in TMN buffer.

5. Cell aliquots (e.g., as prepared from **Section 3.3**) at a total protein concentration of 1 mg/mL.
6. Filtration manifold.
7. 4 mL scintillation counting tubes. For example, Pico Pro Vials^{TM} from PerkinElmer.
8. Liquid scintillant for β-counting. For example, Ultima Gold^{TM} from PerkinElmer.
9. β-Counter. For example, Wallac Liquid Scintillation Counter from PerkinElmer.

2.5. Ligand Culture

1. 1 m*M* atropine (>98%, Sigma-Aldrich) prepared in water. Stock can be aliquoted and stored at –20°C for a few months.
2. 500 μ*M* pirenzipine (>98%) prepared in water. Stock can be aliquoted and stored at –20°C for a few months.
3. 10 m*M* acetylcholine (>99%) prepared in water. The solution should be prepared on the day of use and not stored as a liquid.

3. Methods

3.1. Growth and Maintenance of Sf9 Cells

Cell culture work should be done with aseptic technique within a laminar flow hood.

3.1.1. Growing Cells from Frozen Stocks

Sf 9 cells in serum-free medium can be frozen in 1 mL aliquots of approximately 20 × 10^6 cells/mL (*see* **Section 3.1.3**).

1. Place a sterilized 50 mL glass Schott bottle (or other appropriate sized shaker flask, *see* **Note 1**) into the laminar flow hood.
2. Using aseptic technique, add an appropriate volume of Sf900-II serum-free media to the bottle to provide a final cell concentration of 2 × 10^6cells/mL (e.g., for a frozen aliquot containing 20 × 10^6 cells, add 10 mL of media).
3. Rapidly thaw the frozen cells in a 37°C water bath, this can be done by plunging the vial in and out of the water and inverting the vial in between plunges. The temperature of the cells should be kept below approximately 25°C and the vial should only be plunged into the water bath until the cells are just defrosted.
4. Spray the outside of the vial with 80% v/v ethanol and, in the laminar flow hood, pour the entire contents of the vial into the Schott bottle containing the media. A sterile transfer pipette and media (from the Schott bottle) can be used to transfer any remaining cells from the vial to the bottle.

5. Loosely screw (1 to 2 turns is fine) the lid onto the Schott bottle and place the cells into a 27°C incubator shaking at 130–140 r.p.m.
6. Approximately 48 h after beginning the cell culture, count the cells and determine cell viability (*see* **Note 2**).
7. Once a normal growth rate and high proportion of viable cells is achieved, the culture can be maintained as described in **Section 3.1.2.**

3.1.2. Maintenance of Sf9 cells

In our laboratory, we found it convenient to dilute (passage) cells to 0.5×10^6 cells/mL on Monday, Wednesday, and Friday of each week for maintenance of the *Sf* 9 cell cultures.

1. Before diluting *Sf* 9 cells, heat Sf900-II serum-free medium to 27°C by placing into a 27°C water bath or incubator.
2. Collect the cell culture bottle from the shaking incubator, spray the bottle with 80% v/v ethanol, and place in the laminar flow hood (*see* **Note 3**).
3. Using a sterile transfer pipette transfer a small volume (500 μL is more than sufficient) of cells to a 1.5 mL micro-centrifuge tube. Return the cell culture bottle to the shaking incubator.
4. Remove the cell aliquot from the hood and, on the laboratory bench, transfer 20 μL of cells to a clean micro-centrifuge tube.
5. Add an equal volume (20 μL) of 0.4% v/v Trypan blue to the cells and mix well.
6. Count cells using a hemocytometer, and calculate the percentage of non-viable cells (stained blue) and the density of viable cells (not stained; *see* **Note 4**). In a healthy culture, cell viability should be greater than 95% (*see* **Note 5**).
7. Double (to account for dilution by the Trypan blue addition) the number of total cells counted to give the concentration of cells in the culture.
8. Determine the required final volume of cells required (e.g., for maintenance of the culture only 20–50 mL may be sufficient or, if the culture is being scaled up in preparation for infection and protein expression, 500 mL may be desired) and calculate the required volume of cells needed to prepare the final volume to a cell concentration of 0.5×10^6 cells/mL.
9. Label a sterilized Schott bottle of appropriate size with (at least) the passage number of the cells, that is, the number of times that the cells have been diluted (*see* **Note 6**). Spray the bottle with 80% v/v ethanol and place in the laminar flow hood.

10. In the labeled Schott bottle, combine the required volume of cells and media for a final cell concentration of 0.5 $\times$ 10^6 cells/mL (*see* **Note 7**). Place diluted cells into the shaking incubator set at 27°C.
11. Destroy any unused cells by adding an equal volume of 1% v/v hypochlorite and leaving at room temperature for 24 h. Cells can then be discarded in accordance with established procedures relevant to individual institutions.

3.1.3. Freezing Cells

1. Prepare approximately 200 mL of cells at 2 $\times$ 10^6 cells/mL, for example, by diluting 200 mL of cells to approximately 0.5 $\times$ 10^6 cells/mL, 48 h prior to freezing.
2. In the laminar flow hood, label 20 sterile 2 mL cryo-vials with the date, *Sf* 9 cells, 20 $\times$ 10^6 cells/mL, and the passage number of the cells to be frozen.
3. Centrifuge the cell suspension at 1500 $\times$ g for 10 min in a sterile centrifuge tube (*see* **Note 8**) Discard the supernatant with the exception of 10 mL of the media (supernatant), which should remain with the cell pellet.
4. Add 10 mL of cold (4°C) preservation media and use a sterile transfer pipette to gently resuspend the cells to give a final cell concentration of 20 $\times$ 10^6 cells/mL.
5. Aliquot 1 mL of the resuspended cells into each of the labeled cryo-vials.
6. Place the cells at 4°C for 30 min. Invert the tubes to mix the cells and then place at –20°C for 1 h followed by –80°C for 1 day. Vials should then be transferred to liquid nitrogen for long-term storage.

3.2. Amplification of Recombinant Baculovirus

The amount of virus added to the *Sf* 9 cells for either cell infection or baculovirus amplification is determined by the following equation:

$$\text{Virus required (mL)} = \frac{\text{desired MOI} \times \text{total no. of cells}}{\text{viral titer (PFU)}}$$

where MOI is the multiplicity of infection and PFU is plaque-forming units. For amplification of the recombinant baculovirus it is desirable to inoculate with a low MOI, we use 0.1. Thus, assuming a viral titer of 5 $\times$ 10^7pfu/mL, 2 mL of virus is added to 500 mL of cells that are at a concentration of 2 $\times$ 10^6cells/mL. A low MOI is used for virus amplification as a precautionary measure in the case that there is any non-recombinant virus within the viral population. The lower concentration of virus used, compared to the MOI used during cell infection for protein production, decreases the potential for an increase in any non-recombinant component of the viral population, a problem that will compound with subsequent amplifications.

1. Approximately 48 h prior to the desired day of virus amplification dilute the required volume of *Sf* 9 cells to 0.5×10^6 cells/mL.
2. On the day of virus amplification, count the *Sf*9 cells as described in **Section 3.1**. Ideally cells should be at a concentration of approximately 2×10^6 cells/mL (*see* **Note 9**).
3. Using the equation shown above, calculate the volume of virus required.
4. In the laminar flow hood, draw up the required amount of virus in a syringe, attach a 0.2 μm syringe filter, and filter the virus into the cell culture. Return the cells to the 27°C orbital shaker.
5. Approximately 72 h post-infection count the cells and determine the cell viability. Cell viability should be ≤75% and cells should appear larger than non-infected cells with expanded nuclei occupying much of the cell volume (a key sign of infection). In addition, cells should be at a lower density than what would be expected for healthy cells which double in density in approximately 24 h.
6. Transfer cell culture to a sterile centrifuge tube and centrifuge at $1500 \times g$ for 10 min.
7. Using a syringe and 0.2 μm syringe filter, transfer the supernatant (which contains the virus) to a sterile storage container (*see* **Note 10**).
8. Using a 0.2 μm syringe filter, add fetal bovine serum (FBS) to a final concentration of 2–3% v/v. FBS is thought to aid in preservation of virion proteins as it contains trypsin inhibitors *(12)*.
9. Store the virus at 4°C in the dark.

3.3. Infection of Insect Cells and Expression of GPCR

In our laboratory it is standard to infect *Sf*9 cells for protein production using a MOI of 2. When the receptors are required in large quantities (e.g., for purification attempts) it may be desirable to optimize the MOI for your particular receptor as the expression patterns of different receptors may vary *(4)*. Here, we present data relating to expression of a GPCR in insect cells, specifically a C-terminal, 6 × histidine-tagged mammalian M_2 muscarinic receptor. The method for baculovirus production is not given as it is well described in the manual for the commercially available Bac-to-Bac®system from Invitrogen.

1. Infect the cells as described in Steps 1–4 of **Section 3.2**. When calculating the amount of virus required, remember to use an MOI of 2.
2. Approximately 72 h post-infection (*see* **Note 11**), count the cells and determine cell viability as described in **Section 3.1.2**. Cell viability should be ≤50% at the time of cell harvest as this suggests viral infection and subsequently maximal protein

expression. Cells can be harvested at higher percentage viabilities in order to reduce levels of degraded protein (though this may also reduce the level of functional protein harvested) depending on the type of promoter and MOI used.

3. Centrifuge the infected cell suspension at 1500 × *g* for 10 min and discard the supernatant.
4. If desired, resuspend the cells in incubation buffer. We found that cells may then be frozen at –80°C without loss of receptor activity.
5. Determine the receptor density by radioligand binding assay (*see* **Section 3.4**). An example is shown in **Fig. 1**, where tritiated scopolamine ([^{3}H]-Scopolamine) was used to confirm expression of a 6 × histidine-tagged mammalian M_2 muscarinic receptor. It should be noted that ligand binding is a measurement of expression levels of receptor with a correctly formed ligand binding region and is not a direct measurement of levels of functional receptor (in terms of G protein coupling and signaling abilities), nor total receptor production (including non-functional receptor, which may be determined by Western blot).

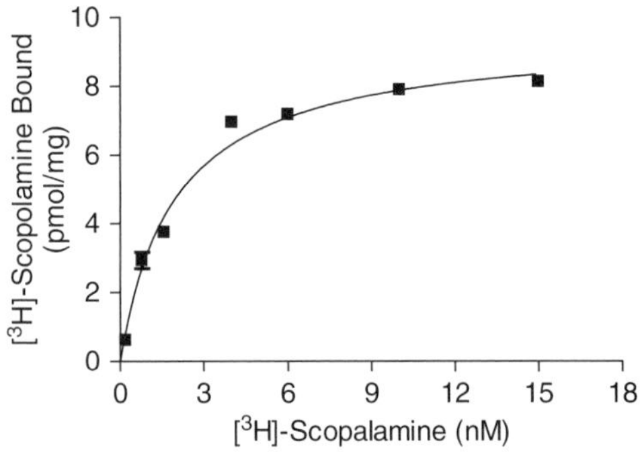

Fig. 1. Detection and quantification of baculovirus-expressed mammalian M_2R muscarinic receptor. [^{3}H]-Scopolamine (antagonist) binding to membranes prepared from *Sf* 9 cells infected with M_2R recombinant baculovirus was measured. Non-specific binding was determined in the presence of 10 μ*M* of the specific antagonist atropine. Analysis confirmed a single [^{3}H]-Scopolamine binding site which had an apparent dissociation constant (K_d) of 2.0 n*M*. Receptor binding sites were saturated at 9.4 pmol/mg of total membrane protein (B_{max}).

3.4. Saturation Ligand Binding Assay

In this section a basic saturation ligand binding assay is described. The reagents listed are for the M_2 muscarinic receptor, but the assay is readily adapted for other receptors. The assay volume and concentration of components can also be modified as appropriate. Here, a final concentration of 0.2 mg of total cellular protein/mL is used for the receptor containing cells (10 μg total protein per 50 μL assay), but this concentration will need to be modified depending on the concentration of receptors within the cell sample. The protein concentration used is determined such fact that the measured β counts (from tritium) for each assay do not exceed 10% of the total counts determined for each assay condition (*see* Steps 9 and 10 below). This is a requirement to ensure that laws of mass action are followed within the binding assay and so allow calculation of B_{max} and apparent K_d. For this reason it is useful to conduct a small-scale version of the assay described below, perhaps using only 2 to 3 radioligand concentrations and single points, to determine whether this requirement is being met. The protein concentration can then be modified accordingly in a subsequent, more thorough assay. Protein concentration and/or radioligand concentration may also need to be modified to ensure that saturation of the ligand binding sites occurs. Furthermore, the time of assay incubation will need to be adapted depending on the receptor–ligand pair being studied. The incubation time should be such that a steady binding state is reached. (This time can be determined by using a single radioligand concentration and varying assay time; plot time against specific binding.)

1. Defrost infected cell aliquots on ice.
2. Label ten 4 mL clear disposable tubes, in duplicate (i.e., a total of 20 tubes) and place on ice.
3. Assays can be prepared as shown in **Table 1**.

   Buffer, cells, and atropine (where applicable) can be combined and then the reaction can be started with addition of the [^{3}H]-scopolamine. Following the table described, even

Table 1
Preparation of sample tubes for the saturation ligand binding assay (all volumes are given in μL)

Tube #	Buffer	Cells	[^{3}H]-Scopolamine(final concentration, *nM*)	Atropine
1a, 1b	60	14	1(0.6)	0
2a, 2b	58.5	14	1(0.6)	1.5
3a, 3b	58	14	3(2)	0
4a, 4b	56.5	14	3(2)	1.5
5a, 5b	53.5	14	7.5(5)	0
6a, 6b	52	14	7.5(5)	1.5
7a, 7b	46	14	15(10)	0
8a, 8b	44.5	14	15(10)	1.5
9a, 9b	31	14	30(20)	0
10a, 10b	29.5	14	30(20)	1.5

numbered tubes will describe the non-specific binding of the [^{3}H]-scopolamine (that which occurs in the presence of excess unlabeled antagonist atropine) and odd numbered tubes will represent the total radioligand binding.

4. Cap tubes and place in a shaking 25°C water bath for 1 h.
5. During the incubation period, place 20 GF/C filters in a tray of TMN buffer. Just prior to the end of the assay incubation period place a single GF/C filter onto each of the manifold filtration localities.
6. Pipette 50 μL of each reaction onto the center of a GF/C filter which has been placed on a filtration manifold. Do not discard the remaining assay mixture in each tube (*see* Step 9).
7. Wash the GF/C filter with 3 × 3 mL of ice-cold TMN buffer.
8. Use forceps to transfer the filter into a labeled 4 mL scintillation counting tube. Leave tubes at room temperature, or place in a heated incubator, until GF/C filters are dry.
9. Label (e.g., 1Ta, 1 Tb, 2Ta, and 2 Tb) an additional twenty 4 mL scintillation tubes and place a GF/C filter in each one.
10. Pipette 5 μL of the remains of each assay onto a dry GF/C filter from Step 9. These tubes will provide the total radioactive counts within each assay.
11. Add 3 mL of scintillant to each tube, cap the tube, and invert a few times to ensure that the GF/C filter is completely submerged in the scintillant.
12. Place tubes in a β-counter, count each tube for 1 min. Measured radioactivity will be produced as counts per minute (c.p.m.) or disintegrations per minute (d.p.m.).
13. To determine the specific radioligand binding, subtract non-specific binding (even numbered tubes) from total binding (odd numbered tubes) for each assay condition.
14. To determine the percentage of specific binding divide the value calculated in Step 13 by the total counts measured for the assay condition (odd numbered tubes) and multiply by 100.
15. To determine molarity of radioligand bound per milligram of total protein a mol/c.p.m. value for the radioligand first needs to be calculated. This can be done from the counts determined in Steps 9 and 10. This value is then applied to the counts determined each assay condition, giving a mol value (usually fmol or pmol) of radioligand binding for the assay. This mol value is then divided by the total protein (mg) in the assay.
16. A program such as GraphPad Prism can be used to determine B_{max} and apparent K_d. Plot the mol/mg value determined in Step 15 against the total concentration of radioligand

in the assay (described in table 1). Commonly, data will fit to a non-linear regression, single site binding equation. This type of analysis was used in **Figs. 1**, **2**, and **3**.

3.5. Time Course of Receptor Expression

1. Infect 300 mL of *Sf*9 cells (in a single bottle) as described in **Section 3.3**.
2. 24 h after infection, remove cells from the shaker and in a laminar flow hood carefully pour 50 mL of cells into a centrifuge tube. Replace the infected culture (~250 mL) in the orbital shaker.
3. Take a small sample (e.g., 50 μL) of the collected cells and determine and record the cell viability as described in **Section 3.1.2**.
4. Centrifuge the 50 mL of cells at 1500 × *g* for 10 min. Discard the supernatant.
5. Resuspend the cells in incubation buffer (~ 2 mL) using a homogenizer. Aliquot the cells into 500 μL aliquots, freeze in liquid nitrogen, and store at –80°C.
6. Repeat Steps 2–4 at 48, 72, 96, and 120 h post-infection.
7. Analyze receptor expression in the cells by radioligand binding assay (*see* **Section 3.4**).
8. A plot of hours post-infection against B_{max} may be useful in determining the time to harvest infected cells for maximum functional (ligand binding site intact) receptor yield. An example is given in **Fig. 2**, which illustrates that the highest

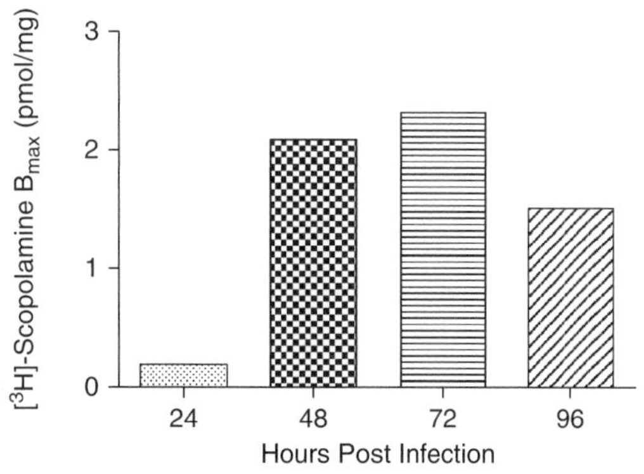

Fig. 2. Time course of expression of 6 × histidine-tagged mammalian M_2 muscarinic receptor in *Sf* 9 cells. [^{3}H]-Scopolamine binding (pmol/mg of total cellular protein) to cells infected with M_2 receptor recombinant baculovirus was measured. Cells were collected at 24 h intervals after baculovirus addition and assayed for specific [^{3}H]-Scopolamine binding. Non-specific binding was determined in the presence of 10 μ*M* of the specific antagonist atropine. B_{max} values were calculated from saturation curves consisting of data points for which the mean ± S.E.M was calculated for three separate experiments. High levels of ligand binding were measured between 48 and 72 h post-infection, with highest levels of functional receptor detected at 72 h post-infection.

level of functional (as defined above) 6 × histidine-tagged mammalian M_2 muscarinic receptor was detected at around 72 h post-infection (MOI=2), when expression was driven by the *polyhedrin* promoter. Again, this is a measure of ligand binding and does not confirm full receptor function such as G protein coupling (receptor-specific functional assays are required for this purpose), nor total (including non-functional receptor protein) receptor expressed.

3.6. Receptor Ligand Addition to Cell Culture

GPCR expression in baculovirus-infected *Sf* 9 cells may be regulated by addition of receptor ligands to the infected cell culture. It may present a simple method for increasing the expression of your receptor of interest. A method to test for ligand modulation of M_2 muscarinic receptor expression is described in this section, but the standard method can be applied to all receptor expression by changing the ligands used to those specific for the receptor being expressed.

1. Infect 1 L of culture as described in **Section 3.3**.
2. 48 h after infection of the cells, determine the cell concentration and viability. If cells are being prepared for infection in more than one bottle, they should be combined in a single bottle prior to counting and the proceeding steps (*see* **Note 12**)
3. In the laminar flow hood, pour 250 mL of the culture into each of 4 × 1 L Schott bottles. Label the bottles (a)–(d).
4. In three separate 5 mL tubes add:
   (a) 12.5 μL of atropine or
   (b) 25 μL of pirenzipine or
   (c) 5 μL of acetylcholine or
   (d) no addition (negative control) (*see* **Note 13**).
5. Add serum-free media to each tube to a final volume of approximately 5 mL.
6. Use a 5 mL syringe and syringe filter to add one ligand (or the control with no ligand) to each of the four Schott bottles. Be sure to label the bottle with the name of the added ligand.
7. Return the cell cultures bottles to the shaking incubator.
8. 72 h post-infection (24 h after ligand addition), collect the cells by centrifugation at 1500 × *g* for 10 min. Discard the supernatant.
9. Use a transfer pipette to resuspend each of the cell pellets in 250 mL of PBS, centrifuge as above to collect the cell pellet. Repeat this step twice.
10. Resuspend the final cell pellets in incubation buffer.
11. Use the ligand binding assay as described in (*see* **Section 3.4**) to determine receptor density (B_{max}) in the cells and compare the effect of the ligand treatments. An example for a 6 ×

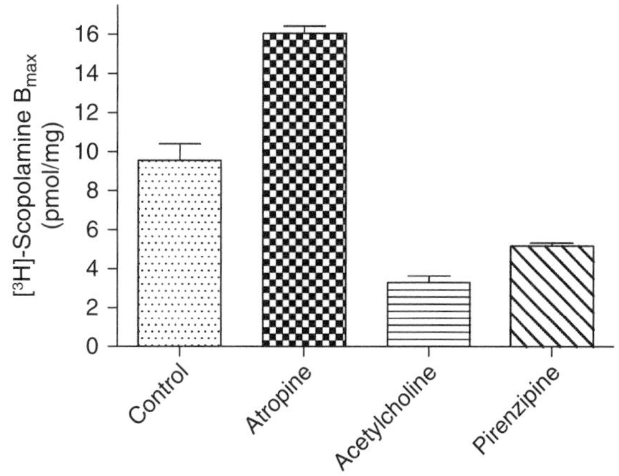

Fig. 3. Effect of ligand addition on expression of 6 × histidine-tagged mammalian M_2 muscarinic receptor in *Sf* 9 cells. Graph shows [^{3}H]-Scopolamine (antagonist) binding to M_2 receptor membranes prepared from ligand-treated, baculovirus infected Sf 9 cells. No ligand treatment (control), $B_{max} \sim 8.4$ pmol/mg. Treatment with the antagonist atropine increased receptor expression, $B_{max} \sim 15.8$ pmol/mg. Treatment with a agonist, acetylcholine decreased receptor expression, $B_{max} \sim 3.3$ pmol/mg. Treatment with a inverse agonist, pirenzipine decreased receptor expression, $B_{max} \sim 5.5$ pmol/mg. Results are representative of one of three complete culture experiments. Replicates represent assay points from a single membrane preparation, mean ± S.E.M., $n = 3$.

histidine-tagged mammalian M_2 muscarinic receptor is shown in **Fig. 3**. In this example, expression was increased by addition of the muscarinic receptor antagonist atropine and was reduced by addition of either the agonist acetylcholine or pirenzipine (each relative to the control which did not have a ligand added).

4. Notes

1. We found glass Schott bottles to be a convenient growth vessel for *Sf* 9 cells. Cell volume should be kept to approximately one-fourth of the bottle volume and the lid should be screwed loosely on the bottle (1–2 turns) to allow sufficient airflow. After bleaching or acid treatment of any unwanted cells, the bottle should be washed with warm water and a harsh detergent such as pyroneg. Bottles should then be autoclaved. Small maintenance cultures of between 10 and 20 mL were routinely maintained in 50–100 mL Schott bottles.
2. Cells grown from a frozen stock will have an initial "lag" period in the first few days after the culture is started and, more than likely, will not begin a normal growth rate

(approximately a double in cell number over 24 h) until after this time. In the first week after beginning the culture it may be best to keep the viable cell concentration at around 2×10^6 cells/mL and then gradually, over the course of a week, bring the final dilution to 0.5×10^6 viable cells/mL as described in the **Section 3.1**.

3. Do not leave the cells in the laminar flow hood for a prolonged period of time as cells will settle during this time causing inaccurate cell count and potentially damaging the cells.
4. Trypan blue cannot penetrate an intact cell membrane, thus cells that are not stained blue are considered viable.
5. Cells which have recently been grown from a frozen stock will have a low viability (<50% is normal); however, this should increase and reach >95% within 2–3 weeks. If this is not the case cells should be discarded and a new culture started. In our laboratory cells were not routinely assessed using Trypan blue staining; if cells demonstrate a 24 h doubling rate this is generally sufficient to demonstrate cell health. Cell viability was assessed, however, prior to and following cell infection with recombinant baculovirus.
6. It is good practice to dilute/passage cells no more than 40 times as normal cell metabolism and health may be compromised. At passage 40 cells should be discarded and a new culture started from frozen stock.
7. A high degree of accuracy is not required for the cell dilution, cells can be poured between Schott bottles and the markers on the bottle used to estimate volume as it is acceptable for cells to be diluted to a density range of between 0.5 and 1 million viable cells/mL.
8. It is convenient to sequentially centrifuge multiple cell aliquots in a single sterile 50 mL tube thus containing all cells in one cell pellet.
9. Dilution of the cells to 0.5×10^6 cells/mL 48 h prior to infection should result in a cell concentration of approximately 2×10^6 cells/mL on the day of infection (as cells double in number in approximately 24 h). Small variations from this value can be dealt with using the equation shown in **Section 3.2** (i.e., the amount of virus or cells can be altered to produce the correct MOI if cell density differs from 2 million cells/mL).
10. For larger culture volumes (> 100 mL), Steritop filters (Milipore) can be attached directly to a Schott bottle to allow automated filtering of the virus containing supernatent via suction through the filter.

11. The post-infection time that cells should be harvested for maximum functional protein yield will vary between receptors. For this reason, it is best to perform a "time course of receptor expression" experiment (*see* **Section 3.5**).
12. To minimize variations in receptor expression, cells should be split from a single source.
13. Generally, nanomolar concentrations of antagonist/inverse agonist and micromolar concentrations of agonist should be sufficient to assess any effect of ligand addition on receptor expression. If an effect is demonstrated for a particular ligand, conditions (such as ligand concentration and time of ligand addition) can be optimized to maximize the observed effect.

References

1. Lynn, D.E. (2007) Available Lepidopteran insect cell lines. In: Murhammer, D. W. (Ed.), *Baculovirus and Insect Cell Expression Protocols* Springer, New York.
2. Vaughn, J.L., Goodwin, R.H., Tompkins, G.J., McCawley, P. (1977) The establishment of two cell lines from the insect Spodoptera frugiperda (Lepidoptera; Noctuidae). *In Vitro* **13**, 213–217.
3. Leifert, W.R., Aloia, A. L., Bucco, O., Glatz, R.V., McMurchie, E.J. (2005) G protein-coupled receptors in drug discovery: nanosizing using cell-free technologies and molecular biology approaches. *J. Biomol. Screen.* **10**, 765–779.
4. Massotte, D. (2003) G protein-coupled receptor overexpression with the baculovirus-insect cell system: a tool for structural and functional studies. *Biochim. Biophys. Acta* **1610**, 77–89.
5. Ciccarone, V., Polayes, D., Luckow, V. (1997) Generation of recombinant baculovirus DNA in *E. coli* using a baculovirus shuttle vector. *Meth. Mol. Med.* **13**, 213–235.
6. Ratnala, V. R., Swarts, H. G., VanOostrum, J., Leurs, R., DeGroot, H. J., Bakker, R. A., et al. (2004) Large-scale overproduction, functional purification and ligand affinities of the His-tagged human histamine H1 receptor. *Eur. J. Biochem.* **271**, 2636–2646.
7. Cherezov, V., Rosenbaum, D.M., Hanson, M.A., Rasmussen, S.G., Thian, F.S., Kobilka, T.S., et al. (2007) High-resolution crystal structure of an engineered human β_2-adrenergic G protein-coupled receptor. *Science* **318**, 1258–1265.
8. Fraser, M.J. (1992) Baculovirus infected insect cell cultures as a eukaryotic gene expression system. *Curr. Top. Microbiol. Immun.* **158**, 131–172.
9. Kojima, K., Hayakawa, T., Asano, S., Bando, H. (2001) Tandem repetition of baculovirus ie1 promoter results in upregulation of transcription. *Arch. Virol.* **146**, 1407–1414.
10. Douris, V., Swevers, L., Labropoulou, V., Andronopoulou, E., Georgoussi, Z., Iatrou, K. (2006) Stably transformed insect cell lines: tools for expression of secreted and membrane-anchored proteins and high-throughput screening platforms for drug and insecticide discovery. *Adv. Virus Res.* **68**, 113–156.
11. Harvey, L., Reid, R.E., Ma, C., Knight, P.J., Pfeifer, T.A., Grigliatti, T.A. (2003) Human genetic variations in the $5HT_{2A}$ receptor: a single nucleotide polymorphism identified with altered response to clozapine. *Pharmacogenetics* **13**, 107–118.
12. Lynn, D.E. (2007) Routine maintenance and storage of lepidopteran cell lines and baculoviruses. In: Murhammer, D. W. (Ed.), *Baculovirus and Insect Cell Expression Protocols.* Springer, New York.

Chapter 9

Radioligand Binding Assays: Application of [^{125}I]Angiotensin II Receptor Binding

Wayne R. Leifert, Olgatina Bucco, Mahinda Y. Abeywardena, and Glen S. Patten

Summary

Angiotensin II (AngII) is an octapeptide hormone with a key role in blood pressure regulation. AngII increases blood pressure by stimulating G protein-coupled receptors in vascular smooth muscle. AngII receptors are therefore an important target in patients with high blood pressure. Strategies to lower high blood pressure (hypertension) include the use of drugs that compete for AngII at the angiotensin II Type 1 receptors (ATR) using ATR antagonists (e.g., irbesartan, valsartan, and losartan). This chapter will demonstrate the subtype specificity of ATR binding and we discuss some of the key experiments that are necessary in optimizing some of the parameters for GPCR screening. The latter protocols include saturation binding to determine K_d and B_{max}, as well as competition/inhibition experiments to determine the IC_{50} of binding. For these experiments we have used rat liver membranes which express ATR (type 1a) in relatively abundant amounts. Additionally, rat liver membrane preparations can be easily prepared in "bulk," frozen away for extended periods (up to 1 year) and used when necessary with no loss of receptor binding activity using the radiolabeled angiotensin II analogue, [^{125}I][Sar^1,I le^8]AngII.

Key words: Angiotensin receptor, Losartan, Radioligand, Saralasin, Liver, Specific binding.

1. Introduction

Radioligand binding assays targeted to G protein-coupled receptors (GPCRs) are a relatively simple but powerful tool for discovering GPCR agonists and antagonists. For many years now, the biochemical and pharmacological identification of GPCRs and their subtypes has been aided by the use of radioligand binding methods *(1, 2)*. A popular technique routinely used is termed the "membrane filtration assay." This type of assay can be literally applied to hundreds of different radioligands. Providing there is easy access to a β-scintillation counter (e.g., for [^{3}H]-labeled ligands) and/or gamma counter (e.g., for [^{125}I]-labeled ligands), the remainder of

Wayne R. Leifert (ed.), *G Protein-Coupled Receptors in Drug Discovery, vol. 552*

Book doi: 10.1007/978-1-60327-317-6_9

equipment required to conduct membrane filtration assays is relatively cheap and minimal. One drawback, however, can be the accumulation of low-level radioactive waste which requires careful monitoring and disposal. Therefore, this assay format is more suitable for low-throughput applications and for screening small sample libraries to characterize receptor ligand binding.

The basic radioligand assay principle is quite simple; however, there are certain rules one should follow to obtain meaningful results (and these will be discussed later in this chapter). Preparations containing the GPCR of interest can be diverse, for example, derived from animal tissue (e.g., red blood cells, liver, and brain) or expressed in cell lines either naturally, stably, or transiently. The primary approach includes the incubation of a specific radioligand with a preparation known to contain the GPCRs of interest (e.g., angiotensin II type 1a receptors (ATRs)) for an optimal time period. The radioligand bound to the receptors can then be determined. Prior to using the preparation containing the GPCRs of interest for screening purposes, "saturation" and "kinetic" assays need to be fully optimized (for temperature, concentration, time, pH, and osmolarity amongst other conditions).

In this chapter we have presented results of radiolabeled [^{125}I]angiotensin II (AngII) binding to ATRs derived from rat liver membranes. Although we present data for the ATR, some of the basic principles used here can be equally applied to a myriad of other radioligands available for GPCR screening. Additionally, with regard to GPCR preparations, we have also used membranes from turkey livers as well as Chinese hamster ovary cells (CHO) overexpressing ATRs with equal success (data not presented). However, some of the advantages of using the rat liver membranes for screening included short preparation time (1 day's work) and a yield sufficient to conduct hundreds of assays saving on time and costs without the need of continually maintaining cell lines. Usually, high throughput is considered an important factor in designing a screening assay (*see (3)* and other chapters in this volume). The screening throughput for this assay as described is quite low; however, when investigating limited sample libraries the membrane filtration assay should be given consideration. Nevertheless, it would be possible to increase the throughput of this assay by various means, if required.

2. Materials

2.1. Isolation Medium for Rat Liver Membranes

1. Isolation medium: 250 m*M* sucrose, 50 m*M* 4-(2-hydroxyethyl)-1-piperazineethanesulfonic acid (HEPES), 1 m*M* ethylenediamine tetraacetic acid (EDTA), final pH adjusted to pH 7.4. Store at 4°C for up to 1 month.

2. Prepare the protease inhibitors (as 1000 × stock solutions) as follows: 20 mg/mL phenylmethyl sulfonyl fluoride (PMSF; Sigma-Aldrich, NSW, Australia) in 100% ethanol, 30 mg/mL benzamidine (Sigma) in 50 m*M* HEPES (pH 7.4), 25 mg/mL bacitracin (Sigma) in 50 m*M* HEPES (pH 7.4), and 30 mg/mL soybean trypsin inhibitor (Sigma) in 50 m*M* HEPES (pH 7.4). Store in 200 μL aliquots at –20°C for up to 6 months (*see* **Note 1**). These should only be thawed once for the rat liver membrane preparations and then the remainder discarded.

2.2. Radioligand Binding Assay

1. Angiotensin II (AngII) (unlabeled, FW 1046.1, acetate form, AusPep, Parkville, VIC, Australia) prepared at 1 m*M* in 50 mM HEPES (pH 7.4) and stored for 1 month at 4°C.
2. Losartan (Cayman Chemical Company, Ann Arbor, MI. USA) 10 m*M* in 90 mM Tris-HCl adjusted to pH 7.4 and stored for 1 month at 4°C.
3. Radiolabeled AngII was in the "saralasin" form, that is, [^{125}I][Sar^1,Ile^8]AngII (PerkinElmer, Waltham, MA, USA) and is herein termed "[^{125}I]-Sar^1-AngII". [^{125}I]-Sar^1-AngII was purchased as 10 μCi lots, at 59.6 days half-life, at 100% remaining, 0.05 mCi/mL, 2200 Ci/mmol gives stock concentration of 22.7 n*M*. It is necessary to ensure that the concentrated form of [^{125}I]-Sar^1-AngII is stored frozen and shielded in a lead pig to prevent accidental radiation exposure. Dilute aliquots down to 1 n*M* using 50 m*M* Tris-HCl (pH 7.4), 1 m*M* glycol-bis(2-aminoethylether)-*N*,*N*,*N*',*N*'-tetraacetic acid (EGTA; Sigma), and 10 m*M* $MgCl_2$ plus 0.2% bovine serum albumin (Sigma, Sydney, NSW, Australia). Store aliquots at –20°C shielded by lead to prevent radiation exposure.
4. PD123319 (AT_2 antagonist; Sigma) or endothelin-1 (ET_1; Sigma) and test samples (from a CSIRO "*in house*" library) were prepared fresh in 10% 90 m*M* Tris-HCl adjusted to pH 7.4 and stored at 20–50 mg/mL at –20°C.

2.3. Wash Buffer and Filtering

1. Wash buffer: 90 m*M* Tris-HCl, 10 m*M* $MgCl_2$, 1 m*M* EDTA adjusted to pH 7.4, prepared in purified water (*see* **Note 2**). Store at 4°C.
2. 25 mm glass fiber type C filter circles (GF/C; Whatman, Maidstone, England).
3. Enhancing solution is 1% polyethylenimine in wash buffer (*see* **Note 3**). Store at 4°C.
4. Filtration manifold apparatus connected to a vacuum pump and liquid trap to contain any unbound radioligand (for disposal) (*see* **Note 4**).

3. Methods

We present here the methods for preparing rat liver membranes to be used for ATR ligand binding studies. Similar pharmacological profiles have been observed using AngII with turkey liver preparations; however, a separate ATR receptor subtype that did not show affinity for saralasin or losartan was observed in turkey liver preparations (Bucco, unpublished results).

3.1. Preparation of Receptors from Rat Liver Membranes

1. Remove an appropriate number of protease inhibitor aliquots from a –20°C or –80°C freezer and allow them to warm to room temperature and then place on ice (except for PMSF, which we allow to warm by holding it in our hands and then placed on the lab bench).
2. Measure out 100 mL of the isolation medium, then add 100 μL each of the protease inhibitors, and mix gently (1000 × dilution of protease inhibitors). Place the incubation medium on ice in an esky.
3. Remove a rat liver (either fresh or one that has been removed previously and rapidly frozen and stored at –80°C) and grind the liver into a powder under liquid nitrogen using a mortar and pestle.
4. Take approximately 1 g tissue and resuspend in 10 mL cold isolation medium (containing protease inhibitors).
5. Homogenize the tissue with a precooled Ultra-Tarrax on low–medium speed for 3 bursts of 10 s giving the sample a short rest on ice in between bursts to ensure the tissue remains cold. We have also used 13 passes of a Dounce glass homogenizer (Wheaton, Millville, NJ, USA) placed in an ice bath, with equal success.
6. Filter the sample through two pieces of nylon gauze to remove any large pieces that have not been dispersed and wash through a further 5 mL of isolation medium through the gauze.
7. Centrifuge the sample at approximately 3000 × *g* (e.g., 4000 r.p.m. using a JA-20 rotor) for 25 min at 4°C.
8. Retain the reddish color supernatant containing the crude membranes and place the sample on ice.
9. Resuspend the pellet in 10 mL cold isolation medium and centrifuge again at 3000 × *g* for 25 min at 4°C.
10. Combine the supernatant from this centrifugation step with the earlier one and centrifuge the pooled supernatants again at 46,000 × *g* (e.g., 20,000 r.p.m. using a JA-20 rotor) at 4°C for 30 min.

11. Discard this supernatant and resuspend the crude membrane pellet in approximately 15 mL isolation medium using a Dounce homogenizer (or similar). The pellet can be transferred to a homogenizer by gently resuspending the pellet using a disposable plastic Pasteur pipette then transferring to a precooled homogenizer on ice.
12. Adjust the final total protein concentration of the crude membrane preparation to approximately 1 mg/mL by determining the total protein concentration on one aliquot using a suitable protein determination method, for example, we use the Bradford (96-well plate) method (Bio-Rad Hercules, CA, USA).
13. Add 800 μL aliquots of the crude membrane preparation to pre-labeled 1.5 mL Eppendorf or 2 mL Sarstedt (screw cap) tubes on ice (*see* **Note 5**).
14. Transfer the remaining aliquots into an appropriate rack and place the rack in a –80°C freezer until use.

3.2. Radioligand ([^{125}I]-Sar^1-AngII) Binding Assay

We present here the methods for [^{125}I]-Sar^1-AngII binding to rat liver membrane preparations; however, it should be noted we have had equal success using turkey liver membranes or CHO cells stably expressing ATR (a gift from Professor Walter Thomas, University of Queensland, Australia).

The method presented here is the basic method that has already been optimized (we also present some very useful data on radioligand binding assay optimization) and is routinely used for screening purposes. Since we were screening samples that were complex mixtures, sometimes containing known toxic agents to whole cells, we decided to screen a small library using the membrane receptor method, as opposed to setting up whole cell-based assays *(4, 5)* where we found a lot of variability in preliminary studies.

1. Label 4 mL clear disposable tubes (duplicates) and place in a rack on ice.
2. The final volume in each tube is 75 μL and can be easily configured to be more or less depending on the circumstances.
3. 45.5 μL ice-cold "wash buffer" is added to each tube.
4. 15 μL of the test samples, buffer (blank) or known inhibitor (controls) such as losartan or unlabeled angiotensin II, are then added to each tube.
5. 7 μL of thawed rat liver membranes (at 1 mg/mL) are then added to each tube to give a final concentration of approximately 100 μg/mL (*see* **Note 6**).
6. The binding reaction is then started by the addition of 7.5 μL of [^{125}I]-Sar^1-AngII. For determining the K_d and B_{max} using a "saturation" binding protocol, final concentrations of

[^{125}I]-Sar^1-AngII used are between 0 and 3000 p*M*. For routine screening purposes we use 0.1 n*M* [^{125}I]-Sar^1-AngII, a concentration that is below the K_d and is an acceptable concentration to use as it still gives enough "counts" bound to allow a good "window" of competition binding *(1, 2, 6)* (*see* **Note** 7).

7. The reaction is allowed to proceed for 50 min for screening purposes and is a time point well above "the steady state" or "equilibrium" of binding which was about 30 min in our experimental conditions at 25°C (this is the optimal incubation temperature determined for this receptor; however, that can vary from 4°C to 37°C depending on the receptor type).
8. To separate the bound radioligand ([^{125}I]-Sar^1-AngII) from free (unbound) radioligand, 3 mL ice-cold wash buffer is added to the tubes and then the contents of the tube are rapidly filtered over the GF/C filters which have been placed on the filtration manifold. The membrane proteins are retained on the GF/C filter along with any bound [^{125}I]-Sar^1-AngII to the angiotensin II receptors in the membrane preparation. Unbound radioligand passes through the filter into the collection chamber.
9. The filters should be washed 3 more times with ice-cold wash buffer to remove any unbound [^{125}I]-Sar^1-AngII, then the filter is gently removed from the filtration apparatus with forceps and placed into a pre-labeled 4 mL plastic (scintillation) vial.
10. To check on background binding of radioligand to filters, set up tubes that contain all the components except the receptor preparation. We find that this background binding to the GF/C filters is very low when using 0.1 n*M* [^{125}I]-Sar^1-AngII as described.
11. We also measure the total counts added to the tubes in a gamma counter such as a Wallac Multichannel or Wallac Clinigamma counter (and for each concentration of [^{125}I]-Sar^1-AngII when doing a saturation binding experiment) as the total counts are required for the calculation of "fmoles" [^{125}I]-Sar^1-AngII bound to receptor and thus the determination of the B_{max} value (see calculations in next section).
12. The tubes containing the GF/C filter with bound receptors and radioligand are then placed in a gamma counter and the radioactivity is determined in counts per minute (c.p.m.).

3.3. Calculation of "Specific Binding"

To determine "specific" angiotensin II receptor binding, that is, binding of the radioligand to the specific receptors, two experiments are carried out in parallel. Assays are considered good if specific binding is >70% and excellent when >90%. For example, one set of tubes contain buffer only (in place of the "test sample") and is usually termed "total binding" and this allows maximal binding of [^{125}I]-Sar^1-AngII to receptor (and non-receptor sites; for example, 2600 c.p.m.). Secondly, the other set of tubes contain a known competing ATR-specific antagonist, such as losartan at a high concentration (e.g., 10 μ*M*), which is able to compete with (0.1 n*M*) [^{125}I]-Sar^1-AngII for ATR binding sites and thus can prevent [^{125}I]-Sar^1-AngII molecules from binding to the receptor sites (e.g., 220 c.p.m.). Note, there is no reason that losartan would necessarily prevent [^{125}I]-Sar^1-AngII binding to other "non-specific" (i.e., non-receptor) sites (such as the GF/C filters, plastic tube, and other proteins, lipids, or carbohydrate moieties in the membrane preparation) as these molecules are structurally very different. Therefore, "specific" binding is a calculated term and is defined as "total binding" minus "non-specific binding" and in this example would be 2600 c.p.m. – 220 c.p.m. = 2380 c.p.m. is due to "specific binding" and this represents: (2380 c.p.m./2600 c.p.m.) × 100 = 91.5% specific binding, therefore 8.5% is non-specific (background) binding.

The above protocol also assumes that the optimum assay time point had also been developed. We have shown under the conditions tested that the 50 min time point of incubation is ideal to establish equilibrium conditions, whereas the maximum [^{125}I]-Sar^1-AngII binding was obtained as early as 30 min.

3.4. Calculation of K_d, B_{max}

The easiest way to calculate K_d and B_{max} from your data is to use a scientific graphing software program, such as GraphPad Prism (*see* http://www.graphpad.com/) or other similar software capable of generating curves and transformations using non-linear models. We have found that Prism is particularly good as the software and associated texts are written by pharmacologists specifically for these types of applications. To determine B_{max} (the maximal density of receptor sites per unit of total protein) we carry out a saturation binding experiment (i.e., 0–3000 p*M* of [^{125}I]-Sar^1-AngII) and express the data on the *y*-axis as fmoles [^{125}I]-Sar^1-AngII bound per mg protein (fmol/mg). This is done by expressing the counts from each [^{125}I]-Sar^1-AngII concentration as a fraction of the "total counts" from **Section 3.2.11** above, then dividing this figure by the protein content in the assay (expressed in mg).

3.4.1. Calculation of B_{max}

For example, let us take an example for a single concentration of [^{125}I]-Sar^1-AngII at 3000 p*M*, which is the highest concentration used on the saturation curve. The total counts (added to the 75 μL reaction) were measured at this concentration (3000 p*M*) and was found to be 814,318 c.p.m. (this is 225 fmol of [^{125}I]-Sar^1-AngII in 75 μL).

The specific number of counts bound at 3000 p*M* was calculated in the experiment (total – non-specific) as 30,949 c.p.m. Therefore, (30,949 c.p.m./814,318 c.p.m.) × 225 fmol = 8.55 fmol of [^{125}I]-Sar^1-AngII was specifically bound to AngII receptors (at 3000 p*M*). Also note than at this concentration only ((30,949 c.p.m./814,318 c.p.m.) × 100) = 3.8% of [^{125}I]-Sar^1-AngII ligand is bound (<10% is ideal as mentioned in **Note 7**).

In the 75 μL assay the total protein amount was 0.0070 mg (i.e., 7.0 μL of 1 mg/mL receptor protein preparation in 75 μL final volume) and then fmol/mg protein = 8.55 fmol/0.0070 mg protein = 1221 fmol/mg.

If this type of calculation is done for each concentration of the saturation curve, the final figure will be similar to that shown in **Fig. 1** When the data are plotted in Prism (for example), there is no need to transform the data into a linear scale, for example, Lineweaver–Burke plot, as Prism automatically calculates K_d and B_{max} from the data entered. K_d denotes the radioligand equilibrium dissociation constant and is the concentration at which half-maximal receptor sites are occupied (i.e., the concentration at $0.5B_{max}$). B_{max} is the maximal density of receptor sites. For the example shown in **Fig. 1**, K_d was found to be 0.516 n*M* and B_{max} was 1270 fmol/mg. Additionally, we also determined K_d and B_{max} for turkey liver membranes prepared in a similar manner and was 0.599 n*M* and 1896 fmol/mg, respectively. Alternatively, we cultured CHO cells stably expressing ATRs and determined the K_d and B_{max} values, which were 0.52 n*M* and 626 fmol/mg, respectively. However, the latter value tended to vary depending on passage number of the CHO cells (work done by Dr Olgatina Bucco).

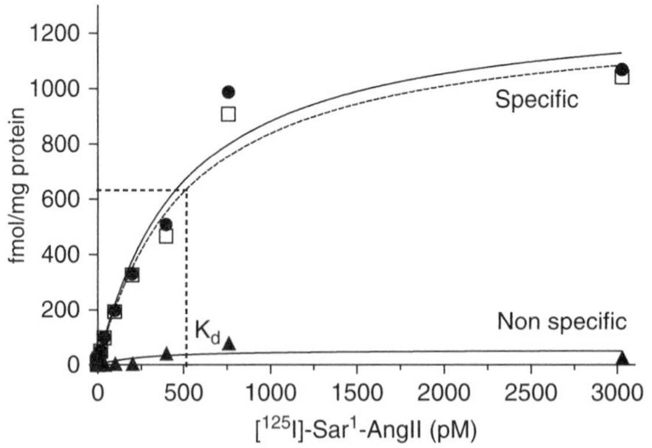

Fig. 1. Saturation binding of various concentrations of [^{125}I]-Sar^1-AngII to rat liver membranes as shown on *x*-axis. "Specific binding" (□) was calculated as total binding (●) minus non-specific binding (▲) and in this representative experiment specific binding was >90% at all concentrations. GraphPad Prism was used to determine the K_d (the concentration at which half-maximal binding occurs) and B_{max} (the maximal density of receptor sites) and were 516 p*M* and 1270 fmol/mg, respectively.

3.5. Calculation of IC_{50}

The IC_{50} value is the concentration of the competitor/inhibitor that competes for half the specific binding. It is a measure of the competitor's potency for interacting with the receptor against the radioligand. In our experiments we use a concentration of [^{125}I]-Sar^1-AngII that is less than the K_d, usually 0.1 n*M*. By carrying out an experiment over a wide concentration range of the antagonist or test sample, the IC_{50} can be calculated (e.g., using Prism) providing the antagonist response generally follows a sigmoid competitive curve, when plotted on a log scale. The classical single-site model usually shows that the antagonist increases from 10 to 90% inhibition over an 81-fold concentration range. Therefore, most of the curve will span 2-log units. In **Fig. 2**, the Hill slope (determined in Prism) was found to be -0.64, which is typical for this type of competitive binding experiment. However, in some

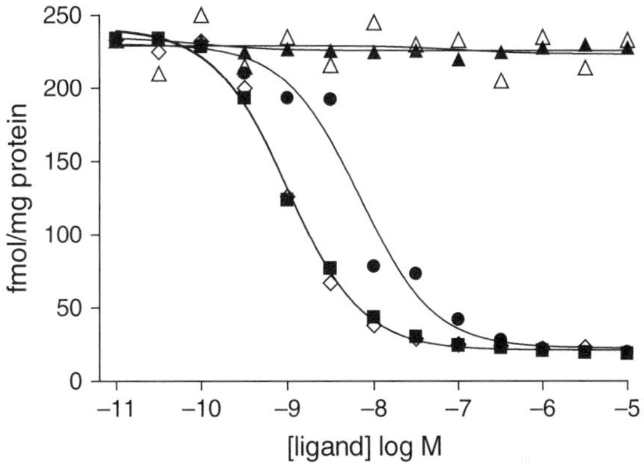

Fig. 2. A representative competition binding experiment using rat liver membranes. [^{125}I]-Sar^1-AngII (1 n*M*) was used in the presence of increasing concentrations of either angiotensin II (■), unlabeled saralasin (Sar^1-AngII, ◊), losartan (a specific angiotensin II type 1a receptor antagonist (●)), PD123319 (an angiotensin II type 2 receptor antagonist (Δ)), or an unrelated GPCR agonist, that is, endothelin-1 (▲). Note that both saralasin and angiotensin II have similar IC_{50} values of 1 n*M*, whereas losartan has an IC_{50} of 6.7 n*M*. The angiotensin II type 2 receptor antagonist (PD123319) and the ET-1 do not compete with [^{125}I]-Sar^1-AngII for binding sites.

circumstances, the slope factor (Hill slope) may be steeper, giving rise to Hill slopes that approach −1.0 or even steeper slopes (e.g., −2.0). It is the latter that one must be weary of, since this indicates that the binding of the "antagonist" does not follow the law of mass action at a single site and indeed is likely to be due to an artefact or some other complex mechanism (*see* **Note 8**) *(7)*. However, as mentioned, the typical dose–response effect of the screened "hits" should give a sigmoid curve over at least 2-log units to satisfy some of the criteria of a potent antagonist. We recorded the IC_{50} for experiments conducted on six separate occasions using angiotensin II (the agonist) or losartan (antagonist) as the competing ligands and obtained IC_{50} values of 1.89 ± 0.40 n*M* and 13.5 ± 2.1 n*M* (mean ± S.E.M., $n = 6$), respectively, and is comparable to that obtained previously *(8)*.

4. Notes

1. PMSF comes out of solution as crystals when placed in the freezer but redissolves when warmed. An alternative to preparing protease inhibitors is to purchase a pre-prepared "protease inhibitor cocktail" mix (obtained from Sigma and others). We have also used the following protease inhibitor combination with success: aprotinin, iodoacetamide, pepstatin A, and PMSF.
2. HEPES or Tris-HCl at pH 7.4 can be used here with final concentrations between 20 and 50 m*M*. NaCl up to 400 m*M* has been tested using the ATR without compromise of binding.
3. The receptor binding assay can sometimes be improved by using polyethylenimine-treated glass fiber filters. A polyethylenimine-treated glass filter has high protein binding capacity.
4. We routinely use a 3-place filtration manifold apparatus (Millipore); however, there are numerous types available (e.g., 6- and 10-place) that allow more filtration experiments to be done. All bottles/liquid traps containing unbound radioligand (^{125}I) should be shielded by lead sheets to prevent excessive exposure to radioactivity. A lead apron can be worn over the lab coat when excessively "hot" (concentrated) ^{125}I-radiolabel is being handled. Radioactivity exposure must be monitored by wearing an appropriate badge that detects levels of exposure to ionizing radiation.
5. Most receptor preparations are stable after a period of freezing and can be stored for long periods without loss in receptor number or binding affinity. Other methods using laborious density gradient procedures (e.g., Percoll) which we have done in our lab have not proved to be superior to this relatively simple "two-step cut" centrifugation procedure. However, clearly different tissue types will require different homogenizing conditions for optimal radioligand binding.
6. For delivering accurate small volumes of liver membranes into the 4 mL tube we find that bending the pipette tip slightly before drawing up the liver membrane preparation then

allows the operator to touch the pipette tip on the inside surface of the tube and this allows better delivery of high protein concentration samples.

7. For GPCR screening studies about $0.2 \times K_d$ is ideal, although any concentration lower than the K_d is generally advisable; however, the highest concentration should probably not exceed 80% of the K_d concentration *(2)*. Furthermore, the rule of thumb is that if >10% of the added radioligand counts are bound, then the tissue concentration is too high and therefore the membrane preparation needs to be diluted further (to maintain appropriate kinetics *(1, 2, 6)*).
8. We have found when screening our "in house" library "hits" that these types of artefacts arose. Sometimes these could be easily explained due to sample pH and salt effects, other times it was less clear.

References

1. Smith, R.G. and Sestili, M.A. (1980) Methods for ligand-receptor assays in clinical chemistry. *Clin. Chem.* **26**, 543–550.
2. Bylund, D.B. and Toews, M.L. (1993) Radioligand binding methods: practical guide and tips. *Am. J. Physiol.* **265**, L421–L429.
3. Fang, M., Jaffrey, S.R., Sawa, A., Ye, K., Luo, X., and Snyder, S.H. (2000) Dexras1: a G protein specifically coupled to neuronal nitric oxide synthase via CAPON. *Neuron* **28**, 183–193.
4. Caballero-George, C., Vanderheyden, P.M., Solis, P.N., Pieters, L., Shahat, A.A., Gupta, M.P., Vauquelin, G., and Vlietinck, A.J. (2001) Biological screening of selected medicinal Panamanian plants by radioligand-binding techniques. *Phytomedicine* **8**, 59–70.
5. Caballero-George, C., Vanderheyden, P.M., Okamoto, Y., Masaki, T., Mbwambo, Z., Apers, S., Gupta, M.P., Pieters, L., Vauquelin, G., and Vlietinck, A. (2004) Evaluation of bioactive saponins and triterpenoidal aglycons for their binding properties on human endothelin ETA and angiotensin AT1 receptors. *Phytother. Res.* **18**, 729–736.
6. Motulsky, H. and Christopoulos, A. (2003) Fitting models to biological data using linear regression and nonlinear regression. GraphPad (USA) http://www.graphpad.-com/prism/Prism.htm.
7. Shoichet, B.K. (2006) Interpreting steep dose–response curves in early inhibitor discovery. *J. Med. Chem.* **49**, 7274–7277.
8. Hines, J., Fluharty, S.J., and Sakai, R.R. (1999) The angiotensin AT(1) receptor antagonist irbesartan has near-peptide affinity and potently blocks receptor signaling. *Eur. J. Pharmacol.* **384**, 81–89.

Chapter 10

[^{35}S]GTPγS Binding in G Protein-Coupled Receptor Assays

Tamara Cooper, Edward J. McMurchie, and Wayne R. Leifert

Summary

The [^{35}S]GTPγS binding assay to measure G protein activation following agonist binding to G protein-coupled receptors (GPCRs) remains a powerful molecular technique to substantiate traditional pharmacological values of potency, efficacy, and affinity. The method described uses membrane preparations of the α_{2A}-adrenergic receptor and purified G protein subunits expressed in *Sf* 9 cells, reconstituted into a functional signaling system. This technology is generic and could be used with other GPCRs to demonstrate initial signaling events following receptor activation. Agonist-stimulated [^{35}S]GTPγS binding is measured in a 96-well plate format using scintillation counting.

Key words: [^{35}S]GTPγS, α_{2A}-adrenergic receptor, G protein activation.

1. Introduction

G protein-coupled receptors (GPCRs) are important pharmacological targets and the range of assay technologies to determine ligand binding and signaling are expanding. However, the [^{35}S]GTPγS binding assay still remains a useful and simple technique to demonstrate receptor activation and is one of the few functional, cell-free assays. Assays measuring ligand binding to the GPCR do not provide the desired information regarding downstream signaling activity of the GPCR (e.g., whether the ligand of interest is an agonist, antagonist, or partial agonist). To provide this information, a functional assay is required which unambiguously measures changes downstream of ligand binding to the receptor. The level of G protein activation following agonist binding to a receptor in a reconstituted system can be measured by monitoring the nucleotide exchange event using radiolabeled,

Wayne R. Leifert (ed.), *G Protein-Coupled Receptors in Drug Discovery, vol. 552*

Book doi: 10.1007/978-1-60327-317-6_10

non-hydrolyzable [^{35}S]guanosine-5′-O-(3-thio)triphosphate ([^{35}S]GTPγS) *(1, 2)*. Upon activation of the receptor by an agonist, the G protein is stimulated to bind [^{35}S]GTPγS which is resistant to hydrolysis by the intrinsic GTPase activity of the Gα-subunit, allowing [^{35}S]GTPγS-labeled Gα-subunits to accumulate following receptor activation. [^{35}S]GTPγS bound to G proteins can be separated from unbound [^{35}S]GTPγS using glass fiber filters and measured using scintillation counting *(1)*. Since by definition, all GPCRs interact with G proteins, nucleotide exchange provides the most upstream generic event available to measure ligand-mediated signaling *(2, 3)*. Using a readout which represents a molecular event in close proximity to receptor activation, such as the nucleotide exchange event described in this assay methodology, is particularly preferential as cell signaling events further downstream can be regulated independent of the GPCR, generating false positives or negatives.

The principles of [^{35}S]GTPγS binding assays have been reformatted to increase throughput by removing the washing steps involved in removing unbound [^{35}S]GTPγS by implementing a scintillation proximity assay *(4)*. Alternatively, where the use of radioactivity is undesirable, europium-labeled GTPγS can replace [^{35}S]GTPγS *(5)*. However, the following method will describe the use of the traditional [^{35}S]GTPγS binding assay which as a minimum output provides pharmacological parameters of efficacy, potency, and affinity.

2. Materials

2.1. Reconstitution of GPCRs and G Proteins

1. Urea-treated *Sf*9 membrane preparations containing the desired GPCR. The expression level of the receptor preparation should be determined prior to use in [^{35}S]GTPγS signaling assay (*see* **Note 1**). We use the α_{2A}-adrenergic receptor as a model GPCR which has been expressed in *Sf*9 cells.
2. Purified G protein subunits (Gα and the Gβγ dimer) (*see* **Note 2**). We use recombinant $G\alpha_{i1}$ and $G\beta_1\gamma_2$subunits purified from *Sf*9 cells.
3. TMN buffer: 50 m*M* Tris-HCl (pH 7.6), 100 m*M* NaCl, 10 m*M* $MgCl_2$ (*see* **Note 3**).
4. TMND buffer: TMN buffer with 1 m*M* DTT (15.4 mg/ 100 mL) added fresh.
5. Guanosine diphosphate (GDP) dissolved at 10 m*M* in TMN buffer and stored in single-use aliquots at –20°C.
6. Adenosine 5′-(β,γ-imido)triphosphate tetralithium salt hydrate (AMP-PNP) dissolved at 10 m*M* in TMN buffer and stored in single-use aliquots at –20°C.

2.2. Other [^{35}S]GTPγS Assay Components

1. [^{35}S]GTPγS (specific activity 1250 Ci/mmol, PerkinElmer Life Sciences) diluted to 40 n*M* in TMN buffer and stored in single-use aliquots at –80°C.
2. Agonist, such as UK14304 for the α_{2A}-adrenergic receptor, dissolved at 17 m*M* in dimethyl sulfoxide and stored in single-use aliquots at –20°C.
3. Antagonists: rauwolscine and yohimbine (α_2-adrenergic receptor specific), prazosin (α-1 adrenergic receptor specific), and propranolol (non-selective β-blocker) dissolved at 10 m*M* in 50% ethanol and stored in single-use aliquots at –20°C.

2.3. [^{35}S]GTPγS Signaling Assay

1. 96-well V-bottom plates (Quantum Scientific, Murrarie, Queensland, Australia).
2. Temperature-controlled orbital shaker for 96-well plates.
3. Opaque, 96-well, 1.2 μm glass fiber type C filter plates (Millipore, North Ryde, NSW, Australia).
4. 96-well plate vacuum manifold.
5. Vacuum pump.
6. Microscint^{TM}20 (PerkinElmer Life Sciences, Waltham, MA, USA).
7. Packard Top Count Microplate Scintillation counter B99041V1 (formerly Packard Biosciences, now PerkinElmer Life Sciences).

3. Methods

[^{35}S]GTPγS binding assays using membrane preparations of receptor were originally described by Hilf et al. *(6)* and more recent studies utilizing [^{35}S]GTPγS binding assays are still largely based on this method with some modifications. Often receptors and G protein are heterogeneously expressed and then reconstituted in the desired combinations *(7, 8)*. Following incubation with [^{35}S]GTPγS and the desired agonists and controls, the unbound [^{35}S]GTPγS is separated using a filtration step through glass fiber filters. This method describes the use of a 96-well plate manifold although lower throughput vacuum manifolds and the required filters and scintillation counting materials are also available. Protein-bound [^{35}S]GTPγS retained on the filters is then measured using scintillation counting.

3.1. Reconstituting GPCRs with G Proteins

GPCRs and G proteins (*see* **Note 4**) are reconstituted with the nucleotides GDP and AMP-PNP at a concentration of 4 × that desired in the [^{35}S]GTPγS binding assay in TMND buffer. The proteins are kept on ice and ice-cold buffers are used.

1. Routinely, we use a GPCR preparation containing 0.08 mg/mL protein concentration (4 × concentrated). Therefore, the final concentration of the membrane preparation in the [^{35}S]GTPγS binding assay is 0.02 mg/mL (unless otherwise indicated).
2. 40 n*M* of G protein subunits are then added so that the final concentration of G proteins will be 10 n*M* and the reconstitution mixes are thoroughly vortexed.
3. The nucleotides GDP and AMP-PNP are then added to 20 and 40 μ*M*, respectively, (*see* **Note 5**) and thorough vortexing is performed.

3.2. Preparing Agonists, Antagonists, and [^{35}S]GTPγS

The desired agonist, antagonists, and [^{35}S]GTPγS are then prepared, all at concentrations of 4 × that desired in the final assay in TMND buffer.

1. To determine the EC_{50} for a particular agonist, a large range of concentrations is generally required that spans several orders of magnitude of dose depending on the efficacy of the agonist. For the α_{2A}-adrenergic receptor we use concentrations of UK14304 that range between 0 and 100 μ*M*. The concentrations used may need optimizing to generate a sigmoidal dose curve that has both bottom and top plateaus with a number of points in between. It is important to perform an assay in the absence of the agonist to determine basal levels of [^{35}S]GTPγS binding as a control assay set.
2. As a control, the antagonist is often included in molar excess compared with the agonist. For the α_{2A}-adrenergic receptor, we routinely use a final assay concentration of 500 μ*M* rauwolscine. The purpose of including an antagonist is to compete with agonist and to demonstrate that [^{35}S]GTPγS binding is specifically being regulated by agonist binding. Doses of antagonist can also be used against a concentration of agonist that stimulates maximal [^{35}S]GTPγS binding to determine IC_{50} values.
3. [^{35}S]GTPγS is diluted in TMND buffer to a concentration of 4 × that desired in the final assay. We routinely use a final concentration of 0.2 n*M* [^{35}S]GTPγS (*see* **Note 6**).

3.3. [^{35}S]GTPγS Binding Assay

1. Add 25 μL of reconstitution mixes into V-shaped wells of a 96-well plate on ice.
2. Add 25 μL of the prepared [^{35}S]GTPγS to the appropriate wells.
3. Add 25 μL of the prepared antagonist or buffer to the appropriate wells.
4. The reaction is then started by the addition of 25 μL of the prepared agonist or 25 μL of buffer to determine basal [^{35}S]GTPγS binding making the final assay volume 100 μL.

5. Plates are then incubated at 27°C with shaking for 90 min.
6. At the conclusion of the incubation period, the desired volume of assay is transferred to the wells of an opaque, GFC filter plate that has been prewet with TMN buffer.
7. The samples are filtered through the plate using a vacuum pump.
8. The wells are washed three times with 200 μL of TMN buffer to remove any unbound [^{35}S]GTPγS.
9. The bottom of the filter plate is then removed to allow the filters to dry (*see* **Note 7**). The plate can be stored until ready for scintillation counting.

3.4. Determining Total Counts and Scintillation Counting

1. Once filters are dry, the base of the plate is sealed appropriately and 40 μL of microscint is added to the wells.
2. Total counts are determined by adding 1 μL of [^{35}S]GTPγS to unused wells containing 40 μL of microscint such that the concentration of [^{35}S]GTPγS is the same as that which was present in the assays. The top of the plate is then sealed appropriately.
3. The amount of bound [^{35}S]GTPγS is then determined using a counter that can detect β-radiation such as the Packard Top Count Microplate Scintillation counter B99041V1 using a 60 s count time.

3.5. Data Interpretation

1. Measuring the total counts from the concentration of [^{35}S]GTPγS present in the assay before bound is separated from free allows the conversion of the data from c.p.m. to fmol bound. Using the total counts, the number of c.p.m. per fmol of [^{35}S]GTPγS can be determined and this is used to convert c.p.m. data to [^{35}S]GTPγS bound (fmol). However, data can also be expressed as fold or percentage increases over basal [^{35}S]GTPγS binding, or as a percentage of the effect produced by an agonist known to have a high efficacy in stimulating a signal response from a given receptor.
2. Data can be graphed as appropriate to illustrate the effects of antagonist and other controls using a software package such as Prism^{TM} (GraphPad Software Inc.). An example of the results produced is shown in **Fig. 1**. The presence of the agonist UK14304 increased [^{35}S]GTPγS binding 5 × above basal and the addition of the antagonist rauwolscine inhibited this response. No increases above background were obtained in the absence of G proteins or receptors.

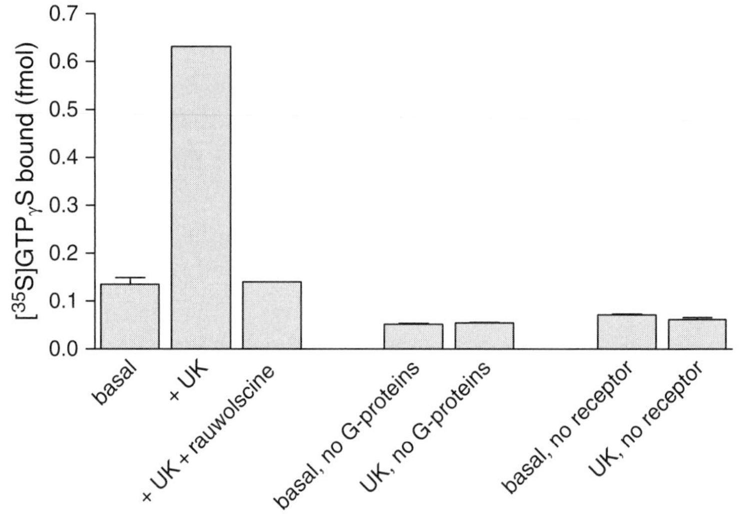

Fig. 1. Agonist-stimulated [^{35}S]GTPγS binding and appropriate controls. Reconstitution mixes were set up ± 0.02 mg/mL α_{2A}-adrenergic receptor membrane preparation (total protein) ± 20 n*M* G protein subunits ($G\alpha_{i1}\beta_1\gamma_2$) in the presence of 0.2 n*M* [^{35}S]GTPγS as indicated. Basal [^{35}S]GTPγS binding was measured in the absence of UK14304 ("UK") and 100 μ*M* UK14304 was used to stimulate [^{35}S]GTPγS binding. Rauwolscine (500 μ*M*; antagonist) was used to compete with UK14304 for binding to the receptors and hence to determine specific signaling. The samples were incubated for 90 min at 27°C and subsequently filtered through GFC filter plates and unbound [^{35}S]GTPγS removed by washing with TMN buffer. [^{35}S]GTPγS bound to the filters was then measured using scintillation counting. Data shown are mean ± S.E.M., *n* = 3.

3. [^{35}S]GTPγS binding stimulated by increasing concentrations of agonist results in a typical sigmoidal response curve that can be fitted to data using an appropriate nonlinear regression. The relative efficacy (E_{max}) (maximal response to an agonist) can be used to distinguish between full and partial agonists; note that metal ion and GDP concentrations are variables that can change the responses. If the data generated has well-defined baseline and maximum response plateaus, the EC_{50} (concentration of agonist generating a response halfway between the baseline and maximum responses) can be determined as a measure of agonist efficacy (**Fig. 2**). Likewise the IC_{50} of an antagonist (that concentration of resulting in 50% inhibition) can be determined (**Fig. 3**). The data can be used to determine rank order potencies of various agonists and antagonists, which can aid in characterizing a receptor particularly with regard to certain receptor subtypes.

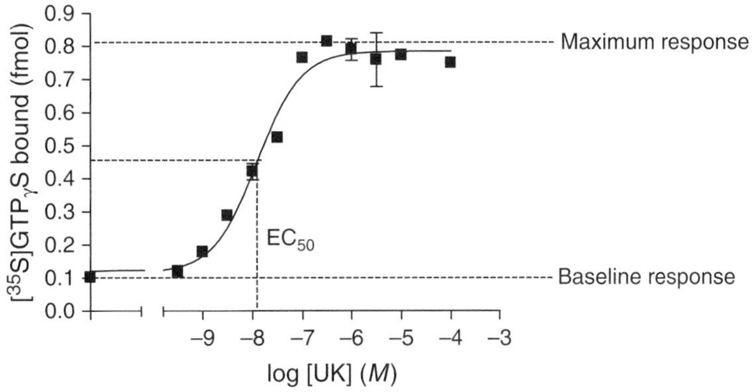

Fig. 2. Concentration–response curve of UK14304-stimulated [^{35}S]GTPγS binding via the α_{2A}-adrenergic receptor and $G\alpha_{i1}\beta_1\gamma_2$. The α_{2A}-adrenergic receptor preparation (0.02 mg/mL) was reconstituted with purified G protein subunits (20 n*M*). [^{35}S]GTPγS (0.2 n*M*) and various concentrations of UK14304 (0–100 μ*M*) were added and the samples were incubated for 90 min at 27°C and subsequently filtered through GFC filter plates and unbound [^{35}S]GTPγS removed by washing with TMN buffer. [^{35}S]GTPγS bound to the filters was then measured using scintillation counting. A sigmoidal curve was fitted using a non-linear regression and an EC_{50} value of 12 n*M* was generated. Data shown are mean ± S.E.M., *n* = 3.

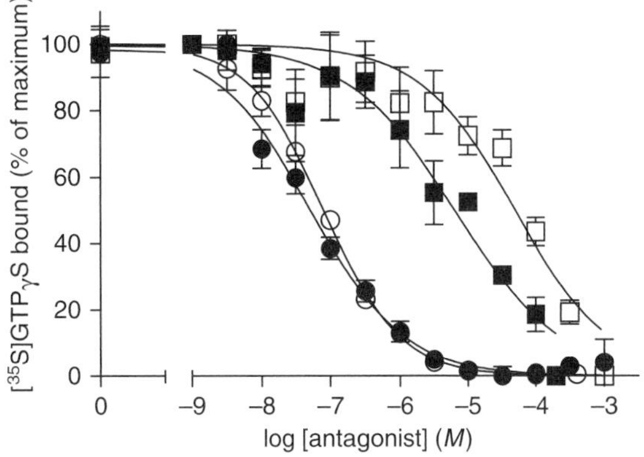

Fig. 3. Antagonist competition curves. To determine IC_{50} values using receptor-stimulated [^{35}S]GTPγS binding, the following antagonists were used at the indicated concentrations: rauwolscine (•), yohimbine (○), prazosin (■), and propranolol (□). The experiment was carried out using 20 n*M* of both Gα and Gβγ combined with 0.1 mg/mL of α_{2A}-aderenergic receptor membranes, 5 μ*M* GDP, 10 μ*M* AMP-PNP ("reconstitution mix"), and 0.2 n*M* [^{35}S]GTPγS in the presence of various concentrations of antagonists and 1 μ*M* UK14304 (agonist) to start the reactions and incubated for 90 min at 27°C. The IC_{50} values for each of the antagonists were determined as 0.051 μ*M* (rauwolscine: selective α_{2A}-adrenergic receptor antagonist), 0.080 μ*M* (yohimbine: selective α_{2A}-adrenergic receptor antagonist), 8.3 μ*M* (prazosin: selective α_1-adrenergic receptor antagonist), and 86.9 μ*M* (propranolol: β_2-adrenergic receptor antagonist). Data shown are mean ± S.E.M., *n* = 3.

4. Notes

1. Membrane preparations containing GPCRs can be prepared as described by Leifert et al. *(9)* and should be stored in single-use aliquots at –80°C to avoid freeze–thaw cycles. The presence of the α_{2A}-adrenergic receptors within the membrane preparations can be measured by radioligand binding assays using [^{3}H]MK912 using excess unlabeled ligand to determine specific binding. The total (membrane) protein concentration is determined using a Bradford assay *(10)*. Membrane preparations are required because [^{35}S]GTPγS does not readily cross cell membranes, although success with permeabilized cells has been achieved in some studies *(11)*.
2. G protein subunits can be purified from recombinant *Sf*9 cells as per Leifert et al. *(9)*. The protein concentrations should be determined using an appropriate method such as that of Bradford *(10)*.
3. All buffers should be prepared with Milli-Q water (resistivity of 18.2 MΩ-cm). Magnesium ions are required to observe agonist-stimulated [^{35}S]GTPγS binding and the concentration can affect the signal-to-noise ratio. Sodium ions also improve the signal-to-noise ratio but are not essential to observe the agonist-stimulated [^{35}S]GTPγS binding *(1)*.
4. This chapter uses the α_{2A}-adrenergic receptor as a model GPCR with the G protein subunits being Gα_{i1}, Gβ_1, and Gγ_2. However, any Gi-coupled receptor that is successfully expressed could potentially be used. Gi-coupled receptors are more suited to [^{35}S]GTPγS binding assays because of the higher GDP/GTP exchange rate of Gi compared to Gs or Gq G proteins. However, Gs and Gq family G proteins have been successfully used in [^{35}S]GTPγS as well as receptor-Gα constructs *(1)*. G proteins or receptor membrane preparations can also be excluded as required for appropriate controls.
5. The concentrations of various reconstitution components which we use routinely are given. However, these should be optimized to achieve the best signal-to-noise ratio for your system. The nucleotides are included to fill empty nucleotide binding sites to decrease the basal signal and increase the signal-to-noise ratio. Estimates of efficacy can also vary with the ratio of receptor to G protein and some studies have employed receptor:Gα fusion proteins to control receptor G protein stoichiometry.

6. The required [^{35}S]GTPγS concentration will need optimization and often depends on the amount of radioactive decay that has occurred so that an adequate number of counts can be obtained. ^{35}S has an approximate half-life of 87 days and appropriate safety precautions and waste disposal regulations should be followed when using this radionuclide.
7. Drying the filters prior to adding scintillant provides for better scintillation counting since water can quench the signal.

Acknowledgments

The authors thank Mrs. Sharon Burnard, Dr. Olgatina Bucco, and Dr. Amanda Aloia for their assistance.

References

1. Harrison, C., and Traynor, J.R. (2003) The [^{35}S]GTPgammaS binding assay: approaches and applications in pharmacology. *Life Sci.* **74**, 489–508.
2. Milligan, G. (2003) Principles: extending the utility of [35S]GTP gamma S binding assays. *Trends Pharmacol. Sci.* **24**, 87–90.
3. Niedernberg, A. Tunaru, S., Blaukat, A., Harris, B., and Kostenis, E. (2003) Comparative analysis of functional assays for characterization of agonist ligands at G protein-coupled receptors. *J. Biomol. Screen.* **8**, 500–510.
4. Ferrer, M., Kolodin, G.D., Zuck, P., Peltier, R., Berry, K., Mandala, S.M., Rosen, H., Ota, H., Ozaki, S., Inglese, J., and Strulovici, B. (2003) A fully automated [35S]GTPgammaS scintillation proximity assay for the high-throughput screening of Gi-linked G protein-coupled receptors. *Assay Drug Dev. Technol.* **1**, 261–273.
5. Frang, H., Mukkala, V. M., Syysto, R., Ollikka, P., Hurskainen, P., Scheinin, M., and Hemmila, I. (2003) Nonradioactive GTP binding assay to monitor activation of g protein-coupled receptors. *Assay Drug Dev. Technol.* **1**, 275–280.
6. Hilf, G., Gierschik, P., and Jakobs, K.H. (1989) Muscarinic acetylcholine receptor-stimulated binding of guanosine 5'-*O*-(3-thiotriphosphate) to guanine-nucleotide-binding proteins in cardiac membranes. *Eur. J. Biochem.* **186**, 725–731.
7. Barr, A.J., Brass, L.F., and Manning, D. R. (1997) Reconstitution of receptors and GTP-binding regulatory proteins (G proteins) in Sf9 cells. A direct evaluation of selectivity in receptor.G protein coupling. *J. Biol. Chem.* **272**, 2223–2229.
8. Francken, B.J., Vanhauwe, J.F., Josson, K., Jurzak, M., Luyten, W.H., and Leysen, J. E. (2001) Reconstitution of human 5-hydroxytryptamine5A receptor–G protein coupling in E. coli and Sf9 cell membranes with membranes from Sf9 cells expressing mammalian G proteins. *Receptors Channels* **7**, 303–318.
9. Leifert, W.R., Bailey, K., Cooper, T.H., Aloia, A.L., Glatz, R.V., and McMurchie, E.J. (2006) Measurement of heterotrimeric G protein and regulators of G protein signaling interactions by time-resolved fluorescence resonance energy transfer. *Anal. Biochem.* **355**, 201–212.
10. Bradford, M.M. (1976) A rapid and sensitive method for the quantitation of microgram quantities of protein utilizing the principle of protein-dye binding. *Anal. Biochem.* **72**, 248–254.
11. Wieland, T., Liedel, K., Kaldenberg-Stasch, S., Meyer zu Heringdorf, D., Schmidt, M., and Jakobs, K.H. (1995) Analysis of receptor-G protein interactions in permeabilized cells. *Naunyn Schmiedebergs Arch. Pharmacol.* **351**, 329–336.

Chapter 11

A Time-Resolved Fluorescent Lanthanide (Eu)-GTP Binding Assay for Chemokine Receptors as Targets in Drug Discovery

Jean Labrecque, Rebecca S.Y. Wong, and Simon P. Fricker

Summary

Chemokines are a family of chemoattractant cytokines involved in leukocyte trafficking, activation, development, and hematopoeisis. Chemokines and their receptors have been implicated in several disease processes, particularly inflammatory and autoimmune disorders and cancer, and are therefore attractive targets for drug development. Chemokine receptors are members of the seven-transmembrane, G protein-coupled receptor (GPCR) family. As such they can be studied using GPCR assays such as ligand binding, G protein activation, and downstream signaling processes such as intracellular calcium flux. In this respect assessing GPCR activation by GTP binding is an important tool to study the early stage of signal transduction. Previously this has been done using the radiolabeled non-hydrolyzable GTP analogue [^{35}S]GTPγS. In order to avoid the problems involved in working with radioactivity, a new non-radioactive version of the assay has been developed using a europium-labeled GTP analogue in which europium-GTP binding can be assayed using time-resolved fluorescence. We have adapted this assay for chemokine receptors. In this chapter, using the chemokine receptor CXCR4 as an example, we describe the steps for assay optimization. In addition we describe adaptation of this assay for the high-throughput screening of chemokine antagonists.

Key words: Chemokine, G protein-coupled receptor, Europium, Time-resolved fluorescence, Drug discovery, Assay optimization, High-throughput screening.

1. Introduction

Chemokines are 8–12 kDa peptides and represent a family of chemoattractant cytokines. They are involved in leukocyte trafficking, activation, development, and play an important role in hematopoeisis *(1)*. There are four classes of chemokines defined by the positioning of the first two of four conserved cysteine residues near the N terminal of the protein. These four classes are CXC where the two cysteines are separated by amino acid X, CC where they are next to one another,

Wayne R. Leifert (ed.), *G Protein-Coupled Receptors in Drug Discovery, vol. 552*

Book doi: 10.1007/978-1-60327-317-6_11

CX_3C where they are separated by three amino acids, and XC. Most of the chemokines come under the first two classes, whereas there is only one member of the CX_3C class and two members of the XC class. Their receptors are seven-transmembrane G protein-coupled receptors (GPCR) of the rhodopsin family. The receptors are classified as CCR1 to CCR10, CXCR1 to CXCR7, CX_3CR1 and XCR1 *(2)*. Many receptors have multiple ligands though some receptors have only the one ligand, as an example the receptor CXCR4 has the single ligand CXCL12, also known as stromal-derived factor-1 (SDF-1). Chemokines and their receptors have been implicated in numerous diseases, particularly inflammatory and autoimmune disorders *(2)*. In addition some chemokines and their receptors such as CXCL12/CXCR4 play a role in cancer biology and progression *(3)*, and CXCR4 and CCR5 have been identified as coreceptors for HIV entry into cells *(4)*.

More than 50% of known drugs are targeted against the GPCR family *(5)*. This, together with the important function of chemokines in immunoregulation, makes the chemokine receptor family an attractive and "druggable" therapeutic target. To date, the only approved drug against a chemokine receptor is maraviroc which is an inhibitor of CCR5 and has been approved for treatment of drug-experienced HIV patients *(6)*. Another chemokine antagonist with demonstrated clinical efficacy is AMD3100 (plerixafor), an inhibitor of CXCR4 that is being evaluated for hematopoietic stem cell mobilization *(7)*.

As chemokine receptors are seven-transmembrane G protein-coupled receptors they can be studied using GPCR assays such as ligand binding, G protein activation, and downstream signaling processes such as intracellular calcium flux. Radiolabeled chemokine binding and agonist-induced intracellular calcium flux are the most widely used. Mobilization of intracellular calcium flux by an agonist is an important route of G protein-associated cell signaling, which modulates many physiological mechanisms *(8)*. The measurement of intracellular variations in calcium concentration using a fluorescent dye constitutes a powerful functional assay, which can be adapted to a high-throughput format for identification of receptor inhibitors as a component of the drug discovery process.

The measurement of agonist-stimulated $[^{35}S]GTP\gamma S$ binding to G protein on cell membranes constitutes an alternative functional GPCR assay. This assay utilizes membranes prepared from cells expressing the appropriate GPCR, and complements cell-based assays, by detecting *in vitro* the earliest component of the signal transduction pathway. In addition, the $[^{35}S]GTP\gamma S$ binding assay can pick up weak stimulation of GPCRs by partial agonists *(9)* and, depending on the conditions used, this assay can detect weak agonist and inverse agonism interactions *(10)*. Hence, proper use of this assay can lead to a better understanding of the mechanism of interaction of compounds with the GPCR.

In the classical GTP binding assay, the stimulation of guanine nucleotide exchange of G proteins in cell membranes is monitored by measuring the binding of a radioactive, non-hydrolyzable GTP analogue, [^{35}S]GTPγS. As with other radiodetection methods, the [^{35}S]GTPγS assay can be adapted to a high-throughput format. On the other hand, because of the inherent limitations associated with working with radioactivity, there is an obvious advantage to adapting the GTP binding assay to a non-radioactive format.

Time-resolved fluorometry is a technology that exploits the unique fluorescence properties of lanthanide chelates. Time-resolved fluorometry assays exhibit advantageous low background and high signal-to-noise ratios *(11)*. Long fluorescence decay after excitation allows time-delayed signal detection (microseconds) to virtually eliminate all natural fluorescent background caused by cells and cell debris, screening compounds, plates, and other reagents (half-life of nanoseconds). A large Stoke's shift (e.g., excitation and emission wavelengths for the Eu-chelate are ~340 nm and ~615 nm, respectively) minimizes cross talk, resulting in a high signal-to-noise ratio. Therefore, because of their excellent temporal and spectral resolution, lanthanide chelate labels can provide highly sensitive assays. PerkinElmer has recently developed a non-radioactive, non-hydrolyzable, europium-labeled GTP analogue, Eu-GTP, for use in GPCR screening assays *(12)*.

In this chapter we describe the Eu-GTP assay adapted for chemokine receptors. We have used this assay as a component of a screening cascade in a chemokine receptor-targeted drug discovery program *(13)*. The assay can be adapted for any chemokine receptor; however, for convenience we used the CXCR4 receptor as an example to demonstrate assay optimization. In addition, we present further modifications which allow this assay to be readily converted into an automated high-throughput screening assay for chemokine receptor inhibitors. Data generated using this assay compares favorably with data generated by the [^{35}S]-GTPγS assay *(14)* but with the advantages and convenience of a non-radioactive assay.

2. Materials

2.1. Cell Line

The CCRF-CEM cell line, which naturally expresses CXCR4, was obtained from the American Type Culture Collection (ATCC; Manassas, VA, USA). Cells were cultured in RPMI containing 1 m*M* sodium pyruvate, 2 m*M* L-glutamine, and 10% fetal bovine serum (FBS) (*see* **Note 1**).

2.2. Reagents and Equipments

1. Dulbecco's phosphate-buffered saline (D-PBS).
2. Delfia GTP binding kit (PerkinElmer) which contains lyophilized europium-labeled GTP (Eu-GTP), lyophilized GDP, 250 m*M* HEPES buffer, GTP wash solution, 50 mg/mL saponin, 1 *M* $MgCl_2$, and 5 *M* NaCl (*see* **Note 2**).
3. Homogenization buffer: 50 m*M* Tris-HCl, 5 m*M* $MgCl_2$, 1 m*M* EDTA, 0.1 m*M* phenylmethylsulfonylfluoride (pH 7.4).
4. CXCR4 ligand SDF-1α (obtained from Phil Owen at the Biomedical Research Center, University of British Columbia).
5. Membrane incubation and filtration performed on AcroWell filter plates (Pall-Gelman, East Hills, NY).
6. Fluorescence measurements were performed on a Wallac Victor II fluorescent plate reader (PerkinElmer).
7. Liquid handling workstations used for high-throughput screening were the Packard Multiprobe II and the Beckman Coulter Biomek FX.
8. Polytron homogenizer.

3. Methods

3.1. Preparation of Membranes

For membrane preparation, CCRF-CEM cells are cultured in spinner flasks at 37°C, 5% CO_2 until the cells reach a concentration of $\sim 2 \times 10^6$ cells/mL. Harvest the cells for membrane preparation at density not greater than 2.5×10^6 cells/mL. It is recommended that the quantity of membrane required for the assay development be estimated in advance so that all the calibration steps can be performed using the same batch of membrane preparation to avoid batch-to-batch variation (*see* **Note 3**).

1. Transfer the CCRF-CEM cells from spinner flasks into 250 mL centrifuge tubes and centrifuge the cells at $100 \times g$ for 20 min.
2. Pour off the supernatant and re-suspend the cells into 18 mL of ice-cold D-PBS per tube. Pool the cells into two 250 mL centrifuge tubes (conical bottom) and re-suspend in a total of 200 mL of ice-cold D-PBS per tube and centrifuge the cells at $100 \times g$ for 20 min. Perform this wash step twice.
3. Aspirate the supernatant and re-suspend each of the cell pellets into 12.5 mL of ice-chilled homogenization buffer and transfer to 50 mL tubes.
4. Homogenize the cells with a Polytron homogenizer with a single burst of exactly 22 s.

5. Bring the volume of each tube to 15 mL by adding ice-chilled homogenization buffer and combine the homogenates of three tubes into one 50 ml tube. Centrifuge the homogenate at 100 × g for 6.5 min (4°C) to eliminate cell debris. It is important not to disturb the three distinct layers obtained from this centrifugation.
6. Collect the top layer containing the membrane fraction. Do not discard the bottom layers (*see* **Note 4**).
7. Add 15 mL of chilled homogenization buffer to the tube containing the remaining two bottom layers. Mix thoroughly but gently to avoid foaming.
8. Centrifuge at 100 × g for 6.5 min (4°C) to eliminate cell debris.
9. Collect the top layer as in Step 6 and pool it with the top membrane fraction obtained from the previous spin (Step 6) (*see* **Note 5**). Centrifuge the membrane fraction (top layer pool) at 45,000 × g for 30 min at 4°C.
10. Aspirate the supernatant and resuspend the membrane pellet in 5–8 mL of homogenization buffer. Homogenize further with a Dounce homogenizer (*see* **Note 6**).
11. Determine the protein concentration using the Bradford assay (Bio-Rad, Hercules, CA). Adjust the protein concentration to 1 mg/mL, aliquot the membrane preparation into 1 mL fractions in cryotubes.
12. Flash freeze the tubes by immersion into liquid nitrogen. Transfer to –80°C for storage until use.

3.2. Eu-GTP Binding Assay Optimization

The following steps are adapted from the PerkinElmer Delfia GTP binding protocol (*see* **Note 7**). In our experience, duplicates are sufficient for each point of the initial titration matrix. Repeats can be performed if either the duplicates are not satisfactory or if a narrower concentration range is required. A baseline control without agonist is included for each point of the titration. All the stock solutions are made in 50 m*M* HEPES from the 250 m*M* HEPES provided in the kit. A final concentration of 5 n*M* SDF-1α is used to activate the receptor (*see* **Note 8**). Once thawed, aliquots of membranes, GDP, and SDF-1α should be kept on ice at all times.

3.2.1. Optimization of GDP and $MgCl_2$ Concentrations

1. The concentrations of GDP and $MgCl_2$ are optimized by cross-titration on a 96-well AcroWell filter plate (Pall Gelman) (*see* **Note 9**). Prepare a concentration matrix with recommended final assay concentrations of 1, 5, and 10 m*M* $MgCl_2$ to be cross-titrated with 0.1, 1, 5, and 10 μ*M* GDP.
2. Thaw the aliquots of CCRF-CEM membranes, GDP, and SDF-1α required for this experiment and keep on ice. Accelerate the thawing by holding the tubes in hands. Warm the 1 *M* $MgCl_2$ from the kit and keep at room temperature (*see* **Note 10**).

3. Make stock solutions in 50 m*M* HEPES buffer: (a) 2.5 × the final assay concentrations of $MgCl_2$ selected for the cross-titration; (b) 5 × the final assay concentration of GDP to be titrated; (c) CCRF-CEM membrane stock solution of 0.4 mg/mL (5 × the final membrane concentration giving a final concentration of 8 μg per well) (*see* **Note 11**); (d) 5 × the final assay concentration of SDF-1α (25 n*M*). Dilute the SDF-1α in polypropylene tubes to avoid sticking; (e) 1 × GTP wash solution made from the 10 × stock provided in the kit. Keep on ice.
4. Add the following components to the wells of an AcroWell filter plate to set up the titration matrix: 40 μL of $MgCl_2$ stock solution, 20 μL of GDP solutions, and 20 μL of SDF-1α (or the no-agonist buffer control). Start the incubation by adding 20 μL of membranes to each well and mix by pipetting up and down twice.
5. Incubate the plate for 30 min at room temperature with slow shaking. During this incubation, prepare a stock solution of Eu-GTP at 10 times (100 n*M*) the final assay concentration (10 n*M*).
6. After 30 min incubation, add 10 μL of 100 n*M* Eu-GTP. Mix by pipetting up and down twice.
7. Incubate the plate for an additional 30 min at room temperature with slow shaking.
8. Wash the plate twice on a vacuum manifold with 200 μL per well of ice-cold GTP wash solution.
9. Read the europium fluorescence at an emission wavelength of 340 nm and an excitation wavelength of 615 nm either up to 30 min after washing or 6 h after the plate has dried.
10. Determine the % of signal over baseline for each condition by calculating the percentage of the plus-agonist signal over the baseline signal (no agonist). Plot the results as a histogram with GDP concentration as the *x*-axis, $MgCl_2$ as the *z*-axis, and the % over basal ratio as the *y*-axis (*see* **Note 12**).

An example of data obtained with CXCR4 is shown in **Fig. 1**. Although 1 m*M* and 5 m*M* $MgCl_2$ give similar signal over baseline ratios, slightly higher specific counts are obtained with 5 m*M* $MgCl_2$. Therefore 5 m*M* $MgCl_2$ was selected for further assay development. Similarly, although 1 μ*M* GDP produces the best signal over baseline ratio, the signal background (non-specific baseline counts) is very high at this GDP concentration (~32000 RFU) and hence 5 μ*M* GDP concentration is recommended as the optimal concentration. Therefore, although the signal over baseline ratio is a good indicator of the signal quality, individual signal, and baseline levels have to be examined separately when choosing optimized conditions.

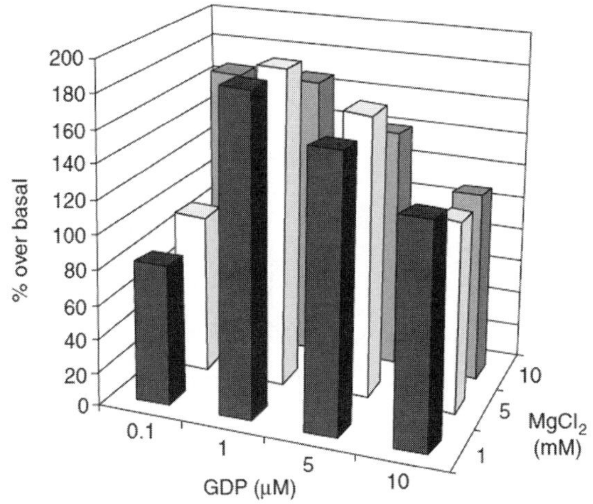

Fig. 1. Optimization of the GDP and $MgCl_2$ concentrations for the CXCR4 Eu-GTP assay.

3.2.2. Optimization of NaCl Concentration

A similar protocol was used to optimize the NaCl concentration using the optimized GDP and $MgCl_2$ concentrations.

1. Select 4–6 concentrations of NaCl for testing in the range of 0–200 m*M* (final assay concentration). Make NaCl stock solutions (5 ×) in 50 m*M* HEPES (use the 250 m*M* HEPES and 5 *M* NaCl provided in the kit).
2. Prepare the stock solutions as described in Steps 2–4 of **Section 3.2.1**, this time preparing a solution containing 2.5 × the optimized concentrations of $MgCl_2$ (12.5 m*M*) and GDP (12.5 μ*M*) as determined in **Section 3.2.1**.
3. Add the following components to the wells of an AcroWell filter plate: 40 μL of $MgCl_2$/GDP 2.5 × stock solution, 20 μL of the NaCl solutions, and 20 μL of SDF-1α (or buffer for control).
4. Start the incubation by adding 20 μL of membranes to each well and mix by pipetting up and down twice and continue as described in Steps 5–11 in **Section 3.2.1**.

In the example shown in **Fig. 2** the titration of NaCl concentrations up to 100 m*M* has no differential effect on the Eu-GTP fluorescent signal. A concentration of 10 m*M* NaCl was chosen based on previous experience with the CXCR4 [^{35}S]GTPγS assay as too high a concentration of NaCl is known to prevent binding of partial agonists in some GPCRs (*see* **Note 13**).

3.2.3. Optimization of Saponin Concentration

Saponin is a mild detergent which can improve the GTP binding to G proteins in certain GTP binding assays.

1. Select the concentrations of saponin to be tested within a range of 0–1000 μg/mL (final assay concentrations).

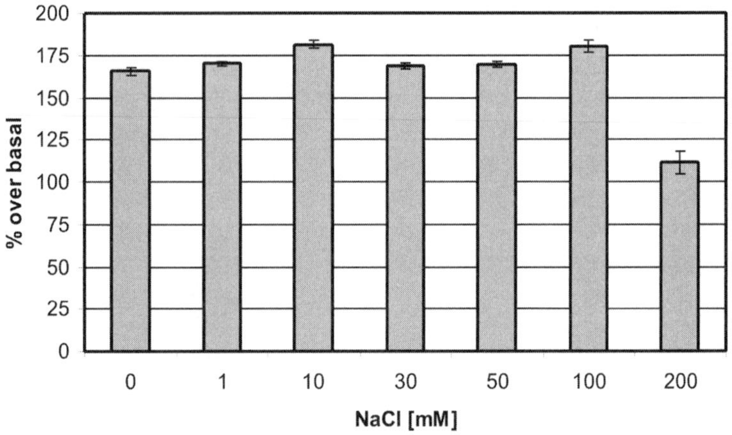

Fig. 2. Optimization of the NaCl concentration for the CXCR4 Eu-GTP assay.

2. Make 5 × saponin stock solutions of the selected concentrations in 50 m*M* HEPES
3. Prepare the stock solutions as described in Steps 2–4 of **Section 3.2.1**, this time using the optimized concentrations of GDP, $MgCl_2$, and NaCl to give a 2.5 × stock consisting of $MgCl_2$ (12.5 m*M*), GDP (12.5 μ*M*), and NaCl (25 m*M*).
4. Add the components in the following order to the wells of an Acrowell filter plate: 40 μL of $MgCl_2$/GDP/NaCl stock solution, 20 μL of saponin solutions, and 20 μL of SDF-1α or 20 μL of buffer to the no-agonist control.
5. Start the incubation by adding 20 μL of CCRF-CEM membranes and continue as described in Steps 5–11 in **Section 3.2.1**.

The optimal signal was obtained with 100 μg/mL saponin and this concentration was used in the subsequent steps of the assay development. The optimal concentrations of all assay components are summarized in **Table 1**.

3.2.4. Temperature Optimization

Following the calibration of the assay components ($MgCl_2$, GDP, NaCl, and saponin), the assay temperature is optimized. In order to do this SDF-1α dose–response curves are performed in parallel at 25 and 30°C.

1. Prepare enough stock solution containing the reagents at 2.5 × the optimized concentrations (12.5 m*M* $MgCl_2$, 12.5 μ*M* GDP, 25 m*M* NaCl, 250 μg/mL saponin in the CXCR4 example given) for two ligand (SDF-1α) dose–response curves of eight concentrations in triplicate.

Table 1
Optimized concentrations for components of the reaction mix

Assay component	Concentration in stock reaction mixture	Final concentration in assay
$MgCl_2$[1]	12.5 m*M*	5 m*M*
GDP[1]	12.5 μ*M*	5 μ*M*
NaCl[1]	25 m*M*	10 m*M*
Saponin[1]	0.25 mg/mL	0.1 mg/mL
Eu-GTP[1]	12.5 n*M*	5 n*M*
Ligand SDF-1α[1]	12.5 n*M*	5 n*M*
CXCR4 membrane[2]	0.4 mg/mL	8 μg/well

[1]Concentrations are based on using 40 μL of a 2.5 × stock solution in a final volume of 100 μL.
[2]Concentration based on using 20 μL of a 5 × stock solution in a final volume of 100 μL

2. Prepare a 2.5 × stock solution (1000 n*M*) of the highest SDF-1α concentration of the dose–response curve (400 n*M* final assay concentration). Keep on ice. From the 1000 n*M* SDF-1α stock solution, prepare serial dilutions of SDF-1α in a 96-well polypropylene plate (*see* **Note 14**).
3. Prepare a stock solution of 0.4 mg/mL CCRF-CEM membranes in 50 m*M* HEPES, keep on ice.
4. Add the following components to the wells of two AcroWell filter plates (one dose–response curve should occupy one plate): 40 μL of $MgCl_2$/GDP/NaCl/saponin master solution, 40 μL of various concentrations of SDF-1α, or the no-agonist control (see **Note 15**). Start the reaction by adding 20 μL of membranes. Incubate one plate at 25°C and the second plate at 30°C with slow shaking for 30 min and continue as described in Steps 6–11 in **Section 3.2.1** to incubate the plates at 25°and 30°C, respectively after adding the EU-GTP.
5. Plot the log dose–response curves using a three-parameter logistic equation (*see* **Note 16**).

An example of the SDF-1α dose–response curves is shown in **Fig. 3**. Very similar EC_{50} values are obtained at 25 and 30°C (1.5 ± 0.3 n*M* and 2.5 ± 0.3 n*M*, respectively). The fluorescent signal is significantly higher at 30°C without a significant increase in the baseline signal indicating that the absolute fluorescent signal is temperature dependent. In these conditions, the EC_{50} was consistently found to be reproducible within twofold with different membrane preparations. On the basis of the enhanced fluorescence signal and the improved temperature control provided by using an incubator, the incubation temperature used for the assay was set at 30°C (*see* **Note 17**).

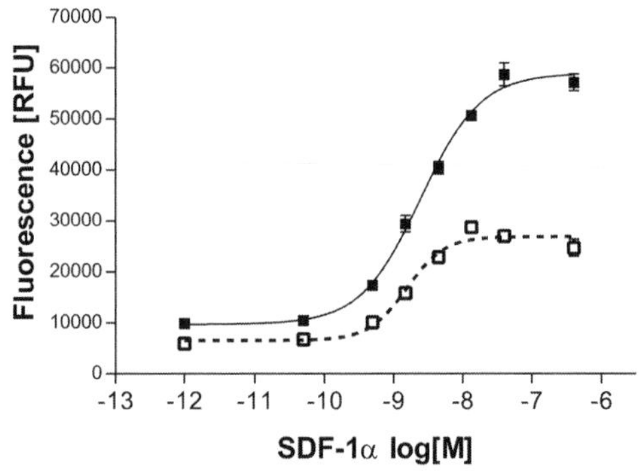

Fig. 3. Optimization of the incubation temperature for the CXCR4 Eu-GTP assay. Two SDF-1α dose–response curves are shown for 25°C (□) and 30°C (■).

3.3. Adapting the Chemokine Receptor Eu-GTP Binding Assay to High-Throughput Screening

As well as the assay optimization described above we recommend the following adaptations if the assay is to be used in a high-throughput screening (HTS) mode.

1) The assay as described above requires two sequential 30 min incubations. To simplify the procedure for HTS we investigated the effect of using a single 60 min incubation.
2) HTS assays usually entail the screening of a large number of compounds over a long time frame (>2 h). We therefore investigated the stability of the reagent mix over time.
3) The cost of reagents is a significant factor in the cost of running HTS. The Eu-GTP reagent is the single most expensive reagent in this assay so we investigated the effect of reducing the amount of Eu-GTP used in the assay.

Throughout these studies we also incorporated robotic liquid handling workstations for dilution of samples on the 96-well plate (Packard Multiprobe II) and dispensing, filtration, and washing (Beckman Coulter Biomek FX). Fluorescent readings were taken on a Wallac Victor II fluorescent plate reader equipped with a plate stacker.

3.3.1. Adaptation of the Assay to Use a Single Incubation

There are two components in the adaptation of the assay to a single step incubation. The first is to compare a single incubation versus the sequential two-step incubation procedure. The second is to test starting the incubation by addition of membrane instead of Eu-GTP. This requires adding the Eu-GTP in the incubation premix thus avoiding the necessity of adding small volume aliquots of this reagent to every well. This should both reduce the number of pipetting events and improve reproducibility by eliminating a pipetting step with inherent inaccuracies because of the small volume (particularly as in a later stage we want to reduce the amount of this reagent). These modifications are tested by comparing the ligand dose–response curve under the different conditions as outlined below.

1. Prepare stock solutions as described in **Section 3.2.4** for two SDF-1α dose–response curves.
2. Follow the two-step incubation procedure in **Section 3.2.4** using the optimum assay conditions for one dose–response curve.
3. For the second dose–response curve add all the components as in **Section 3.2.4**, but add 10 μL of 10 n*M* Eu-GTP immediately and incubate for 60 min at 30°C.
4. At the end of both incubations (60 min total for each) read the europium fluorescence and plot the log dose–response curves as described previously.

The SDF-1α EC_{50} values obtained from the two incubation procedures are very similar: 3.9 ± 0.9 n*M* for the two-step incubation and 2.5 ± 0.7 n*M* for the single 60 min incubation. These data indicate that the assay can be performed with a single incubation thus making it more compatible for HTS.

The above procedure requires pipetting a small volume of the most expensive reagent (Eu-GTP) to each assay well. To avoid this, and thus further simplify the procedure, the Eu-GTP was added in a single pipetting step to the pre-incubation mix. The membrane was excluded from the pre-incubation mix, and the assay started by addition of membrane.

1. Prepare a stock solution containing the reagents at 2.5 × the optimized concentrations (12.5 m*M* $MgCl_2$, 12.5 μ*M* GDP, 25 m*M* NaCl, 250 μg/mL saponin, and 25 n*M* Eu-GTP) and 2.5 × ligand (SDF-1α) sufficient for two dose–response curves of eight concentrations in triplicate.
2. To each well of a 96-well plate add 40 μL of the stock reaction mix and 40 μL of 50 m*M* HEPES buffer (*see* **Note 18**).
3. Start the incubation by the addition of 20 μL of the CXCR4 membrane preparation and incubate for 60 min at 30°C as described above.
4. Measure fluorescence and plot the log dose–response curves as described previously.

A comparison of the SDF-1α EC_{50} values starting the incubation with Eu-GTP compared with Eu-GTP in the incubation pre-mix and starting the incubation with membrane gave values of 1.3 ± 0.2 n*M* versus an EC_{50} of 1.5 ± 0.2 n*M*. In addition the signal level obtained with the two procedures was similar. On the basis of these data the Eu-GTP was included in the pre-mix and the incubation was started by the addition of membrane for the subsequent steps in the assay development.

3.3.2. Reaction Mixture Stability

1. Prepare enough SDF-1α for two dose–response curves as described in **Section 3.2.4**.
2. Prepare a stock solution of the reaction mix containing 12.5 m*M* $MgCl_2$, 12.5 μ*M* GDP, 25 m*M* NaCl, 250 μg/mL saponin, and 25 n*M* Eu-GTP.
3. Keep the stock reaction mix on ice. At various time points take 40 μL aliquots and add to the wells of a 96-well plate with 20 μL of the CXCR4 membrane preparation, 20 μL SDF-1α, and 20 μL of 50 m*M* HEPES buffer.
4. Incubate for 60 min at 30°C and followed by fluorescence measurement as described previously.
5. Plot the log dose–response curves as described previously and compare the EC_{50} values from each pre-incubation period to determine the stability of the stock solution while stored on ice.

Figure 4 shows the SDF-1α dose–response curves performed with reaction mixes that have been pre-incubated on ice for various lengths of time. The calculated EC_{50} values were constant for pre-incubation periods up to 45 min, indicating that the stock reaction mix was stable for that time period. All subsequent compound screening assays were completed within this time frame.

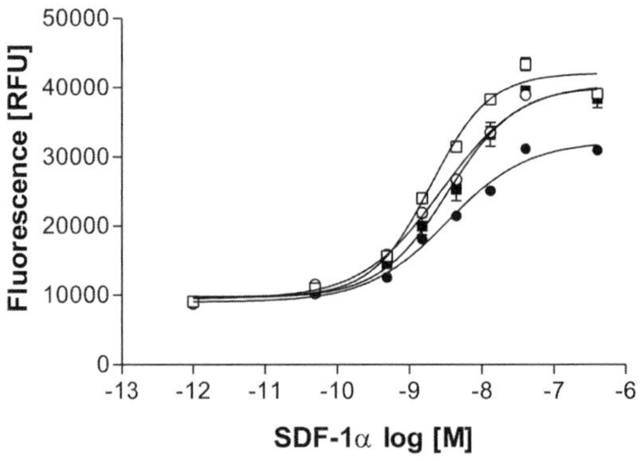

Fig. 4. Stability of the stock reaction mix when stored on ice. SDF-1α dose–response curves are shown for different pre-incubation times; 10 min (■), 20 min (□), 45 min (○), and 60 min (●).

3.3.3. Reducing the Concentration of Eu-GTP in the Reaction Mixture to Improve the Cost-Efficiency of the Assay

1. Prepare two SDF-1α dose–response curves as described in **Section 3.3.1**, with the addition of Eu-GTP in the master solution. Prepare one of these curves with suggested final concentrations of 10 n*M* Eu-GTP and 5 n*M* Eu-GTP (*see* **Note 19**).
2. Make sufficient quantities of two (2.5 ×) stock solutions of the reaction mix as described in Step 2 of **Section 3.3.2**, except that one has 25 n*M* Eu-GTP and the other has 12.5

n*M* Eu-GTP in 50 m*M* HEPES. Prepare a stock solution of 0.4 mg/mL CEM membranes in 50 m*M* HEPES and keep on ice.

3. To each well add 40 μL of the stock reaction mix, 20 μL of SDF-1α, and 20 μL of 50 m*M* HEPES buffer.
4. Start the reaction by adding 20 μL of membranes and incubate at 30°C with slow shaking for 60 min.
5. Measure fluorescence and calculate the EC_{50} from the log dose–response curve.

In the case of the CXCR4 assay, a decrease in the baseline fluorescent signal of 10,000–15,000 RFUs was observed when the concentration of Eu-GTP is reduced from 10 to 5 n*M* (**Fig. 5**). However, the maximum % signal to baseline ratio only decreased from 400% (10 n*M* Eu-GTP) to 350% (5 n*M* Eu-GTP) and the response was still considered suitable for agonist and antagonist screening assays. A comparison of the Z′, a screening coefficient which incorporates both assay signal dynamic range and data variation *(15)*, for the two conditions gave similar values of 0.92 for 10 n*M* Eu-GTP and 0.94 for 5 n*M* Eu-GTP. On the basis of this we decreased the concentration of Eu-GTP to 5 n*M* for our screening protocol, resulting in a twofold improvement of cost-efficiency (*see* **Note 19**).

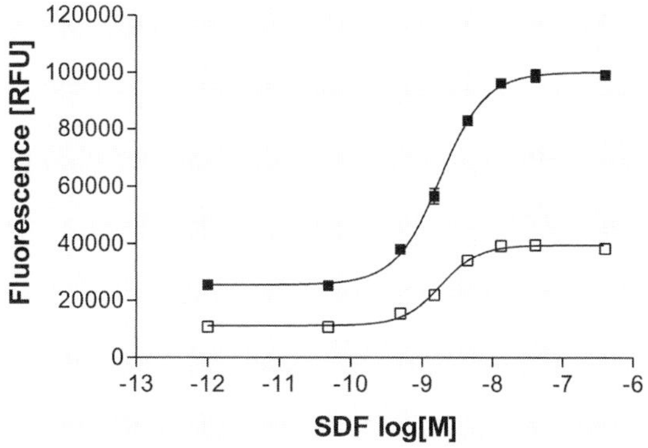

Fig. 5. Effect of reducing the concentration of Eu-GTP. Two SDF-1α dose–response curves are shown for 5 n*M* Eu-GTP (□) and 10 n*M* Eu-GTP (■). The SDF-1α EC_{50} values remain unchanged though a decrease in the fluorescence signal is observed.

3.3.4. Screening for Receptor Antagonists

In the examples given above we use the ligand dose–response to optimize the assay. The aim of these modifications to the assay is to use it to screen inhibitors. In order to utilize the assay for this purpose the 40 μL buffer included in the assay mix can be replaced with dilutions of test compound (*see* **Note 18**). The dose–response of the CXCR4 antagonist AMD3100 under optimized conditions is shown in **Fig. 6**. Under these conditions the IC_{50} of AMD3100 was determined to be 30 ± 2.9 n*M*, with a Z′ factor in the range of 0.86–0.90.

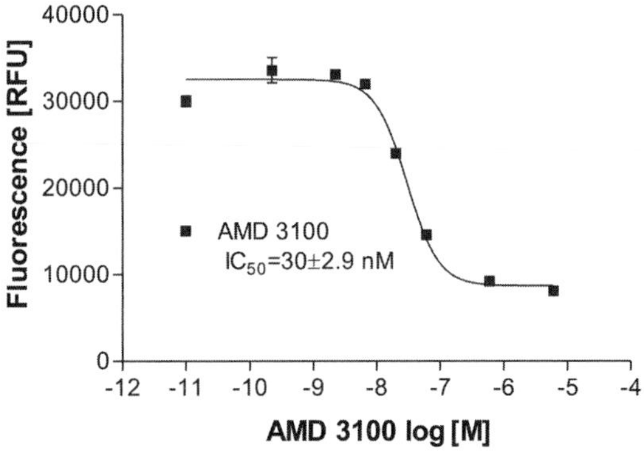

Fig. 6. Inhibition of Eu-GTP binding to CXCR4-CCRF-CEM membranes by AMD3100.

4. Notes

1. This assay can also be used for other chemokine receptors. The assay for CXCR4 utilizes membranes prepared from a cell line which naturally expresses the CXCR4 receptor. However, for other chemokine receptors it may be necessary to use transfected cells expressing the cloned receptor. As an example we have used this assay with CCR5 expressed in HEK293 cells. It should therefore be noted that optimization is required for each receptor membrane system as conditions will be different depending upon the receptor and the cell type.
2. The GDP and Eu-GTP provided in the PerkinElmer kit are lyophilized and must be dissolved in 50 m*M* HEPES made from the 250 m*M* HEPES included in the kit. After dissolving these reagents, distribute them into small aliquots and freeze them at –20°C as soon as possible. These aliquots should be thawed only once since GDP and Eu-GTP are unstable upon repeated freezing and thawing.
3. For our CCR5 Eu-GTP binding assay, membranes are prepared from adherent HEK293/CCR5 cells. The culture of these cells is done in triple decker tissue culture flasks from Invitrogen to maximize culture surface. For membrane preparation, these cells are detached using Versene, washed with PBS, and homogenized as for the CCRF-CEM cells.
4. Be careful not to contaminate the supernatant with the middle layer while collecting it. It should also be noted that the three layers resulting from the low-speed centrifugation are not observed from homogenates of all cell types. For instance, in the membrane preparation from the HEK293/CCR5 cells,

only one typical small bottom pellet is obtained. In this case, the supernatant is simply collected by avoiding this small pellet.

5. The Steps 7–9 are very important to increase the membrane recovery. A limited amount of membranes can be recovered from the first spin from the supernatant since a significant amount of membranes is trapped into the other centrifugation layers. It is also difficult after the first centrifugation to collect the membrane fraction adjacent to the interface between the membrane supernatant and the middle layer.
6. The Dounce homogenizer has to be kept on ice to keep the membrane fraction chilled. Apply six to eight slow and constant piston movements in order to allow the entire fraction to pass through the piston/tube interface. After the homogenization some aggregates may remain. They should be disrupted as much as possible by gentle aspiration–expiration using a Pasteur pipette. If the aggregates are too big, start with another type of pipette with a larger opening.
7. http://las.perkinelmer.com/Catalog/FamilyPage.htm?CategoryID=DELFIA+GTP-binding+Kit
8. 5 n*M* SDF-1α was chosen because it corresponds to the $EC_{50}$of SDF-1α in the CXCR4 [^{35}S]GTPγS assay *(14)*. We found that this concentration produced sufficient signal for the calibration of the concentration of the assay components. On the other hand, 10 n*M* RANTES was used for ligand concentration in the CCR5 Eu-GTP assay, again based on our in-house CCR5 [^{35}S]GTPγS assay conditions.
9. The AcroWell filter plate developed by Pall Gelman incorporates a patented low fluorescent background membrane and sealing process with a filter plate design compatible with robotic systems.
10. Take the following precautions when thawing frozen stock solutions. Do not overheat the GDP and membrane tubes in your hand. Stop heating them in your hand at the point when a small amount of frozen material remains in the tubes. For the membranes, mix the contents by gently drawing the liquid up and down 2–3 times (not more) with a pipette. If the $MgCl_2$ has crystallized at 4°C, warm it up to dissolve it (in your hand or in a 37°C water bath).
11. We observed that the vacuum plate filtration was significantly slower at membrane concentrations higher than 8 μg per well. This concentration was used throughout as it provided sufficient signal for the assay development. In the case of the CCR5 Eu-GTP assay, using the membranes from the HEK293/CCR5 cells, the membrane concentration could be increased to10 μg per well.

12. The % signal over baseline (% over basal) ratio is a good indicator of signal quality since it represents the proportion of real signal over the noise. The noise can be due to the Eu-GTP binding to G proteins without agonistic activation of GPCRs. In order to determine how much noise is due to G protein spontaneous activation, a control with an excess of GTPγS (provided in the kit) can be performed. The GTPγS will compete for all the GTP binding sites.
13. In the case of the CCR5 Eu-GTP assay development, the titration of NaCl concentration produces the typical differential effect on the fluorescent signal that is expected for this kind of calibration. The apparent absence of a NaCl effect on the CXCR4 Eu-GTP is an atypical observation.
14. Always use polypropylene tubes or plates to dilute SDF-1α as it is a positively charged protein and readily sticks to other materials. An example of serial dilution on a 96-well plate is shown in **Table 2** starting with a stock solution of 100 μ*M* SDF-1α. Prepare the first dilution (N1) in an Eppendorf tube and then transfer to the polypropylene plate. Use 40 μL of the 2.5 × solution in the assay which has a final volume of 100 μL per well.
15. A 20 μL is used to make up the volume to 100 μL. This volume of buffer can also be used to add inhibitors to the assay.
16. Dose–response curves were analyzed using Graphpad Prism 3.0 with the non-linear regression (variable slope) formula or XLFit add-in for Microsoft Excel. Replicate experiments were compared by calculating mean values and using the *t*-test where appropriate.

Table 2
An example of serial dilution on a 96-well plate

No	Volume of 100 μ *M* SDF-1α (μL)	Volume of buffer (μL)	Concentration of stock 2.5 × (n*M*)	Final SDF-1α concentration in well (n*M*)
1	6	594	1000	400
2	30 previous	270	100	40
3	100 previous	200	32.5	13
4	100 previous	200	11.0	4.4
5	100 previous	200	3.75	1.5
6	100 previous	200	1.225	0.49
7	30 previous	270	0.123	0.049
8	–	270	0.000	0

17. The instructions in the Delfia assay kit use incubation at room temperature. However, experience with the [^{35}S]GTPγS assay has shown that the temperature has to be optimized for different cell types and G protein interactions. We initially calibrated the concentrations of the components ($MgCl_2$, GDP, NaCl, and saponin) at room temperature, optimizing temperature later in the assay development. In the case of the CCR5 Eu-GTP binding assay development, we increased the incubation temperature to 37°C early in the assay development in order to obtain a sufficient signal.
18. The aim of these modifications is to adapt the assay for the screening of inhibitors. To this end, the 40 μL buffer was included in the assay mix so that it can be replaced with dilutions of test compound.
19. Though it was possible to reduce the Eu-GTP concentration for the CXCR4 assay it was found that this was not practical for the CCR5 assay using membranes from the HEK293/CCR5 cells due to the lower signals.

References

1. Broxmeyer, H.E. (2008) Chemokines in hematopoiesis. *Curr. Opin. Hematol.* **15**, 49–58.
2. Viola, A., Luster, A.D. (2008) Chemokines and their receptors: drug targets in immunity and inflammation. *Ann. Rev. Pharmacol. Toxicol.* **48**, 171–197.
3. Balkwill, F. (2004) Cancer and the chemokine network. *Nat. Rev. Cancer* **4**, 540–550.
4. Moore, J.PKitchen, S.GPugach, P Zack, J.A (2004) The CCR5 and CXCR4 coreceptors – central to understanding the transmission and pathogenesis of human immunodeficiency virus type 1 infection *AIDS Res. Hum. Retroviruses* **20**, 111–126.
5. Pierce, K.L Premont, R.T Lefkowitz, R.J. (2002) Seven-transmembrane receptors. *Nat. Rev. Mol. Cell. Biol.***3**, 639–650.
6. Meanwell, N.A Kadow, J.F. (2007) Maraviroc, a chemokine CCR5 receptor antagonist for the treatment of HIV infection and AIDS. *Curr. Opin. Investig. Drugs* **8**, 669–681.
7. Cashen, A.F Nervi, B DiPersio, J. (2007) AMD3100: CXCR4 antagonist and rapid stem cell-mobilizing agent. *Future Oncol.* **3**, 19–27.
8. Rink, T.J. (1990) Receptor-mediated calcium entry. *FEBS Lett.* **268**, 381–385.
9. Niedernberg, A Tunaru, S Blaukat, A Harris, B Kostenis, E. (2003) Comparative analysis of functional assays for characterization of agonist ligands at G protein-coupled receptors. *J. Biomol. Screen.* **8**, 500–510.
10. Alper, R.H Nelson, D.L. (1998) Characterization of 5-HT1A receptor-mediated [^{35}S]GTPgammaS binding in rat hippocampal membranes. *Eur. J. Pharmacol.* **343**, 303–312.
11. Selvin, P.R. (2002) Principles and biophysical applications of lanthanide-based probes. *Ann. Rev. Biophys. Biomol. Struct.* **31**, 275–302.
12. Frang, H Mukkala, V.M Syysto, R., et al. (2003) Nonradioactive GTP binding assay to monitor activation of g protein-coupled receptors. *Assay Drug Dev. Technol.* **1**, 275–280.
13. Labrecque, J Anastassov, V Lau, G Darkes, M Mosi, R Fricker, S.P. (2005) The development of an europium-GTP assay to quantitate chemokine antagonist interactions for CXCR4 and CCR5. *Assay Drug Dev. Technol.* **3**, 637–648.
14. Fricker, S.P Anastassov, V Cox, J et al. (2006) Characterization of the molecular pharmacology of AMD3100: a specific antagonist of the G protein coupled chemokine receptor, CXCR4. *Biochem. Pharmacol.* **72**, 588–596.
15. Zhang, J-H Chung, T.D.Y Oldenburg, K.R. (1999) A simple statistical parameter for use in evaluation and validation of high throughput screening assays. *J. Biomol. Screen.* **4**, 67–73.

Chapter 12

Use of the DiscoveRx Hithunter cAMPII Assay for Direct Measurement of cAMP in Gs and Gi GPCRs

Joe Bradley and David McLoughlin

Summary

G protein-coupled receptors (GPCRs) are druggable targets of great interest to the pharmaceutical industry. Generally, functional cell-based assays can be employed to detect agonists (inverse, partial, and full) in addition to allosteric and classical orthosteric antagonists. Several different homogenous assay systems can be used to monitor the signaling cascades of GPCRs. This chapter details the authors' collective experience of using the DiscoverX Hit Hunter cAMPII kit from GE Healthcare/DiscoverX Corporation for the direct quantification of cAMP levels in Gs and Gi GPCRs.

Key words: cAMP, cAMPII, Gs, Gi, HTS, DiscoverX, GPCR, EFC.

1. Introduction

Following stimulation GPCRs signal through predominantly one of three main G protein-linked pathways Gq, Gs, and Gi, respectively. All three pathways are of major interest to the pharmaceutical industry, with many assay kits and technologies in use, or in development, to monitor signaling through a variety of methods and end points *(1)*. Some assay formats rely on endogenous downstream events such as ERK or B-arrestin activity *(2)*. These are often common to all three pathways and hence can monitor multiple signaling routes in parallel. Others such as calcium-sensitive dyes, LANCE and DiscoverX Hithunter cAMPII monitor activity at an early stage before significant downstream amplification has occurred (compared to reporter gene assays), but are usually limited to monitoring one activation pathway per assay.

Wayne R. Leifert (ed.), *G Protein-Coupled Receptors in Drug Discovery, vol. 552*

Book doi: 10.1007/978-1-60327-317-6_12

The DiscoverX cAMPII assay utilizes enzyme complementation fragment (ECF) technology. ECF employs an enzymatic method to amplify the signal generated by cAMP release without having to rely on intrinsic protein production *(3)*. One advantage of this system is that it does not require cellular transfection other than that of the receptor of interest, unlike reporter gene formats. ECF has also found use in other homogenous formats used for measuring intracellular events such as protein trafficking, kinase and protease activity, and nuclear hormone receptor binding *(4)*.

The basis of ECF technology centers on two fragments of β-galactosidase (β-gal) enzyme, the enzyme acceptor (EA), and the enzyme donor (ED). When these two fragments are mixed, they bind to form an active β-gal enzyme that enables hydrolysis of a substrate to give a detectable luminescent signal. In order to link β-gal activity to cellular cAMP levels, the smaller of the two fragments (ED) is labeled with cAMP. A separate cAMP antibody competes with the EA fragment to prevent formation of an active enzyme complex. Change of cellular cAMP levels (as a response to GPCR modulation) will affect the levels of free antibody available to bind to the ED (**Fig. 1**). The greater the concentration of free cAMP, the more antibody that is bound to it, thus leaving the ED to form an active β-gal enzyme complex and hydrolyze the substrate to produce a luminescent signal. Full details of the use of this system can be found at http://www.discoverx.com/technology.html#invitro.

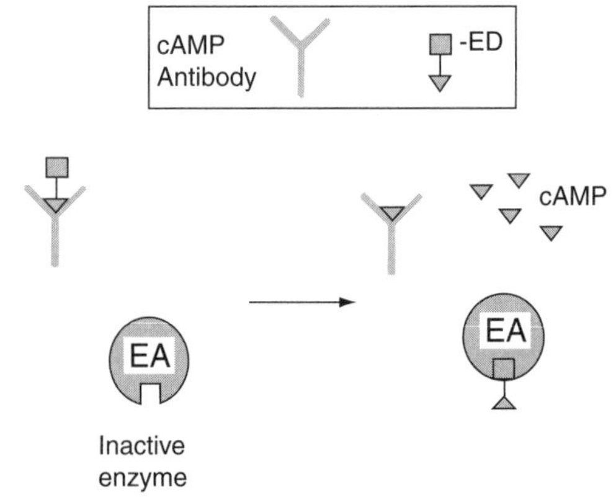

Fig. 1 In the absence of cAMP the antibody binds to the ED fragment preventing an active EA/Ed complex from forming.

The DiscoverX cAMP II assay can be configured using adherent cells. However, it is more commonly executed with a non-adherent cell suspension added to a microtiter plate at the point of assay. The use of non-adherent assay formats provides an opportunity for execution in a single working day. Furthermore, the non-adherent assay format provides a good starting point for miniaturization to low-volume 384- or 1536-well formats, as evaporation issues are reduced. That being said, the non-adherent cell suspension approach may require more cells per well than adherent cell formats. Furthermore, cell suspensions are typically harder to handle on fully automated systems. Hence the non-adherent cell approach is more suited to semi-automated screening. The adherent cell-based format normally requires cells to be plated one day prior to investigation. To reduce the effect of evaporation cells are plated in media volumes greater than those using cellular suspensions. However, as cells multiply overnight, cell seeding densities in adherent assays are a third to a quarter of the amount per well in comparison to those in suspension assay formats. Furthermore, in the non-adherent assay format, the lack of a cellular addition step aids execution on a fully automated system. As is often the case, the most appropriate method will depend on assay performance and local laboratory logistics. **Table 1** summarizes the benefits and disadvantages of both approaches. The authors' typically employ the suspension cell approach primarily for the benefits of miniaturization to low-volume 384 and single-day assay.

Table 1
The benefits and disadvantages of suspension versus adherent cells

Suspension assay		Adherent assay	
Pro	**Con**	**Pro**	**Con**
Single-day assay	Higher cell plating density (more flasks required)	Reduced cell plating density (less flasks required)	Larger volume of medium in plates offsets flask savings.
Reduced evaporation, especially in low-volume 384- and 1536-well formats.	Less suited to full automation – problems maintaining and dispensing a uniform cell suspension over long periods	1536 miniaturization compatible	Low-volume 384 difficult due to increased evaporation rates (high surface area to low volume)
More amenable to miniaturization		Full automation compatible	2 day assay

2. Materials

Materials and methods will vary depending on the cell line and construct used. The protocol below describes a typical CHO non-adherent cell-based assay in a 50 μL volume expressing a Gs-coupled receptor (*see* **Note 1**).

1. Growth medium: Dulbecco's modified Eagle's medium (DMEM:F12 (1:1); Gibco, Paisley, UK) supplemented with 10% fetal bovine serum (FBS; PAA Pasching, Austria), 400 μg/mL Geneticin (Gibco), and Glutamax (Gibco).
2. Dimethyl sulfoxide (DMSO).
3. Forskolin.
4. Phosphate-buffered solution without Ca^{2+} and Mg^{2+} (PBS; Gibco).
5. Cell dissociating solution (CDS; Sigma-Aldrich Company Ltd., Dorset, England).
6. Isobutylmethylxanthine (IBMX).
7. 384-well polypropylene plates (Matrix, Cheshire, UK).
8. 384-well white plates (Lumitrac 200; Griener, Stonehouse, Great Britain).
9. DiscoverX Hithunter cAMP II Assay kit containing: cAMP lysis buffer, cAMP EA-Ab reagent, cAMP ED reagent, cAMP standard, Galacton Star, Emerald II, substrate diluent (GE Healthcare).
10. 384-well plate capable luminescence reader (*see* **Note 2**).
11. 37°C/5%CO_2 incubator.
12. Automated cell counting system (e.g., Cedex).
13. Liquid handling system (e.g., Matrix Platemate).
14. Microvolume dispenser (e.g., Multidrop micro).

3. Methods

3.1. Preparation of Cells

1. Cells are grown in growth medium and harvested when they reach 70–80% confluence. Cells are harvested by pouring off the medium and washing 3 times with pre-warmed PBS.
2. The PBS is poured off and enzyme free cell dissociation buffer added to the cells, which are then incubated for 5 min in a 37°C/5%CO_2 incubator.
3. Once the cells have detached, pre-warmed growth media is added and cells are resuspended by gentle pipetting to achieve a single cell suspension. Cell density and viability is then measured on a Cedex.
4. Following centrifugation at 200 × g RCF for 4 min the cells are resuspended to 2×10^6 cells/mL in PBS (*see* **Note 3**) containing 1.5 m*M* IBMX (*see* **Note 4**) (500 μ*M* FAC, final assay concentration).

3.2. Assay Assembly

1. 5 μL of test compound or controls (as appropriate) are transferred to a 384-well plate using a Matrix Platemate. Compounds can be prepared in water, PBS, or pre-delivered in the plates as a nanoliter spot of 100% DMSO (*see* **Note 5**).
2. To initiate the assay add 5 μL of the cell suspension to the 384-well assay plate using a multidrop micro (10,000 cells/well). Cells and compounds should be left for 15 min at room temperature to allow slow-onset compounds to bind. Depending on the well geometry, dispensing accuracy, and volume of test compound, centrifugation of the plates at 200 × g RCF for 1 min may be required to ensure adequate mixing.
3. Add 5 μL of agonist at EC50 to the cells using a Multidrop micro. For a Gi-coupled receptor an appropriate concentration of forskolin (to stimulate baseline cAMP levels) is also added at this time. Again, depending on the well geometry and dispensing accuracy, centrifugation of the plates may be required to ensure adequate mixing.
4. Incubate the plates for 90 min at room temperature (*see* **Note 6**). Finally add 20 μL of reagents Rl and R2 (details of preparation are shown in **Section 3.3**) from the DiscoverX kit (*see* **Notes 7, 8, 9**).
5. The plates are then incubated for approximately 6 h before reading (*see* **Notes 10, 2, 11**).

3.3. DiscoverX Kit Preparation

1. Substrate working solution: gently mix 1 part Galacton Star/5 parts Emerald II/19 parts substrate diluent (*see* **Note 12**).
2. Reagent 1: cAMPII ED/substrate mix: gently mix 1 part cAMP II-ED reagent and 1 part substrate working solution (R1).
3. Reagent 2: cAMPII EA-Ab/lysis mix: gently mix 1 part cAMPII EA-Ab reagent and 1 part lysis buffer (R2).

3.4. cAMP Level Determination/Kit Sensitivity

The level of cAMP within the cell, along with the assay kit's intrinsic sensitivity to cAMP can be determined by performing a cAMP calibration curve.

1. Dilute the kit supplied cAMP to 30 μ*M* (10 μ*M* FAC) and then prepare a series of 1 in 3 dilutions to a FAC of 0.1 n*M*.
2. Transfer the cAMP to an assay plate in place of the test compound, instead of cells dispense PBS. Perform the rest of the assay as shown in **Section 3.2** (*see* **Note 13**).

4. Notes

1. Gi-coupled receptors involve a suppression of the levels of cAMP rather than activation. As such the basal levels of cAMP need to be raised before the agonist-induced reduction. Typically an EC50 concentration of forskolin is used. Increasing the concentration of forskolin will often improve assay quality by increasing the working window but lower assay sensitivity to the agonist and compounds.
2. Our reader of choice for luminescent assays is the GE Leadseeker, although other CCD single channel readers such as the Viewlux are also reported to have similar performance. Once calibrated correctly these CCD readers tend to be faster, especially in 1536 and produce higher quality data than PMT readers. However, modern PMT readers still produce good quality data, are more widespread, and for most low- to medium-throughput users provide a more cost-effective solution.
3. Cell growth medium containing Phenol Red may quench signal and reduce assay quality for DiscoverX assays. However, if you replace medium with PBS cells may tend to be more prone to cell aggregation or "clumping." To reduce "clumping" gently pipette and agitate the cells when in solution. In general, the less time between cell suspension preparation and its use the better! Constant agitation with a magnetic stirring flea may also reduce cell settling and clumping during dispensing.
4. The presence of IBMX in the assay will raise the basal level of cAMP within the cell. For a typical cell line this will lead to a higher signal level, but also a higher cell background, often negating any overall change in assay window or Z'. However, assays with a small window and Z' in the 0–0.4 range can sometimes benefit through reduced assay variability.
5. When testing compounds prepared in a particular solvent it is important to assess signal responses to increasing solvent levels. Typically CHO cell lines are tolerant to 1% DMSO.
6. Incubation times and conditions. Typical incubation times vary between 30 and 90 min, but it is important to choose an incubation time that suits your pharmacology as well as window/Z' *(5)* requirements. For short incubation periods, especially at 37°C, we found that strong spatial trends occur because of differential heating between edge and center wells. This spatial trend can be reduced by placing an assay plate directly onto the metal shelf of an incubator during the

incubation phase of the experiment, in doing so heat transmission to the plate is maximized. Placing plates in stacks may lead to significant edge effects as the plates positioned in the center of a stack are insulated by those either side *(6)*. During large high-throughput screening (HTS) runs the sheer amount of room temperature plastic introduced to a 37°C incubator can in itself cause significant drop in temperature, which takes time to recover. In order to avoid all these differential temperature effects, we often tend to run assays for relatively long incubation periods (60–120 min) at room temperature. This avoids uneven plate heating, with the added benefit of simplifying the schedule when running in a semi-automated format.

7. Although termed a “lysis buffer,” this is better thought of as a membrane permeability buffer allowing the cellular cAMP and cAMP antibody to mix. We often see only moderate amounts of lysis occurring. For some assays Z′s are improved by replacing the lysis buffer with PBS (especially at low volumes). We hypothesize that this is due to decreased detergent levels improving dispensing accuracy at low volumes.
8. The use of a freeze–thaw cycle to improve “lysis” efficiency has been seen to improve assay window and Z′ in *some* assays. However, great care should be taken when using this technique. The process can introduce significant spatial trends via non-uniform heating and cooling of edge wells affecting biological kinetics. It has been most effective on non-mammalian cell lines such as yeast or bacteria, or those with low cAMP levels (see notes on IBMX). It is thought to improve membrane permeability to cAMP via enhanced lysis. Freeze–thaw is usually carried out after the addition of Reagent 1 and Reagent 2. Following addition of reagents, immediately freeze the plates at –80°C and then thaw at 37°C. It is important not to stack plates on top of each other to aid even freeze–thawing. Do not thaw too many plates at one time as this may effect the incubator temperature (defrosting will obviously effect the ambient temperature inside your incubator). We find this freeze–thaw technique is not suited to the HTS environment because of the large numbers of plates run and the additional manual steps involved. In our experience, we observe that the freeze–thaw methodology has proved to introduce more signal variability than size of signal improvement reported. However, for some low-throughput assay formats, our internal data (not reported) clearly demonstrates the assay improvements that can be gained.
9. Typically once defrosted we find the assay kits are stable for 3 or 4 days at 4°C before the signal starts to decrease. This may not immediately cause a decrease in Z′, rather a decrease in

absolute counts. The rate of signal degradation and effect on Z′ over time appears to be batch dependent. Typically we advise to use kits within 1 week of opening.

10. When stacked for several hours prior to reading, plates often stick together causing reader automation failure. A potential cause is the presence of small amounts of "splashed" reagents that act as a form of "glue." Occasionally plates or wells "froth," possibly due to bacterial contamination in combination with the high detergents concentration and this can also cause plates to stick. Where possible seal plates before stacking or use lidded plates with an automated delidder before reading to prevent sticking issues.
11. The time required between addition of Reagent 2 and detection via an assay reader is highly assay dependent. Typically it varies between 4 and 16 h; however, plates can normally be read for up to 24 h after experiment, if well evaporation has been controlled.
12. The Emerald II in the kits is a bright yellow/green color. If a decrease in intensity or brightness is seen between batches, extra care should be taken to check assay performance.
13. The DiscoverX cAMPII kit is luminescence based and in theory should be less susceptible to compound interference. In reality it is actually an enzymatic generated signal and compounds have several sites in which they may interact to provide a false signal. These include inhibiting the β-gal itself, the complementation event, or by preventing the antibody binding to the ED fragment. Therefore it is critical to check for these interactions against the biochemical components of the assay before hit follow up. The necessary components for this optimization are provided in the kit as part of the cAMP level quantification reagents.

Acknowledgments

We thank Dan Rodrigues and Chris Williams for their help in preparing this manuscript.

References

1. Williams, C. (2004) cAMP detection methods in HTS: selecting the best from the rest. *Nat. Rev. Drug Discov.* **3**, 125–135.
2. McLoughlin, D., Bertelli, F., and Williams, C. (2007) The A, B, Cs of G protein-coupled receptor pharmacology in assay development for HTS. *Exp. Op. Drug Discov.* **2**, 603–619.
3. Eglen, R. (2002). Enzyme fragmentation complementation: a flexible high throughput

screening assay technology. *Assay Drug Dev. Technologies* **1**, 97–104.

4. Eglen, R. (2002) A homogenous enzyme fragment complementation cyclic AMP screen for GPCR agonists. *J Biomol. Screen.* **7**, 515–525.
5. Zhang, J.H., Chung, T.D., and Oldenburg, K.R. (1999) A simple statistical parameter for use in evaluation and validation of high throughput screening assays. *J Biomol. Screen.* **4**, 67–73.
6. Gribbon, P., Lyons, R., Laflin, P., Bradley, J., Chambers, C., Williams, B. S., Keighley, W., and Sewing, A. (2005) Evaluating real-life high-throughput screening data. *J Biomol. Screen.* **10**, 99–107.

Chapter 13

Use of Aequorin for G protein-Coupled Receptor Hit Identification and Compound Profiling

Stephen J. Brough and Parita Shah

Summary

G protein-coupled receptors (GPCRs) represent the largest class of targets in drug discovery, one-third of all marketed drugs are active at GPCRs and drugs targeted at GPCRs are marketed in virtually every therapeutic area. GPCRs can be classified by virtue of their coupling to second messenger signaling systems. In the last decade functional evaluation of Gαq-coupled GPCRs has been enabled by advances in fluorescence dye-based methodologies and detection instrumentation. Investigations into the bioluminescence of jelly fish in the early 1960s isolated the photoprotein aequorin that required only the addition of calcium to generate a luminescent signal. The recent development of sensitive detection platforms with integrated fluidics for liquid handling has revived interest in bioluminescence as an alternative to chemical fluorophore-based detection for characterizing the pharmacology of this target class. In this chapter we describe a detailed methodology for the development and execution of bioluminescence apoprotein aequorin-based screens for hit identification and structure–activity relationship compound profiling and highlight the opportunities and challenges associated with this technique.

Key words: Aequorin, G protein, 7-transmembrane, Receptor, Luminescence, High-throughput screen, Structure–activity relationship, Metabotrobic, mGluR5, Glutamate.

1. Introduction

During the past 15 years high-throughput screening (HTS) has become a central engine of drug discovery. Pharmaceutical and biotechnology companies have established the infrastructure to screen large libraries of chemically diverse molecules against drug targets, using automated screening platforms *(1, 2)*. In parallel a huge range of assay technologies have been enabled which share a number of common features; the assays are typically homogeneous (require no wash steps), amenable to sub-100 μL assay volumes,

Wayne R. Leifert (ed.), *G Protein-Coupled Receptors in Drug Discovery, vol. 552*

Book doi: 10.1007/978-1-60327-317-6_13

tolerant to solvents such as dimethyl sulfoxide (DMSO) and relatively cheap and simple to configure *(3)*. These assays rely upon the use of recombinant proteins or cell lines as the source of the biological material because of the ability to generate a virtually limitless supply of consistent, high-quality material *(4)*.

G protein-coupled receptors (GPCRs) represent the largest single class of targets in drug discovery. Approximately one-third of all marketed drugs are active at GPCRs and drugs targeted at GPCRs are marketed in virtually every therapeutic area *(5)*. GPCRs can be classified by virtue of their coupling to second messenger signaling systems *(6)*. GPCRs coupling to, and signaling through, the Gαs family of G proteins result in an increase in intracellular cyclic AMP (cAMP), while coupling to, and signaling through, the Gαi/o family of G proteins results in a reduction in intracellular cAMP. Finally, GPCRs which couple to, and signal through, the Gαq family of G proteins result in an increase in cytoplasmic calcium *(7)*. These changes can be measured and used as a surrogate of receptor activity. In the last decade, functional evaluation of Gαq-coupled GPCRs has been enabled by advances in fluorescence dye-based methodologies and detection instrumentation *(8)*.

Many marine coelenterates contain a small protein that requires only the addition of calcium to generate a luminescent signal *(9)* and six calcium-activated photoproteins have been identified (aequorin, clytin, obelin, berorin, mitrocomin, and mnemopsin). All of these photoproteins exist as complexes of an apoprotein, a chromophore cofactor, and oxygen. There is a high degree of homology between the photoproteins and all contain a highly conserved calcium-binding site. The aequorin bioluminescent calcium-sensitive photoprotein originally isolated from the jelly fish *Aequorea victoria* was cloned in 1985 *(10)* and has been expressed in mammalian cells to allow the configuration of assays for both GPCR and ion channel screening. The apoprotein is activated by the binding of the chromophore cofactor coelenterazine and has three high-affinity binding sites for calcium. Binding of calcium induces a conformational change resulting in an oxidative decarboxylation reaction producing coelenteramide and a flash luminescence signal at 469 nm. Aequorin has several advantages over traditional dye-based techniques for measuring calcium: it has low affinity for calcium (K_d=10 μ*M*) and a large dynamic range which makes it a good sensor in the biological calcium concentration range; unlike traditional calcium-sensitive chemical fluorophores, it is not cytotoxic and not activated by other cations; and tagged apo-aequorin protein can be targeted to specific sites within the cell *(11)*. The aequorin signal is generally produced between 0.1 and 5 s post-agonist addition and the signal decays to baseline within 30–60 s (**Fig. 1**). The rapid kinetics of the agonist response means that it is essential to have a luminescence detector with built-in liquid handling capabilities to enable simultaneous compound addition and signal detection capability.

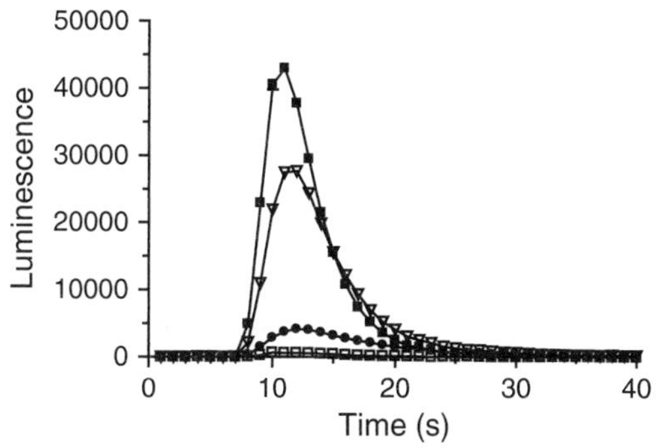

Fig. 1. A typical temporal profile of luminescence response recorded on the Lumilux™ to glutamate (e.g., responses of 1, 10, and 100 μ*M* (mean ± S.E.M., *n*=16) can be seen) in cells expressing human mGluR5 and the aequorin protein. A baseline read is taken for 5 s, followed by addition of 10,000 cells per well using the integrated cell dispenser to a 384-well plate containing 0.5 μL of glutamate, pre-diluted with 20 μL of buffer online. The change in luminescence is captured over a further 35 s. The chart demonstrates the rapid kinetics of the flash luminescence response.

The PerkinElmer (www.perkinelmer.com) Lumilux™ is one of a number of platforms currently available for the development luminescent plate-based assays in 384- or 1536-well microtiter plate format (Hammamatsu FDS6000™, Cybio Lumax™, and MDS Sciex FLIPRtetra™). The integrated pipettor and cooled charge-coupled device (CCD) camera allow simultaneous addition and signal detection from every well of an assay plate with the ability to acquire and display images in real time. In addition the internal cell handling system enables screening with suspension or adherent cells. These features also enable the standalone, walk away capability vital to concerted hit identification campaigns.

In this chapter we describe a detailed methodology for the development and execution of bioluminescence apoprotein aequorin-based screens for hit identification and subsequent pharmacological characterization through structure–activity relationship (SAR) compound profiling using as a model system an assay to detect antagonists of the human metabotrobic glutamate mGluR5 receptor, with high-throughput screening being performed in a 1536-well plate format and subsequent SAR performed in a 384-well plate format, and highlight the opportunities and challenges associated with this technique.

2. Materials

2.1. Biological and Chemical Reagents and Solutions

1. Chinese hamster ovary (CHO) cells stably expressing apo-aequorin and human metabotrobic glutamate receptor mGluR5 (Euroscreen SA, Brussels, Belgium) under the control of receptor expression induction agent doxycycline (Clontech, Mountain View, CA, USA).

2. Cell culture medium: Ham's F12 (Gibco, Paisley, Scotland) with 10% fetal bovine serum (FBS; Clontech).
3. Phosphate-buffered saline (PBS; Invitrogen, Paisley, Scotland).
4. DMSO (Fisher Scientific, Loughborough, Leicestershire, UK).
5. Bovine serum albumin (BSA; fatty acid, nuclease, and protease free; Calbiochem, San Diego, CA).
6. Pluronic F-68 (Gibco Invitrogen, Paisley, Scotland).
7. Coelenterazine (Invitrogen): 500 μM in 100% ethanol. Store at –20°C, protect from light.
8. Ethanol.
9. Base buffer: Hank's balanced salt solution (Sigma, Poole, UK) supplemented with 20 mM HEPES and 4.16 mM $NaHCO_3$, to pH 7.4 with NaOH.
10. Loading buffer: base buffer supplemented with 0.1% BSA and 0.1% pluronic acid F68 solution.
11. Dilution buffer: base buffer supplemented with 0.1% pluronic acid F68 solution is used to dilute cells and compounds.
12. Pharmacological standards: L-glutamic acid (Sigma) and fenobam (Tocris Bioscience, Bristol, UK) or MPEP (6-methyl-2-(phenylethynyl)pyridine; Sigma).

2.2. Hardware

1. Lumilux (PerkinElmer, Waltham, MA): These studies were configured with either 1536 dispensing head (for hit identification) with tip-blotting station (PerkinElmer, Waltham, MA) or 384 dispensing head (for compound profiling); however, the models can be used for either screening paradigm as throughput demands.
2. Cell viability analyzers: Cedex (Innovatis AG, Bielefeld, Germany).
3. Centrifuge: Any supplier capable of reaching 400 × g and supporting 50 mL centrifuge tubes.
4. Stuart Model SM27 battery-operated magnetic stirrer (Bibby Scientific, Stone, Staffs, UK) or Stuart Bibby Model SB2 Windmill Rotator (Bibby Scientific, Stone, Staffs, UK).
5. Multidrop (ThermoScientific, Waltham, MA): Multidrop384 for additions to 384-well plates or MultidropCombi nL for additions to 1536-well plates.
6. Low-volume liquid handlers: Echo550 liquid handler (Labcyte, Sunnyvale, CA) for dispensing low nanoliter reagent volumes into 1536-well plates or Biomek FX (Beckman Coulter, High Wycombe, Buckinghamshire, UK). Used for preparation of serial dilutions of compounds.

2.3. Plasticware

1. Frozen cell aliquots are stored in 5 mL polypropylene cryogenic vial, self-standing with round bottom (Corning, Corning, NY) or 1.4 mL flat bottom tubes, sterile (Nunc, Fisher Scientific, Loughborough, Leicestershire, UK).
2. 50 mL centrifuge tube (Becton Dickinson, Franklin Lakes, NJ, USA) or 15 mL centrifuge tube (Becton Dickinson, Franklin Lakes, NJ).
3. 125 mL disposable spinner flasks (Corning, Corning, NY, USA) or 500 mL disposable spinner flasks (Corning) or CelstirInstruments glass spinner flask (Wheaton Science, Millville, NJ, USA).
4. Lumilux P7 Tips (PerkinElmer, Waltham, MA, USA) for 1536-well pipettor or Lumilux P30 Tips (PerkinElmer) for 384-well pipettor.
5. Compounds are prepared in Echo550 qualified 1536 compound source plates (Corning) or 384-well v-bottom polypropylene plates (Greiner, Kremsmunster, Austria).
6. Assay ready plates: black-walled clear-bottomed 1536-well plate (Greiner, Kremsmunster, Austria) or black-walled clear-bottomed 384-well plate (Greiner).

3. Methods

3.1. Cell Thawing Protocol

1. Chinese hamster ovary (CHO) cells expressing human mGluR5 under the control of doxycycline provided as frozen, preinduced aliquots at 6×10^7 cells per mL and stored at –140°C prior to use. All assays described below use cryopreserved cells (*see* **Note 1**) prepared by GlaxoSmithKline Cell Fermentation Group (*see* **Note 2**).
2. Culture medium pre-warmed to 37°C in a water bath.
3. Thaw the vial of cells rapidly in beaker containing pre-warmed (37°C) sterile water until only a small ice chip remains visible. Use gentle agitation to mix the cells. Upon thawing, remove the vial from the water bath, swab with disinfectant solution, and wipe dry.
4. Using a serological pipette, transfer cells to an appropriate container (*see* **Section 2.3**, Step 2). Take care to gently pipette the cell suspension down the side of the container and avoid generating foam.
5. Add pre-warmed (37°C) culture medium drop wise with mixing to resuspend the cells to a nominal cell concentration of 2×10^6 cells/mL. It is important that this order of addition is followed to avoid osmotic shock because of the rapid release of DMSO from the cells.

6. Centrifuge the cell suspension at 300 × g for 5 min for 15–50 mL centrifuge tubes or 10 min for 250–500 mL centrifuge tubes. Discard the supernatant and resuspend the cell pellet in a spinner flask in an appropriate volume pre-warmed (37°C) cell culture medium.
7. Place spinner flask on a magnetic stirrer and incubate at 37°C, 5% CO_2 for 60 min (*see* **Note 3**). Ensure lid is loose and stirrer is at a moderate speed (60–90 r.p.m.). Decant cell suspension to centrifuge tube. Rinse cell stirrer with small volume of PBS. Centrifuge at 300 × g for 5 min.

3.2. Cell Loading Protocol

1. Remove supernatant and resuspend cells in an appropriate volume of assay buffer. Assess cell count and viability.
2. Owing to different final assay concentration of cells/mL in the two assay formats it is necessary to dilute cells to 5×10^6 cells/mL for hit identification or 2.5×10^6 cells/mL for compound profiling in loading buffer (*see* **Note 4**). The presence of pluronic acid in the loading buffer leads to an improved uniformity and quality of cell suspension over time.
3. Add coelenterazine to final concentration of 5 μ*M*. Wrap cell suspension vessel in foil to protect from light. All cell counters have upper limit for accuracy, as such, the cells should be resuspended somewhere between 1×10^5 and 1×10^7 per mL for all count steps. Loading at a higher cell density can increase the signal window in an assay (*see* **Note 5**).
4. Incubate cells for 4–20 h (*see* **Note 6**) at room temperature with mixing, either in a spinner flask or on a windmill rotator. Maintain temperature below 25°C. As cell stirrer or windmill speed can be critical for assay performance (this must be determined on a case-by-case basis) groups would benefit from using consistent equipment during assay development and implementation.

3.3. Plate Preparation

1. Assay ready compound plates (*see* **Note 7**) are prepared for 1536-well hit identification assays as follows. Compounds are supplied in assay ready plates as 50 nL stamp outs of 1 m*M* stock solutions in 100% DMSO in 1536-well black optical bottom plates. Control wells for the normalization of data and calculation of robust statistics such as Z′ are referenced to maximum, minimum, and mid-point pharmacological effect. To achieve this, low control (minimum effect at blocking $4 \times EC_{50}$ concentration of standard agonist glutamate) wells (column 11, 12 rows A–AF) receive a 50 nL stamp out of DMSO. High control (maximum effect at blocking $4 \times EC_{50}$ concentration of standard agonist glutamate) wells (column 35, 36 rows A, B, E, F, etc., to AC, AD) receive a 50 nL stamp

out of standard mGLuR5 antagonist fenobam. Mid control wells (column 35, 36 rows C, D, G, H, etc., to AE, AF) receive a 50 nL stamp out of standard mGLuR5 antagonist fenobam at a concentration which should reproducibly provide 50% inhibition of the standard agonist glutamate response. High and mid controls are alternated down the plate in blocks of four as noted in the well references. These plates are stored at –20°C until required.

2. Assay ready agonist plates (used to calculate EC_{50}, and appropriate $4 \times EC_{50}$ concentration of agonist to block in antagonist format assays) are prepared for 1536-well hit identification assays as follows. A 384-well plate containing 11 point, threefold serial dilutions of the standard agonist glutamate concentration–response curves (**Fig. 2**) is prepared in 100% DMSO with a top concentration of 1 m*M*. 50 nL of this is stamped out into 1536-well black optical bottom assay ready microtiter plates using an Echo550 Liquid Handler. The plates are sealed and stored at –20°C until required.

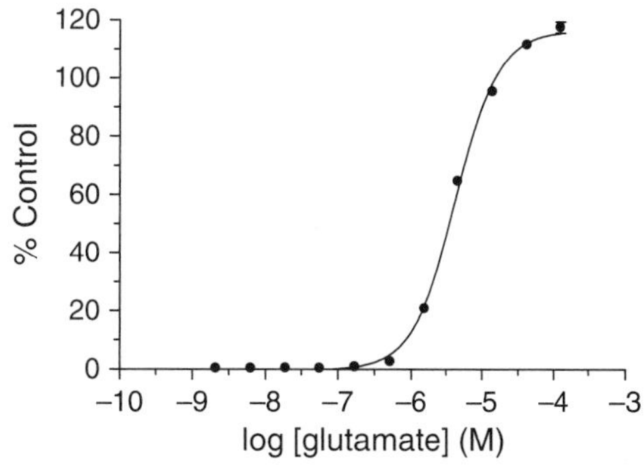

Fig. 2. Typical concentration–response curve of standard agonist glutamate (mean_± S.E.M., n=16) in cells expressing human mGluR5 and the aequorin protein. Area under curve (AUC) data generated on the Lumilux™ is normalized to a maximal concentration of glutamate (100% activation) and DMSO (0% activation).

3. Assay ready compound plates (*see* **Note 7**) are prepared for 384-well compound profiling assays as follows. Compound dilution plates are supplied with samples (at 10 m*M*) in columns 1 and 13. Eleven-point, threefold serial dilutions are prepared in 100% DMSO with a top concentration of 1 m*M* skipping columns 6 and 18. DMSO (0.5 µL) is transferred to 384-well black optical bottom assay ready compound plates using the Biomek FX Liquid Handler. Control wells for the normalization of data and calculation of robust statistics such as Z′ are referenced to maximum and minimum pharmacological effect. To achieve this, low control (minimum effect) wells (column 6 rows A–P) receive a 0.5 µL stamp out of

DMSO. High control (maximum effect) wells (column 18 rows A–P) receive a 0.5 μL stamp out of standard mGluR5 antagonist MPEP. These plates are stored at –20°C until required.

4. Assay ready agonist plates (used to calculate EC_{50}, and appropriate $4 \times EC_{50}$ concentration of agonist to block in antagonist format assays) are prepared for 384-well compound profiling assays as follows. A 384-well plate containing 11-point, 3-fold serial dilutions standard agonist glutamate concentration–response curves is prepared in 100% DMSO with a top concentration of 1 m*M*. 0.5 μL of this is stamped out into in 384-well black optical bottom assay ready plates using the Biomek FX Liquid Handler. The plates are lidded and stored at –20°C until required.

3.4. Assay Steps for Hit Identification Screening

1. On the day of assay, compound plates (prepared following Step 1 in **Section 3.3**) are removed from storage, allowed to thaw for 30 min, and centrifuged for 1 min at 300 × g prior to buffer and cell addition.
2. Immediately prior to assay cells are counted and diluted to 5×10^6 cells per mL in dilution buffer (*see* **Note 8**). Cells are kept in suspension by placing spinner flask on a magnetic stirrer set at a slow-to-moderate speed.
3. Tubing on the Multidrop Combi nL is washed with deionized water. Dilution buffer is primed through the tubing and 2 μL of dilution buffer is dispensed to all wells of the compound plates. The tubing is emptied and washed with deionized water. Cell suspension (at 5×10^6 cells per mL) is decanted into the pressurized Combi nL dispensing unit. The tubing is primed with cell suspension and 2 μL is added to every well of the plates giving a final cell density of 5000 cells per well to produce "assay ready" compound plates.
4. Compound dilution and cell addition steps are conducted on a Combi nL and only additions where the resulting luminescence changes are captured are made within the Lumilux. When this protocol is used 16 plates are "batched" for buffer and cell addition to ensure a consistent time between additions (*see* **Note 9**).
5. Following 30 min incubation at room temperature from the first buffer addition to the batch of 16 assay ready compound plates (prepared following Step 1 in **Section 3.3**) and agonist (in dilution buffer) are loaded into the appropriate locations within the Lumilux enclosure and disposable tips are loaded onto the Lumilux pipettor. Wash bottles are filled with deionized water and waste bottles are emptied.

6. For each plate changes in luminescence are followed over a 40 s time course with the addition of 2 μL of a pre-determined approximate $4 \times EC_{50}$ concentration of glutamate at a height of 0.5 mm at 10 μL/s after 8 s (*see* **Note 10**). The Lumilux tips are washed with 4 cycles of 3 μL H_2O.
7. For hit identification campaigns agonist potency is assessed during assay development and monitored for consistency. A fixed, pre-determined approximate $4 \times EC_{50}$ concentration of standard agonist is used. If the recorded EC_{50} is not consistent it can be evaluated on each screening day, as is done for compound profiling.
8. It is critical to monitor and optimize the number of tip wash cycles and the volume used, particularly in 1536-well assays. There is a balance of carry over of compound, build up of residual fluid in tips, and capillary action of residual into the pipettor head over a prolonged run (*see* **Note 11**).
9. Full diversity hit identification campaigns test compounds at a single high concentration for their ability to stimulate the receptor (if searching for agonists) or attenuate the response to a reference agonist (if seeking to identify antagonists).
10. Prior to the campaign, tests examine the stability and consistency of responses to single concentrations of reference agonists and antagonists as controls (**Fig. 3**). This will allow the user to define measures such as Z′ and coefficients of variation (CV) across 1536-well plates. Subsequently, two standardized small compound validation sets reflecting the

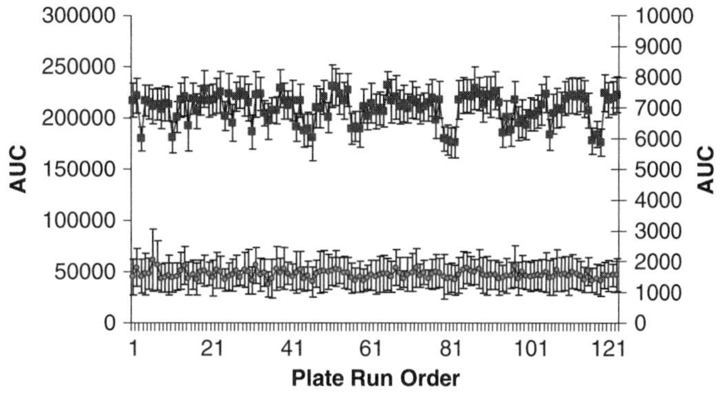

Fig. 3. Graph demonstrating typical high and low area under curve (AUC) values generated for a 1536-well hit identification run of 121 plates. Each 1536-well plate contains 64 wells containing DMSO (high control) and 32 wells containing a maximal concentration of standard mGluR5 antagonist fenobam (low control) as described in **Section 3.3** step 1 (assay ready compound plates). Upon $\sim 4 \times EC_{50}$ glutamate addition to the 1536-well plate the DMSO controls generate the signal and the wells containing standard antagonist denote full inhibition of the glutamate response. Each data point represents a single plate in a 1536-well run.

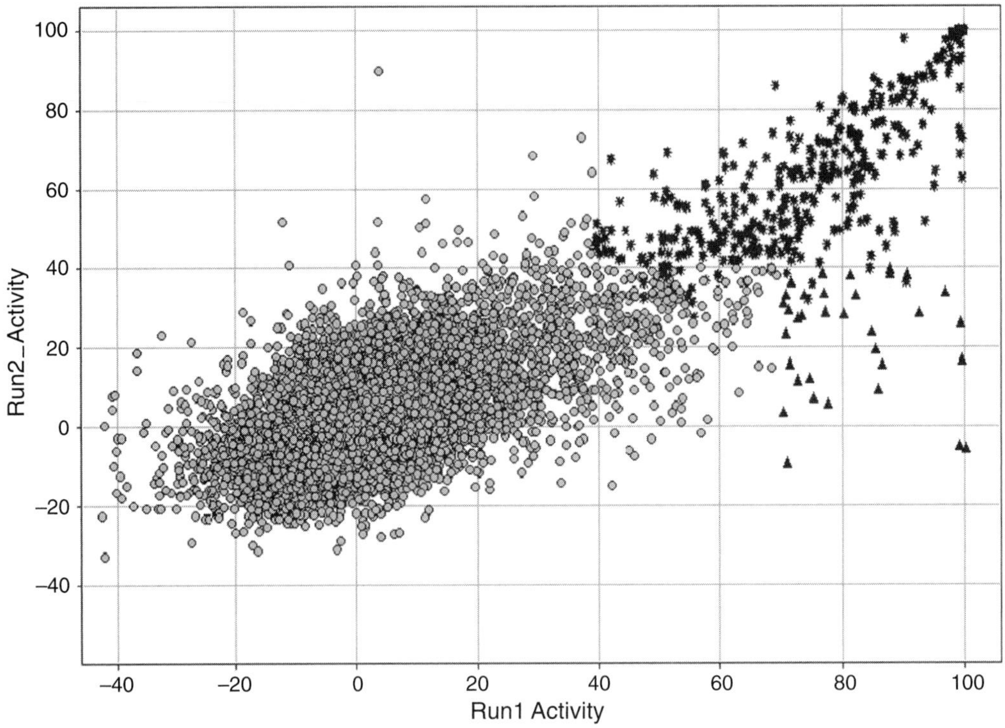

Fig. 4. Correlation of % inhibition results for a 10,000 compound assay validation set tested at 10 μ*M* on two independent test occasions in the mGluR5 1536-well hit identification assay. Area under curve (AUC) data are generated on the Lumilux™ for each compound and the values are normalized to minimum (DMSO) and maximum (maximal concentration of standard mGluR5 antagonist fenobam) following stimulation with an ~4 × EC_{50} concentration of glutamate on each 1536-well plate.

diversity of the corporate collection are exposed to the assay as replicates between and within days (**Fig. 4**). This allows an early determination of whether the assay is fit for purpose for hit identification and allows the robustness of the screen in a production format to be defined. The analysis encompasses inter- and intra-assay reproducibility, hit rates, false-positive rates, and false-negative rates, statistically derived activity cutoff measures in addition to tracking signal stability and assay pharmacology over the duration of extended runs. Typically we find hit rate to be ~2%, false-positive and false-negative rates <1%, cutoff for defined "active" <50%, 80% confirmation rate on retest or inter-assay correlation coefficient of >0.8.

11. The final round of benchmark testing uses a standard 10,000 compound robustness set screened at 10 μ*M* in three separate experiments. We observed a good correlation of percent inhibition values for each compound on two separate occasions (**Fig. 4**) with low false-positive and false-negative rates and

an average hit rate of 4% based on an activity threshold of 38% inhibition (*see* **Note 12**). During this testing, the coefficient of variance (CV) for an 4 × EC_{50} concentration of agonist across a whole 1536-well plate was measured and ranged between 6 and 8%, which is broadly in line with the CV for 1536-well liquid handling, meaning there is virtually no biological variability apparent.

12. For this hit identification campaign 1.7 million compounds were screened at 10 μ*M* in 1300, 1536-well plates with a throughput of 130 plates per day with 4 screening experiments a week due to the requirement to load cells overnight to generate acceptable signal window during a 6 h screening run. During a typical run, Z′ values of greater than 0.7 were observed indicating excellent assay quality. Typical signal to background for a screening run (**Fig. 3**) gives a signal window of approximately 100:1 (minimum requirement for 1536-well assay is 20:1). A "mid control" (which should track at 50% inhibition of the agonist response) of standard mGluR5 antagonist fenobam was tracked on every 1536-well plate throughout the campaign to monitor assay sensitivity. The percent inhibition of this control was calculated by normalizing the AUC values to the high and low controls. Typical data ranged 52±8% inhibition.

3.5. Assay Steps for Compound Profiling Structure–Activity Relationship Screening

1. Immediately prior to assay cells are counted and diluted to appropriate final cell density (usually 7.5 × 10^6 cells per mL) in dilution buffer (*see* **Note 8**).
2. An initial plate full of agonist concentration–response curves (created following Step 4 in **Section 3.3**) is used to calculate agonist potency (**Fig. 2**) and subsequently determine an appropriate glutamate concentration to include in antagonist studies (typically 4 × EC_{50}).
3. Disposable tips are loaded onto the Lumilux pipettor. Tubing serving the integrated cell dispenser is rinsed with deionized water. Cell suspension, assay ready compound plates (prepared following Step 3 in **Section 3.3**), dilution buffer, and agonist in dilution buffer (required for antagonist determinations) are loaded into the appropriate locations within the Lumilux enclosure.
4. For assays directed at detecting agonists the method entails: Tips are pre-wet in dilution buffer with a simple aspirate and dispense of 20 μL of dilution buffer prior to the first compound plate dilution step. Assay ready agonist compound plate (prepared following Step 4 in **Section 3.3**) receives 20 μL dilution buffer. Suitable settings for buffer addition are height of 2 mm, mix of 10 μL × 3 at height of 2 mm. For each plate changes in luminescence are followed over a 40 s

time course with the addition of 20 μL of cells (final cell density of 10,000 cells per well) at a height of 2.8 mm and speed of 50 μL/s after 5 s (*see* **Note 10**). The Lumilux tips are washed with 3 cycles of 20 μL H_2O (*see* **Note 13**).

5. The measurement of antagonism on the Lumilux follows a similar methodology: Plates containing concentration–response curves to the compounds of interest (prepared following Step 3 in **Section 3.3**) are placed in stacks in the Lumilux enclosure. The protocol then carries out the following steps: Tips are pre-wet in dilution buffer with a simple aspirate and dispense 20 μL of dilution buffer prior to the first compound plate dilution step. Batches of four assay ready compound plates (prepared following Step 3 in **Section 3.3**) receive 20 μL dilution buffer. Suitable settings for buffer addition are height of 2 mm, mix of 10 μL × 3 at height of 2 mm. Subsequently, 20 μL of cells (final cell density of 10,000 cells per well) are added to the compound plate. The capture of the resulting change in luminescence over a 40 s time course (with cell addition at time point 5) is optional and reflects any agonist or intrinsic efficacy of compounds in the assay system (*see* **Note 14**). Suitable settings for cell addition on Lumilux are height of 2.8 mm (*see* **Note 10**) and speed of 50 μL/s. Wash tips in H_2O with 3 cycles of 20 μL between addition of dilution buffer and cells.
6. Defining the protocol in batches of four allows the setting of a static 15 min incubation at room temperature prior to the addition of 20 μL of four times the pre-defined EC_{50} concentration of glutamate agonist prepared in dilution buffer at a height of 2.8 mm (*see* **Note 10**) and speed of 50 μL/s. Changes in luminescence are followed over a 40 s time course with the addition after 5 s. The Lumilux tips are washed with 3 cycles of 20 μL H_2O.
7. Using these wash protocols allow the same set of disposable tips to be used for over 100 plates.
8. Fit-for-purpose determinations during assay development examine whether receptor pharmacology in the aequorin format matches that reported in the literature. In the case of mGluR5 we are in the fortunate position of having a large array of well-characterized agonists, antagonists, and allosteric modulators, both positive and negative, with which to characterize the reagent and benchmark compound activity across formats (384- and 1536-well) to ensure data consistency and fidelity.
9. In addition a "training set" of 60 compounds from a well-established in-house fluorescence-based calcium mobilization assay were profiled in the 384-well luminescence assay

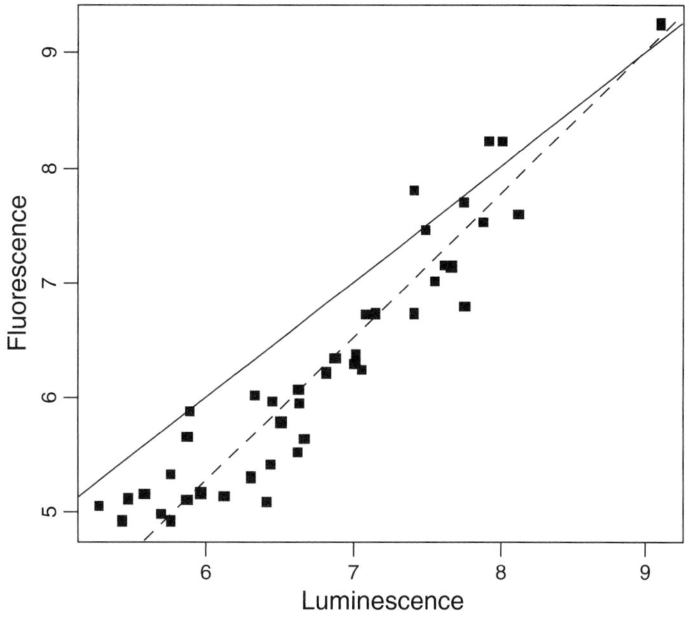

Fig. 5. Correlation of calcium luminescence (*x*-axis; *see* **Section 3.4** for assay protocol) and fluorescence (*y*-axis) pIC_{50} responses for a standard training set of compounds tested in the 384-well mGluR5 compound profiling assay. The *solid line* is line of unity and the "hashed line" is the line of best fit.

format. These data (**Fig. 5**) allowed us to compare the pharmacology of the reagent in direct head-to-head fluorescence and luminescence assays from the same master compound dilution plate ruling out all sources of variation but assay format and reagent. These data allowed us to measure other indicators of assay quality such as Z′ and pharmacological reproducibility (as defined by standard deviations) in addition to softer quality metrics such as curve fit, plate, and whole-assay failure rates.

10. Over 30 test occasions (145 plates) the average Z′ for the 384-well compound profiling screen in the aequorin bioluminescent format is 0.78 ± 0.09. Six pharmacological standard compounds tracked show a standard deviation of less than 0.2 log units (**Fig. 6**). Over the same period only three screening plates (3% of tested IC_{50}s) failed assay quality control (**Fig. 7**). We have performed 2400 11-point IC_{50} determinations on 650 unique chemical compounds. The data is analyzed by a four-parameter logistic fit, initially with no constraints. Of the compounds tested 31% were inactive, 43% fitted to the primary model without constraints, 23% were rescued by a constrained model, and only 3% of curves failed to fit (*see* **Note 15**).

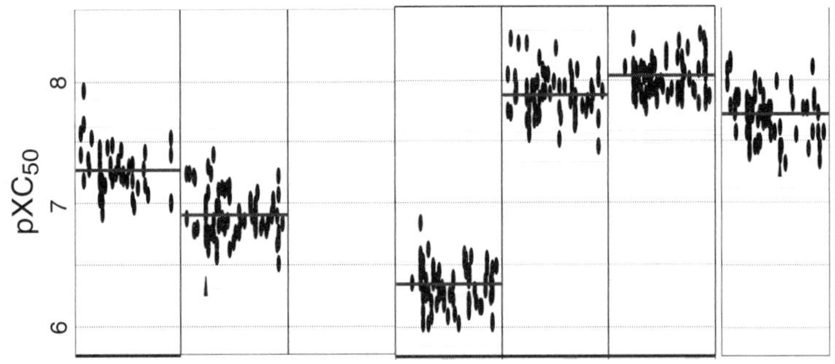

Fig. 6. Graph tracking pIC_{50} values for a range of standard mGluR5 antagonist compounds tested over 3 months of biweekly compound profiling using two distinct frozen cell batches. Each of the six panels represents data generated for a single standard compound. The "lines" indicate the mean pIC_{50} _± 3_S.D.

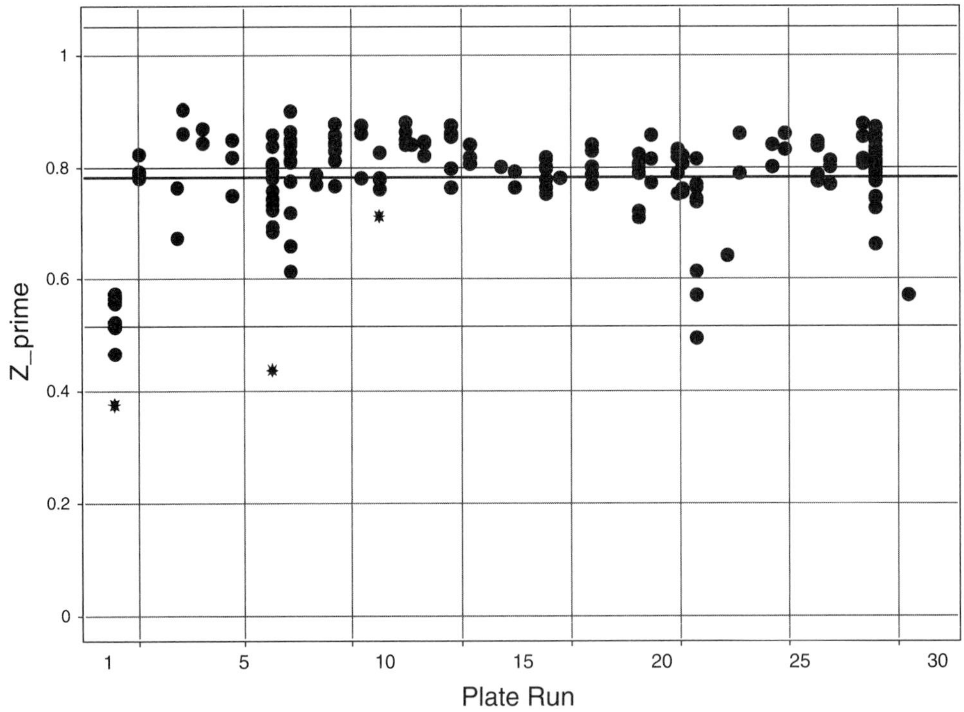

Fig. 7. Chart of robust Z′ over 3 months of biweekly compound profiling using two distinct frozen cell batches. Z′ is calculated for each plate based on the signal window between column 6 (DMSO) and column 18 (a maximal concentration of an mGluR5 antagonist MPEP) as described in (compound plate section 3.3 step 3) following stimulation with an $\sim 4 \times EC_{50}$ concentration of glutamate. Each point represents a single 384-well plate.

3.6. Data Analysis

1. Data are exported as the area under curve (AUC) for the full time course (*see* **Note 10**).
2. The generation of robust statistics *(12)* around pharmacologically relevant high ($4 \times EC_{50}$ standard mGluR5 agonist glutamate) and low controls (standard mGluR5 antagonist fenobam) are defined each in 16 wells of the 384-well plate or

32 wells (high) and 64 wells (low) of a 1536-well plate (*see* **Section 3.3**, Steps 1 and 3 for details on plate preparation and layout) allow the calculation of Z' as a surrogate of assay quality *(13)*.

3. Hit identification data – based on the robust mean ± 3 S.D. is further analyzed using a statistically determined activity flag algorithm within proprietary GlaxoSmithKline software.
4. Compound profiling data is analyzed using a four-parameter logistic fit of data normalized to internal high and low controls *(14)*.
5. Aequorin/Lumilux screening costs 25% as much per IC_{50} as compared to a traditional fluorescence-based method (excluding technology license costs, operator time, or instrument purchase/service costs). In addition, owing to the simpler assay methodology, the luminescence format requires less scientist's time.

4. Notes

1. Cells in continuous culture allow a window of 15–20 usable passages for screening campaigns. However, the use of assay ready cryopreserved cells in these studies eradicates this concern.
2. When using large batches of frozen cells it is vital to ensure that batch-to-batch variation is minimized such that assay performance and reagent pharmacology remain consistent.
3. When using assay ready cryopreserved cells there is little direct evidence that cell viability post-loading has a direct impact on luminescence counts, but there is no doubt that in some cases the inclusion of the "post-thaw" (Step 7, **Section 3.1**) where cells are incubated for 1 h at 37°C in media after defrosting and before cell loading does afford improved viability and generation of an acceptable signal from otherwise dim, relatively low signal reagents. This is often necessary with cells types that are particularly sensitive to DMSO or endogenous ligands which may be present in the freezing media.
4. The contents of the cell culture media, loading and dilution buffer must be examined for any potential to adversely affect signal magnitude or receptor pharmacology. For example, while pluronic acid F68 is beneficial for compound solubility with this reagent, this must also be established in every case.

5. Using the Lumilux an "area under curve" measurement of 40,000 flash luminescence counts is the minimum acceptable signal level for a reagent to be considered robustly fit for purpose of a hit identification or long-term compound profiling campaign. This signal must be stable over time both in terms of test occasion to test occasion (vital for concerted SAR campaigns) and over time within a test occasion (vital for prolonged hit identification plate runs).
6. Optimal cell loading and post-dilution signal stability (typically 4–6 h) times vary, and while this reagent gives identical signal magnitude and pharmacology whether loaded for anything from 3 to 24 h, this must be determined on a case-by-case basis as optimized loading times can range from 90 min to 30 h.
7. As with any assay using intact live cells, sensitivity to the solvent DMSO must be characterized, and the assay must be robustly resistant to a final assay concentration to be able to screen compounds at sufficiently high concentrations for hit identification purposes. Generally aequorin assays tolerate final concentrations of DMSO in excess of 1% which is regarded as a benchmark of acceptability.
8. We have observed a relationship between cell number and response. 1536-well hit identification screening efforts use 1000 to 5000 cells per well while for 384-well assays an acceptable signal is usually generated by 2500 to 15,000 cells per well. Varying cell density can impact observed pharmacology, thus when a cell density is selected it must be closely adhered to.
9. Lack of signal stability over prolonged plate runs (fully automated plate runs can take 4 h to run 50 plates) can be alleviated by loading a single large batch of cells and diluting this in several smaller batches.
10. It is well established that target pharmacology and assay performance can be impacted by pipettor height and speed and addition volumes. Whilst these settings are appropriate for this target they may require modification for other targets or applications.
11. The Lumilux 1536-well head can wash tips between transfers. However, we have implemented a screening strategy where only those additions where the change in luminescence is to be measured are made by the Lumilux pipettor. Great care must be taken to ensure that liquid is not retained in the tips after any transfer or washing step. We have instituted a tip blotting step in the 1536 pipettor protocols to ensure the tips are fully dried after the tip washing cycle.

12. When screening a target where little or no tool compounds are available to evaluate pharmacology, it is possible to proceed with caution using the results of the standard robustness compound set to validate assay performance.
13. Within the Lumilux cells are added to plates from a self-emptying trough filled from a reservoir by means of a peristaltic pump. Certain cell types tolerate this step better than others, and it must be determined on a case-by-case basis. Its effect over a long plate run can be alleviated by diluting pre-loaded cells in several smaller batches.
14. It is important to accurately track the potency of standard agonist on every test occasion across time, and take this into account in defining the day-to-day agonist concentration ($4 \times EC_{50}$) for antagonist screening. For assay ready cryopreserved cells the standard deviation of agonist pEC_{50} over time is typically less than 0.2 log units.
15. Close tracking of a number of surrogates of assay quality: Z′, standard compounds, signal magnitude, cell viability (post-thaw and post-loading), allow the early identification of trends and highlight issues before they negatively impact assay performance.

Acknowledgments

The authors acknowledge the expertise and dedication of members of the Departments of Biological Reagents and Assay Development and Screening and Compound Profiling who made this body of work possible.

References

1. Posner, B. A. (2005) High-throughput screening-driven lead discovery: meeting the challenges of finding new therapeutics. *Curr. Op. Drug Disc. Dev.* **8**, 487–494.
2. Gribbon, P. and Andreas, S. (2005) High-throughput drug discovery: what can we expect from HTS? *Drug Disc. Today* **10**, 17–22.
3. Walters, W. P. and Namchuck, M. (2003) Designing screens: how to make your hits a hit. *Nat. Rev. Drug Disc.* **2**, 259–266.
4. Moore, K. and Rees, S. (2001) Cell-based versus isolated target screening: how lucky do you feel? *J. Biomol. Scr.* **6**, 66–74.
5. Hopkins, A. L. and Groom, C. R. (2002) The druggable genome. *Nat. Rev. Drug Disc.* **1**, 727–730.
6. Lefkowitz, R. J. (2004) Historical review: a brief history and personal retrospective of seven-transmembrane receptors. *Trends Pharm. Sci.* **25**, 413–422.
7. Berridge, M. J. (1993) Inositol triphosphate and calcium signalling. *Nature* **361**, 315–325.
8. Sullivan, E., Tucker, E. M., Dale, I. L. (1999). Measurement of $[Ca^{2+}]_i$ using the Fluometric imaging plate reader (FLIPR). In: Lambert, D.G. (ed.), *Calcium Signaling Protocols*, pp. 125–136. New Jersey: Humana Press.

9. Shimomura, O. and Johnson, F. H. (1970) Calcium binding, quantum yield, and emitting molecule in aequorin bioluminescence. *Nature* **227**(5265), 1356–1357.
10. Inouye, S., Noguchi, M., Sakaki, Y., Takagi, Y., Miyata, T., Iwanaga, S., Miyata, T., and Tsuji, FI. (1985) Cloning and sequence analysis of cDNA for the luminescent protein aequorin. *Proc. Nat. Ac. Sci. USA* **82**(10), 3154–3158.
11. Rizzuto, R., Brini, M., and Pozzan, T. (1993) Intracellular targeting of the photoprotein aequorin: a new approach for measuring, in living cells, Ca^{2+} concentrations in defined cellular compartments. *Cytotechnology* **11**(Suppl 1), S44–S46.
12. Royal Society of Chemistry – Analytical Methods Committee. (1989). Robust statistics – how not to reject outliers. *Analyst*, **114**, 1693–1697.
13. Zhang, J-H., Chung, D. Y., and Oldenberg, K. R. (1999) A simple statistical parameter for use in evaluation and validation of high throughput screening assays. *J. Biomol. Screen.* **4**, 67–73.
14. Bowen, W. P., and Jerman, J.C. (1995) Non-linear regression using spreadsheets. *Trends Pharmacol. Sci.* **16**, 413–417.

Chapter 14

BacMam: Versatile Gene Delivery Technology for GPCR Assays

Elizabeth A. Davenport, Parvathi Nuthulaganti, and Robert S. Ames

Summary

BacMam viruses are modified baculoviruses that contain mammalian expression cassettes for viral gene delivery and transient expression in mammalian cells. They are easily, inexpensively, and rapidly generated and provide a versatile solution for G protein-coupled receptor (GPCR) cell-based assay development. Using BacMam technology, target gene expression levels are easily controlled and simultaneous delivery of multiple genes is possible, for example, coexpression of a receptor and a G protein or a reporter gene. BacMam viruses are compatible with the GPCR cell-based assay formats typically used in high-throughput screening and provide an unparalleled level of experimental flexibility that is simply not possible when using stable recombinant cell lines.

Key words: BacMam, Modified baculovirus, Transient expression, Viral transduction, G protein-coupled receptors, GPCR, Cell-based assay.

1. Introduction

High-throughput screening (HTS) has become the primary approach for new lead discovery in the pharmaceutical industry and currently more than half of all screens are performed using cell-based assays *(1)*. Increasing screening throughput of compound collections of in excess of 1 million discrete chemical entities and a trend toward HT G protein-coupled receptor functional rather than binding assays necessitates a steady supply of high-quality, assay ready cells. In addition to the cells and assays used for the primary HTS target, there is also a requirement of cell-based assays for the key selectivity target(s) as well as rodent orthologues needed for down stream lead optimization and SAR

Wayne R. Leifert (ed.), *G Protein-Coupled Receptors in Drug Discovery, vol. 552*

Book doi: 10.1007/978-1-60327-317-6_14

screening. We have implemented BacMam virus gene delivery as means of rapidly generating robust and reproducible cell-based assays to support our GPCR screening activities.

We have recently reviewed our experiences with the technology and have documented the advantages we perceive in using BacMam-based transient gene delivery in lieu of stable cell lines to support cell-based drug discovery assays *(2–4)*. Data obtained with BacMam-expressed receptors are consistent with data obtained with stable cell lines *(5)*, but there are inherent advantages of BacMam as assays can be developed faster using transients than using stable cell lines. In addition, receptor expression levels can be easily controlled by titrating the amount of virus added to the host cells. BacMam has successfully been used to generate cell-based assays of GPCRs from each of the three main families of receptors and receptors, which are either G_i, G_q, or G_s coupled *(5)*. Recently, BacMam-expressed receptors have been used to support cell-based assays for several of GSK's GPCR lead optimization programs; notably fluorescent imaging plate reader (FLIPR) assays for characterization of Urotensin II receptor antagonists *(6)*, CCR5 receptor antagonists *(7)*, NK3 receptor antagonists *(8)*, GPR40 receptor antagonists *(9)*, as well as underpinning cAMP accumulation and GTPγS binding assays for an H3 antagonist program *(10)*. Several reports have also reported success with BacMam-transduced cells in support of high-content β-arrestin–green fluorescent protein translocation GPCR assays *(11–13)*.

Details of the BacMam transfer vectors and methods for virus production have been described previously *(14, 15)*. It is not our intent in this chapter to describe functional assay methodology but rather to present methods for how one would go about using a BacMam virus encoding a GPCR of interest to transduce cells for use in a GPCR cell-based assay described elsewhere in this volume. While the procedures we describe will be exemplified with FLIPR assays, the procedures used to transduce the host cells and optimize the transduction conditions will be readily applicable to other assay formats.

2. Materials

2.1. Biological Reagents, Buffers, and Kits

1. GPCR BacMam and G protein chimera BacMam (titer $\sim 1 \times 10^8$) are generated as described *(14, 15)* and stored at 4°C in the dark.
2. U-2 OS (ATCC, Rockville, MD), Grip Tite 293 MSR (Invitrogen, Carlsbad, CA), HEK-293 (ATCC), CHOK1 (ATCC) cells, or other transducible mammalian host cells *(16)*.

3. Dulbecco's modified Eagle's medium (DMEM)/F12 cell medium supplemented with 10% gamma-irradiated and heat-inactivated fetal bovine serum (FBS; JRH Biosciences, Lenexa, KS).
4. Trypsin (JRH biosciences).
5. Target-specific ligands: ADP, histamine, acetylcholine (Sigma, St. Louis, MO).
6. FLIPR ligand dilution buffer: Hank's Buffered Salt Solution (HBSS) with calcium, magnesium, and 20 m*M* HEPES (pH 7.4; Invitrogen) and supplemented with 0.1% Bovine serum albumin (BSA; Sigma).
7. Probenecid stock: 285 mg probenecid in 1 mL 1 *M* NaOH (Sigma). Stock must be prepared fresh daily. Do not store.
8. FLIPR assay buffer: HBSS containing 2.5 m*M* probenecid (Sigma).
9. Brilliant Black-Fluo-4 kit (Molecular Devices Corporation, Sunnyvale, CA).
10. 2 m*M* Fluo-4 stock (1000 ×): 1 mg Fluo-4 (Molecular Devices Corporation) in 450 μL 20% Pluronic Acid (Sigma).
11. 50 m*M* Brilliant Black Stock (100 ×): 2 g Brilliant Black in 46 mL distilled H_2O.
12. Brilliant Black/Fluo-4 loading buffer: FLIPR assay buffer containing 500 μ*M* Brilliant Black and 2 μ*M* Fluo-4.

2.2. Plasticware

1. Sterile 15 mL (Corning, Lowell, MA) and 50 mL (BD Falcon, Franklin Lakes, NJ) conical tubes.
2. T75 and T150 tissue culture-treated cell culture flasks (Corning).
3. Sterile reagent troughs (Corning).
4. 384-well black, clear bottom TC-treated plates (Greiner, Monroe, NC, USA) and 384-well Black, clear bottom poly-D-lysine-coated plates (Greiner).
5. 384-well white polypropylene plates (Greiner).

2.3. Equipment

1. 37°C water bath.
2. Hemocytometer or other cell counting/viability instrumentation, such as CEDEX cell counter (Innovatis, Malvern, PA) or Vi-cell (Beckman coulter, Fullerton, CA).
3. Centrifuge and rotor for 15 and 50 mL tubes.
4. 8- and 12-channel (50/850 μL) multi-channel pipettor (Matrix Technologies, Hudson, NH).
5. Humidified tissue culture incubator.
6. Flexstation, FLIPR, or FLIPR Tetra instrument (Molecular Devices Corporation).

3. Methods

3.1. BacMam-Transduced Cellular Systems for Robust and Reliable Functional Assays

In both basic research and drug discovery, the ability to quickly develop specific, high-quality assays is a competitive advantage. For drug discovery efforts utilizing cellular systems, such as GPCR functional assay screening, BacMam reagents may be utilized to quickly compare multiple assay formats as well as a range of potential host systems during the initial phase of assay development. An early critical step in assay development, whether utilizing endogenous receptor, stable cell line, or transient system such as BacMam, is the characterization and choice of cellular host systems. Identification of a host system with no (or low) endogenous functional activity of target specific ligand is essential for development of a specific engineered cellular system. Besides allowing quick identification and reliable transient expression of GPCR targets for identification and characterization of agonists and antagonists, BacMam allows for changes in target expression levels which enable characterization of partial agonists/antagonists *(2, 7)*.

For drug discovery work, the development of streamlined assay protocols with low false-positive and false-negative hit statistics, and excellent correlation of well-to-well, plate-to-plate, and day-to-day experimental results leads to high-quality data and lower costs because of fewer failed plates. During assay development, we measure efficacy (background, signal, and signal-to-background ratio), agonist and antagonist potency (pXC_{50}), and Z' *(17)* from low and high signal control wells. Through multiple iterations assays are optimized for HTS and compound profiling. The methods below describe how to define and optimize a target-specific system utilizing a GPCR target BacMam to produce a robust and reliable assay.

3.2. Preparation of BacMam Transductions

The optimization of the BacMam transduction concentration, transduction time, and host cell line are important steps for the use of BacMam technology for GPCR assays. Transduction of mammalian cells can be performed in tissue culture flasks as described previously *(15)* or within the assay plate. To prepare for a FLIPR intracellular calcium assay, we recommend BacMam transduction directly in the assay plate. Below protocol will outline the process for initial optimization of BacMam concentration for a G_q protein-coupled receptor, assuming testing of duplicate 384-well plates in a traditional FLIPR assay for two BacMams per assay plate.

Host cells (i.e., HEK-293, CHO, U-2 OS) are maintained in Corning T150 culture flasks. Cells are cultured in DMEM/F12 medium and are split twice a week at 1:5 or 1:10 as needed depending on the host cells.

3.2.1. Basic BacMam Transduction Protocol

1. Recover host cells (HEK-293, CHOK1, or U-2 OS) from tissue culture flasks via trypsin treatment and add cells to conical centrifuge tubes (*see* **Note 1**).
2. Centrifuge cells (e.g., 100 × *g*) to remove medium and resuspend cells in growth medium to a density of approximately 1 × 10^6 cells/mL.
3. Determine cell density and viability by Trypan blue exclusion via hemocytometer (or other cell counting instrument such as CEDEX or Vi-Cell).
4. Resuspend cells to a final density of 3 × 10^5 viable cells/mL (*see* **Note 2**).
5. Combine cells and GPCR BacMam into four 15 mL conical tubes as described in **Table 1**.

Table 1
Single transduction BacMam titration table to optimize target BacMam concentration

[BacMam] (%)	Host cell volume (mL)	BacMam volume (μL)
0	10	0
1	10	100
3	10	300
6	10	600

To test a range of volume-to-volume ratio of target BacMam to cells in duplicate plates, mix 10 mL of host cells (3 × 10^5 cells/mL) with BacMam volumes specified in the third column in 15 mL conical tubes. In secondary tests, one can refine or expand the range of concentrations tested, depending on the host cells and results from the initial experiment.

6. Gently mix cells and BacMam mixture by hand.
7. Transfer cells and BacMam to sterile reagent trough.
8. Using multichannel pipette, dispense 50 μL (1.5 × 10^4 cells per well) of cell and BacMam mixture to 384-well plates as shown in **Fig. 1**.
9. Incubate cell transduction plates 18–24 h in humidified 37°C tissue culture incubator (*see* **Note 3**).

3.2.2. GPCR Functional Assay and Data Analysis

1. Load cells with appropriate FLIPR dyes as Brilliant Black-Fluo-4 Kit protocols:
   a. Aspirate medium from wells.
   b. Add 20 μL loading dye.
   c. Incubate cells at 37°C, 5% CO_2 for 1 h.

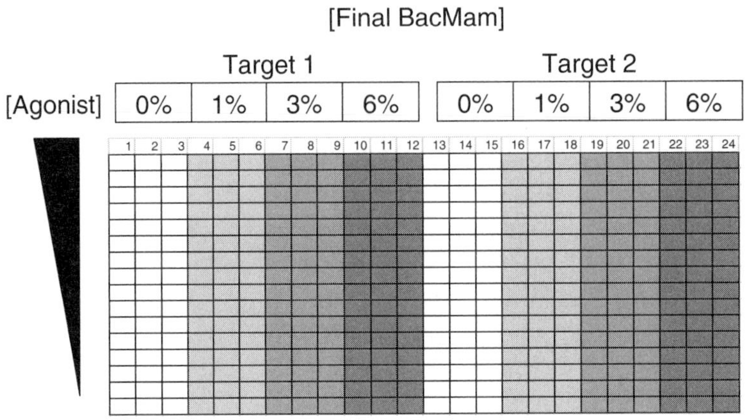

Fig. 1. A plate map of cells transduced with a range of BacMam concentrations. Agonist dilutions are prepared in 384-well polypropylene plates with high concentration in row A, 1:3 dilutions through row O, and no agonist control in row P. The plate can accommodate two targets in this format.

2. Prepare threefold concentration of serially diluted ligand in FLIPR ligand dilution buffer (1:2 or 1:3 dilutions with 12 points) in 384-well polypropylene plate (*see* **Note 4**).
3. Dose cells with 10 μL per well target-specific ligand as shown in **Fig. 1** Platemap.
4. Read on FLIPR instrument as per standard protocols.
5. Graph data (for FLIPR max–min) and calculate pEC_{50} as exemplified in **Fig. 2** in which agonist dose–response curves were obtained on FLIPR from U-2 OS cells transduced with varying concentrations of a BacMam encoding the rat P2Y1 receptor.

3.2.3. Interpretation of Results

From the results presented in **Fig. 2**, at the concentration tested there was no response to ADP agonist in untransduced U-2 OS cells and the potency of ADP was similar regardless of BacMam concentration. However, the most efficacious response was observed upon transduction with 1% BacMam (*see* **Note 5**).

3.3. Optimizing Cotransduction Conditions: Receptor and G protein

There are times when more than one BacMam must be introduced into host cells in order to create a biological system that is functionally responsive (*see* **Note 6**). For example, G_i-coupled receptors can be evaluated in FLIPR assays through coexpression of chimeric G proteins. Also, new cell-based assay methods for measuring intracellular calcium levels or cAMP concentrations for G_i-and G_s-coupled receptors expressed in suspension cells are becoming more common place. These assay formats are amenable to BacMam

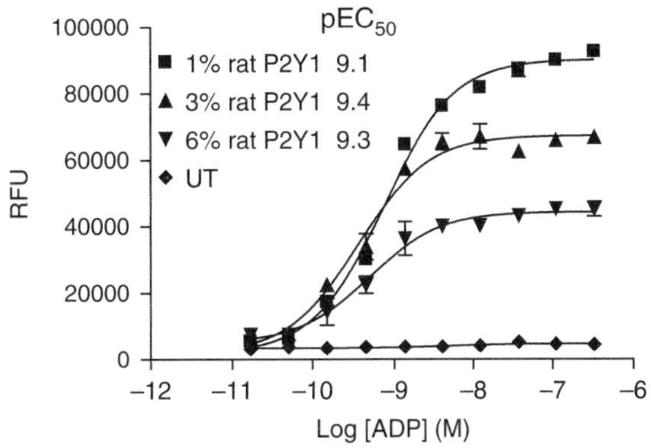

Fig. 2. Initial titration of rat P2Y1 BacMam in U-2 OS cells. U-2 OS cells (3×10^5 cells/mL) were transduced with 0%, 1%, 3%, and 6% rat P2Y1 BacMam for 20 h at 37°C (UT, untransduced U-2 OS cells). Transduced cells dosed with ADP agonist were read on FlexStation using Calcium 3 kit (MDC) protocol. In this experiment, the most robust results were obtained with U-2 OS cells transduced with 1% BacMam. This assay was further optimized to reduce the final BacMam concentration to lower than 1% (data not shown).

delivery as well. For example, aequorin protein may be coexpressed with GPCR target via dual transduction BacMam approach (*see* **Note 7**).

3.3.1. Dual Transduction Protocol: Target and Chimeric G Protein BacMams

1. Follow Steps 1–5 in **Section 3.2.1**.
2. Mix cells, target-specific BacMam, and chimeric G protein BacMam as described in **Table 2** (*see* **Note 8**).
3. Proceed with remaining steps in **Sections 3.2.1** and **3.2.2** (*see* **Note 9**).

3.3.2. Interpretation of Dual Transduction (GPCR + G Protein Chimera) Experiments

As depicted in **Fig. 3a**, changes in the target BacMam concentration will result in a range of potencies and efficacies. Since the lowest concentration of BLT-1 BacMam with the highest efficacy was 0.5% (in the presence of 0.5% $G_{\alpha 16}$) in U-2 OS, this concentration was utilized for future optimization studies. BLT1 BacMam was also cotransduced with a range of chimeric G protein G_{qi5} concentrations (data not shown) in the same experiment. In **Fig. 3b**, data for 0.5% BLT1 BacMam alone versus cotransduction with 0.5% G_{qi5} or $G_{\alpha 16}$ are plotted. Note that BLT1 alone had low efficacy and potency, while coupling with chimeric G proteins resulted in a marked increase in efficacy in response to LTB4 treatment. Dual transduction of chimeric G protein Gα16 with BLT1 resulted in the highest potency response to ligand and therefore was the reagent selected for further assay optimization steps.

Table 2
Dual transduction BacMam titration table to optimize target BacMam concentration and choose optimal chimeric G protein BacMam

Target		G protein chimera		Host cells
[BacMam] (%)	Volume (μL)	BacMam [%]	Volume (μL)	Volume (mL)
0	0	0.50	50	10
0.10	10	0.50	50	10
0.50	50	0.50	50	10
1	100	0.50	50	10
3	300	0.50	50	10
6	600	0.50	50	10

To identify the best coupling agent for the target, use the table above to set up dual transductions with multiple chimeric G proteins in parallel. For initial testing of dual transductions, vary the GPCR target BacMam concentration while keeping the chimeric G protein BacMam concentrations constant. Once the optimal target concentration is determined, the G protein BacMam concentration is optimized by fixing the target BacMam concentration at the optimal level and varying the G protein concentration.

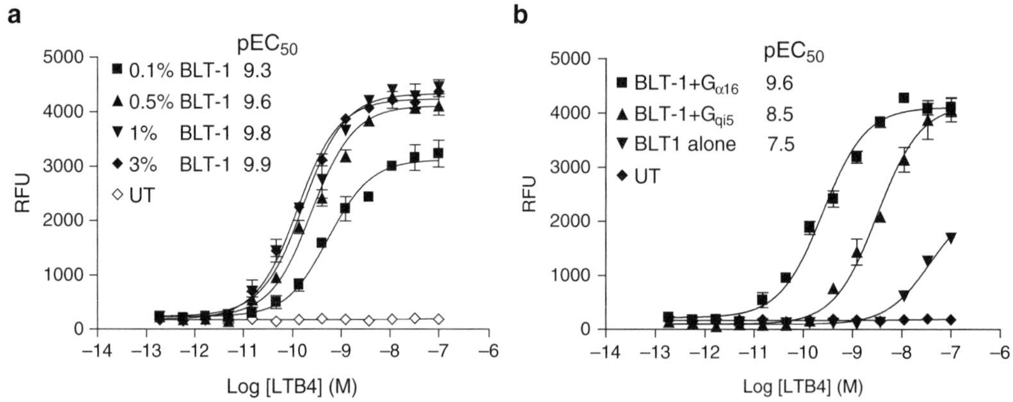

Fig. 3. **(A)** Initial optimization of dual transduction conditions. A range of BLT-1 BacMam concentrations (0%, 0.1%, 0.5%, 1%, and 3%) were transduced in U-2 OS cells (3×10^5 cells/mL) in the presence of 0.5% chimeric G protein $G_{\alpha16}$ BacMam (UT, untransduced U-2 OS cells). Cells were incubated 20 h at 37°C, loaded with dye, dosed with LTB4 agonist, and then read on a FLIPR Tetra using Fluo-4 Brilliant Black no-wash FLIPR protocol. Results demonstrated that 0.5% BLT-1 BacMam was the lowest concentration required for optimal efficacy and potency. Further assay development was continued with 0.5% BLT-1 BacMam-transduced cells. **(B)** Determination of best chimeric G protein BacMam for optimal target performance. Dual transductions were prepared as described in **Table 2**. Duplicate plates were prepared by mixing U-2 OS cells (3×10^5 cells/mL) with 0.5% BLT-1 BacMam alone or in combination with 0.5% $G_{\alpha16}$ or 0.5% G_{qi5} BacMam (UT, untransduced U-2 OS cells). As per outlined protocol, cells were incubated for 20 h at 37°C. Following dye load and treatment with LTB4 agonist, as per Fluo-4 Brilliant Black no-wash FLIPR protocol, plates were read on FLIPR Tetra. Results demonstrated that U-2 OS cells cotransduced with BLT-1 and $G_{\alpha16}$ BacMams had similar efficacy but greater potency than cells cotransduced with BLT1 and G_{qi5} BacMams.

3.4. Optimizing Transduction Conditions: Varying Host Cells

The use of untransduced cells (no BacMam control) is an important control to determine the endogenous response to the test ligand in the host cells. If there is a weak response in the target-transduced host cells or potent and efficacious response to the ligand in the host cells in the absence of transduced target, proceed with BacMam transductions in a larger host cell panel.

3.4.1. Characterizing BacMam Expression in a Range of Host Cells

1. Trypsinize different host cells, such as U-2 OS cells, CHOK1 cells, or HEK-293 cells (*see* **Note 10**).
2. Proceed with steps outlined in **3.2.1** and **3.2.2** (*see* **Notes 2** and **11**).

In **Fig. 4**, U-2 OS and HEK MSRII cells were cotransduced with 0.5% BLT1 and 0.5% $G_{\alpha16}$ BacMams. While the LTB4 agonist potencies were quite similar, U-2 OS cells had a more efficacious response to the ligand, which is highly desirable for development of a robust and reliable cellular assay.

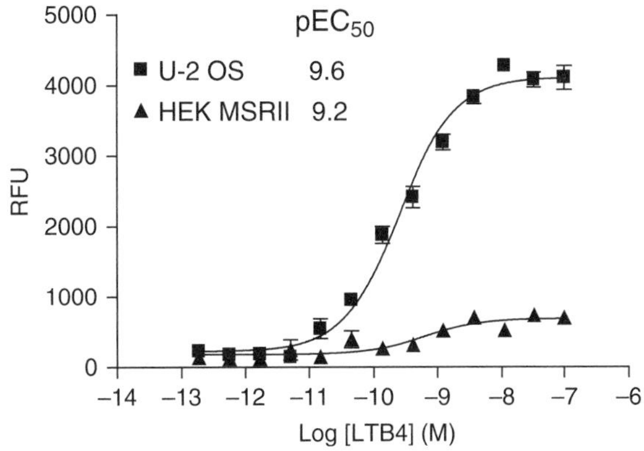

Fig. 4. Testing host cell lines for optimal target expression. U-2 OS and HEK MSRII (HEK-293 cells engineered to express macrophage scavenger receptor) cells (3×10^5 cells/mL) were cotransduced with 0.5% BLT1 and 0.5% $G_{\alpha16}$ BacMams for 18 h at 37°C. As per Fluo-4 Brilliant Black no-wash FLIPR protocol, cells were loaded with dye, dosed with LTB4 agonist and plates were read on FLIPR Tetra. Results demonstrated that LTB4 had higher potency and efficacy in U-2 OS cells transduced with BLT1 and $G_{\alpha16}$ compared to HEK MSRII cells cotransduced with the same BacMams.

3.5. Transduction of Frozen Host Cells

Cryopreserved host cells are an excellent alternative to freshly maintained cells and may be substituted for freshly maintained cells without alterations to the base transduction protocol. In most cases, frozen cells utilized as transduction hosts have similar performance to freshly maintained cells in FLIPR assays (**Fig. 5**) (*see* **Note 12**).

1. Prewarm medium to 37°C.
2. Remove cryopreserved cells from liquid nitrogen.

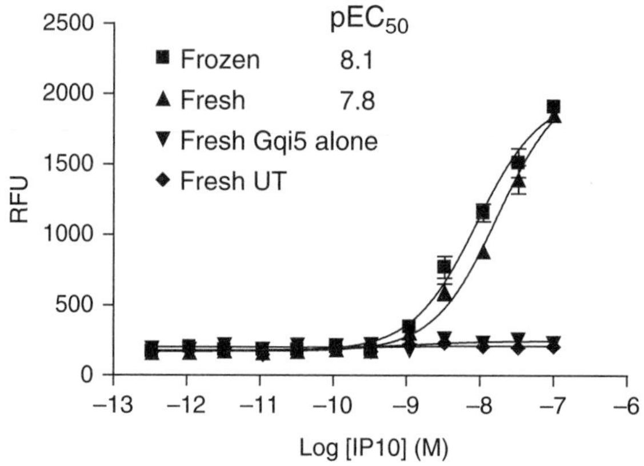

Fig. 5. Functional performance of freshly maintained versus frozen stocks of host cells. Freshly maintained and thawed frozen U-2 OS cells (3×10^5 cells/mL) were cotransduced with 1% mCXCR3 and 0.5% G_{qi5} G protein chimera BacMam (UT, untransduced cells). Following 18 h transduction at 37°C, cells were loaded with dye as per standard Fluo-4 Brilliant Black no-wash FLIPR protocol and dosed with IP10 ligand. Similar IP10 efficacy and potency were observed from transductions prepared with freshly maintained and frozen U-2 OS cells.

3. Thaw frozen cell aliquots rapidly with agitation in 37°C water bath.
4. Continue with Step 2 of the BacMam transduction procedure in **Sections 3.2.1** and **3.2.2** (*see* **Note 13**).

4. Notes

1. U-2 OS cells are a good starting place for BacMam-based GPCR assays as these cells are highly susceptible to BacMam transduction and lack many of the endogenous receptors present on HEK-293 and other mammalian host cells typically used for cell-based GPCR assays *(18)*.
2. Optimal host cell concentration will vary, depending on the characteristics of the host cell and the assay readout. Cell density may be optimized once functional response is confirmed. For 384-well transductions for FLIPR assays, 1.0×10^4 cells per well is often optimal transduction cell density for U-2 OS cells while higher cell densities (1.5×10^4 to 2.0×10^4 cells per well) are generally best for HEK-293-derived and CHO-derived host cells for 24 h end-point read.
3. For many GPCR targets, 24 h transduction time results in optimal expression and excellent functional response. As with transient transfections, incubation time required for optimal

functional response is target specific. If signal window is low, test functional response following 48 and 72 h transduction time. BacMam concentration, transduction time, cell density, cell host line, and target GPCR are codependent variables, so changes in transduction time will often require re-optimization of some or all of the other experimental variables.

4. For each cell line, a specific ligand for an endogenous receptor may be included as an additional control (e.g., histamine for U-2 OS cells, muscarine or acetylcholine for HEK-293 cells and ADP for CHO cells).
5. At completion of the initial reagent validation experiment, there are several kinds of follow-up experiments that can be initiated to improve the assay in terms of reproducibility and agonist-induced efficacy and potency. For example, in **Fig. 2**, 1% BacMam results in the most efficacious response. We repeated the basic transduction protocol for this target, with further refinements to transduction levels (0.1%, 0.5%, 1%, 2%) and measured not only efficacy and potency via dose response, but also additional wells for Z' controls (16 no ligand wells and 16 EC_{100} wells for agonist assays or DMSO first addtion with 16 buffer and 16 EC_{80} second addtion for antagonist assays (9)). From this experiment, the final optimized BacMam concentration was 0.1%, which was the concentration with the greatest efficacy, most potent response, and lowest variation as determined by Z' calculation.
6. Multiple BacMams may be introduced to cells simultaneously. We have introduced as many as five BacMams into host cells concomitantly. It must be noted, however, that individual host cells will have some transduction limit. Also, extreme overexpression of some targets may have deleterious effects on cell health or functional performance.
7. For suspension assay formats, BacMam transductions may be performed in culture flasks or cell stacks. Following the 24–48 h transduction time, cells are harvested and used directly as per the aequorin or cAMP detection protocols.
8. $G_{\alpha 16}$ and G_{qi5} are commonly used G protein chimeras. Refer to **Table 2** to set up separate transductions in parallel with the target in combination with each chimeric G protein. Other G protein chimeras or accessory proteins may also be cotransduced as additional variables.
9. If background is observed because of G protein coupling to endogenous GPCRs, optimize the G protein BacMam concentration by fixing the target BacMam concentration at the lowest dose that results in highest efficacy and potency and cotransduce a range of G protein BacMam concentrations as described in **Table 2** for the optimization of target BacMam concentration.

10. When using HEK-293 cells in FLIPR assays, utilize poly-D-lysine-coated assay plates to improve well-to-well reproducibility. Alternatively, HEK-293 cells that are engineered to express macrophage scavenger receptor II (MSRII) *(19)*, such as the commercially available GripTite cells (Invitrogen), retain the high transduction efficiency of HEK-293 cells, yet display superior adherent properties. For these reasons, HEK-293 cells expressing MSRII are an excellent choice host cell for BacMam-transduced FLIPR assays and other adherent cell assays requiring wash steps.
11. HEK-293 and U-2 OS cells are excellent choices for first host cell panel, due to their excellent transduction efficiencies. A secondary panel of transducible host cells might include Saos-2, SH-SY5Y, CHOKI, BHK, Cos-1 and CV-1 cells, for example.
12. Cells to be used for FLIPR, aequorin, or cAMP measurements may also be transduced in flasks or cell stacks, harvested, and used directly or frozen for later use. If the transduced frozen cells are to be utilized for FLIPR assays, test effect of transduction time (24, 48, and 72 h) on freshly transduced cells prior to freezing cells. If there is a decline in efficacy or potency at 72 h, for example, keep the total time (transduction time plus the time cells are in assay plate) to 48 h, or where performance is optimal for transduction of fresh cells. For suspension assays formats such as cAMP measurement or aequorin, cells that are transduced, harvested, frozen, and then thawed for assay may require a thaw recovery time for best assay performance. For post-thaw recovery, use growth medium with gentle stirring and test various recovery times (15 min to several hours) and temperatures (37°C, room temperature, and 4°C).
13. The use of untransduced cells (no BacMam control) is important to determine the endogenous responses to ligand. If the G protein chimera is cotransduced with the target, then the G protein chimera transduced cells without the target is used as an additional control.

References

1. Fox, S., Farr-Jones, S., Sopchak, L., Boggs, A., Nicely, H.W., Khoury, R., et al. (2006) High-throughput screening: update on practices and success. *J. Biomol. Screen.* **11**, 864–869.
2. Kost, T.A., Condreay, J.P., Ames, R.S., Rees, S., Romanos, M.A. (2007) Implementation of BacMam virus gene delivery technology in a drug discovery setting. *Drug Discov. Today* **12**, 396–403.
3. Condreay, J.P., Ames, R.S., Hassan, N.J., Kost, T.A., Merrihew, R.V., Mossakowska, D.E., et al. (2006) Baculoviruses and mammalian cell-based assays for drug screening. *Adv. Virus. Res.* **68**, 255–286.
4. Ames, R.S., Kost, T.A., Condreay, J.P. (2007) BacMam technology and its application to drug discovery. *Expert Opin. Drug Discov.* **2**, 1669–1681.

5. Ames, R., Fornwald, J., Nuthulaganti, P., Trill, J., Foley, J., Buckley, P., et al. (2004) BacMam recombinant baculoviruses in G protein-coupled receptor drug discovery. *Receptors Channels* **10**, 99–107.
6. Behm, D.J., Stankus, G., Doe, C.P., Willette, R.N., Sarau, H.M., Foley, J.J., et al. (2006) The peptidic urotensin-II receptor ligand GSK248451 possesses less intrinsic activity than the low-efficacy partial agonists SB-710411 and urantide in native mammalian tissues and recombinant cell systems. *Br. J. Pharmacol.* **148**, 173–190.
7. Kenakin, T., Jenkinson, S., Watson, C. (2006) Determining the potency and molecular mechanism of action of insurmountable antagonists. *J. Pharmacol. Exp. Ther.* **319**, 710–723.
8. Sanger, G.J., Tuladhar, B.R., Brown, J., Aziz, E., Sivakumar, D., Furness, J.B. (2007) Modulation of peristalsis by NK3 receptor antagonism in guinea-pig isolated ileum is revealed as intraluminal pressure is raised. *Auton. Autacoid. Pharmacol.* **27**, 105–111.
9. Briscoe, C.P., Peat, A.J., McKeown, S.C., Corbett, D.F., Goetz, A.S., Littleton, T.R., et al. (2006) Pharmacological regulation of insulin secretion in MIN6 cells through the fatty acid receptor GPR40: identification of agonist and antagonist small molecules. *Br. J. Pharmacol.* **148**, 619–628.
10. Medhurst, A.D., Atkins, A.R., Beresford, I.J., Brackenborough, K., Briggs, M.A., Calver, A.R., et al. (2007) GSK189254, a novel H3 receptor antagonist that binds to histamine H3 receptors in Alzheimer's disease brain and improves cognitive performance in preclinical models. *J. Pharmacol. Exp. Ther.* **321**, 1032–1045.
11. Garippa, R.J., Hoffman, A.F., Gradl, G., Kirsch, A. (2006) High-throughput confocal microscopy for beta-arrestin-green fluorescent protein translocation G protein-coupled receptor assays using the Evotec Opera. *Methods Enzymol.* **414**, 99–120.
12. Hoffman, A.F., Garippa, R.J. (2007) A pharmaceutical company user's perspective on the potential of high content screening in drug discovery. *Methods Mol. Biol.* **356**, 19–31.
13. Oakley, R.H., Hudson, C.C., Sjaastad, M.D., Loomis, C.R. (2006) The ligand-independent translocation assay: an enabling technology for screening orphan G protein-coupled receptors by arrestin recruitment. *Methods Enzymol.* **414**, 50–63.
14. Merrihew, R.V., Kost, T.A., Condreay, J.P. (2004) Baculovirus-mediated gene delivery into mammalian cells. *Methods Mol. Biol.* **246**, 355–365.
15. Fornwald, J.A., Wang, D., Lu, Q., Wang, D., Ames, R.S. (2007) Gene expression in mammalian cells using BacMam, a modified baculovirus system. In: Murhammer, D.W., (ed.), *Methods in Molecular Biology, Baculovirus and Insect Cell Expression Protocols.* Humana Press, Totowa, New Jersey, pp. 95–114.
16. Organelle Lights^{TM} reagents. 2007. http://www.invitrogen.com/content.cfm?pageid=11890
17. Zhang, J.H., Chung, T.D., Oldenburg, K.R. (1999) A simple statistical parameter for use in evaluation and validation of high throughput screening assays. *J. Biomol. Screen.* **4**, 67–73.
18. Ames, R., Nuthulaganti, P., Fornwald, J., Shabon, U., van der Keyl, H., Elshourbagy, N. (2004) Heterologous expression of G protein-coupled receptors in U-2 OS osteosarcoma cells. *Receptors Channels* **10**, 117–124.
19. Robbins, A.K., Horlick, RA. (1998) Macrophage scavenger receptor confers an adherent phenotype to cells in culture. *Bio Techniques* **25**, 240–244.

Chapter 15

Yeast Assays for G Protein-Coupled Receptors

Simon J. Dowell and Andrew J. Brown

Summary

The functional coupling of heterologous G protein-coupled receptors (GPCRs) to the pheromone-response pathway of the budding yeast *Saccharomyces cerevisiae* is well established as an experimental system for ligand identification and for characterizing receptor pharmacology and signal transduction mechanisms. A number of groups have developed yeast strains using various modifications to this signaling pathway, especially manipulation of the G protein alpha subunit Gpa1p, to facilitate coupling of a wide range of mammalian GPCRs. The attraction of these systems is the simplicity and low cost of yeast cell culture enabling the assays to be set up rapidly in academic or industrial labs without the requirement for expensive technical equipment. Furthermore, haploid yeasts contain only a single GPCR capable of activating the pathway, which can be deleted and replaced with a mammalian GPCR providing a cell-based functional assay in a eukaryotic host free from endogenous responses. The yeast strains used for this purpose are highly engineered and may be covered by intellectual property for commercial applications in some countries. However, they can usually be obtained from the host labs for research purposes covered by a Material Transfer Agreement and/or licence where appropriate. The protocols herein assume that such strains have been acquired and begin with introduction of the heterologous GPCR into the engineered yeast cell. Assays are configured such that agonism of the GPCR leads to induction of a reporter gene and/or growth of the yeast. A number of parameters may be optimized to generate robust experimental formats, in high-density microtiter plates, that may be used for ligand identification and pharmacological characterization.

Key words: Yeast, GPCR, Assay, Chimeric G protein, Pheromone-response pathway, 7-transmembrane, Receptor, High-throughput screen, Structure–activity relationship, Compound profiling.

1. Introduction

The pheromone-response pathway of *Saccharomyces cerevisiae* has long been studied as a model for G protein-coupled receptor (GPCR)-mediated signal transduction and has elucidated many

Wayne R. Leifert (ed.), *G Protein-Coupled Receptors in Drug Discovery, vol. 552*

Book doi: 10.1007/978-1-60327-317-6_15

regulatory mechanisms that are conserved in evolution *(1, 2)*. Haploid yeast cells secrete peptide pheromones that bind to GPCRs on yeast of the alternative mating type, leading to activation of heterotrimeric G proteins composed of Gpa1p (G_α), Ste4p (G_β), and Ste18p (G_γ). $G_{\beta\gamma}$ transduces the signal to a mitogen-activated protein (MAP) kinase cascade leading to cell cycle arrest, mediated by the cyclin-dependent kinase inhibitor Far1p, and induction of mating genes such as *FUS1*, to prepare the haploid cells for mating. The regulator of G protein signaling (RGS) protein Sst2p is a principal negative regulator of the pathway.

In early developments of an assay system for heterologous GPCRs it was shown that some mammalian GPCRs could couple directly to the yeast heterotrimeric G protein *(3, 4)*. Subsequently, systems were improved through a number of steps including: deletion of *SST2* to sensitize the pathway, deletion of *FAR1* to prevent cell cycle arrest enabling a positive readout for agonism, and the development of chimeric G proteins *(1)*. Several reporter genes have been described, typically utilizing the *FUS1* promoter which is induced by activation of the pheromone-response signal transduction pathway. These include *HIS3* (His3p; *(3)*), *lacZ* (β-galactosidase; *(5)*), and EGFP (enhanced green fluorescent protein; *(6)*). The methods described herein are based on the GlaxoSmithKline system *(7, 8)* utilizing the *HIS3* reporter.

2. Materials

2.1. Yeast Culture and Maintenance

1. YPD: 1% Bacto-yeast extract (Difco), 2% Bacto-peptone (Difco), 2% dextrose in distilled water. For plates, 2% Bacto-agar (Difco) is added. The medium is autoclaved at 121°C for 15 min and stored at room temperature. Plates are stored at 4°C. For general information on yeast media and selection, *see* Sherman *(9)*.
2. WHAUL powder (*see* **Note 1**): 1.2 g L-arginine (HCl), 6.0 g L-aspartic acid, 6.0 g L-glutamic acid (monosodium), 1.8 g L-lysine, 1.2 g L-methionine, 3.0 g L-phenylalanine, 22.5 g L-serine, 12 g L-threonine, 1.8 g L-tyrosine, and 9.0 g L-valine. Solid ingredients are combined and mixed by grinding in a clean dry mortar and pestle until homogeneous. The mixture is stored desiccated at room temperature.
3. 10× YNB: 6.7 g yeast nitrogen base without amino acids (Difco) is dissolved in 100 mL milliQ H_2O, filter sterilized (0.2 μm pore size), and stored at 4°C.
4. 40% glucose solution in water, filter sterilized (0.2 μm pore size) and stored at room temperature.

5. 100× Histidine: 2 mg/mL L-histidine (Sigma, Poole, UK) solution in water, filter sterilized (0.2 µm pore size) and stored at 4°C.
6. WHAUL medium (pH 7): 1.1 g of WHAUL powder is dissolved in 750 mL deionized H_2O. For agar plates, 20 g Bacto-agar is added. The pH is adjusted to 7.0 with NaOH and the volume adjusted to 850 mL. The solution is autoclaved at 121°C for 15 min. The following supplements are added to the broth or melted agar: 100 mL 10 × YNB, 50 mL 40% glucose.
7. WHAUL medium pH 5.5: as for WHAUL pH7.0 except the pH is adjusted to 5.5.
8. WHAUL+His: 10mL 100 × histidine is added per liter of WHAUL medium (pH 5.5).

2.2. Yeast Transformation

1. 1 *M* LiAc: 1 *M* lithium acetate, filter sterilized (0.2 µm pore size) and stored at room temperature.
2. 50% PEG: 50 g PEG3350 is dissolved in distilled water to a final volume of 100 mL, filter sterilized (0.45 µm pore size) and stored at room temperature.
3. 10× TE: 0.1 *M* Tris-HCl (pH 7.5), 0.01 *M* EDTA.
4. LiAc-TE: 5 mL 1 *M* LiAc, 5 mL 10 × TE, 40 mL H_2O.
5. LiPEG-TE: 5 mL 1 *M* LiAc, 5 mL 10 × TE, 40 mL 50% PEG.
6. ssDNA: 200 µL aliquots of single-stranded DNA (Salmon Testes DNA; Sigma-Aldrich, Dorset, England) are prepared in microfuge tubes, boiled for 10 min, cooled immediately on ice, and frozen at –20°C. For best transformation efficiency, aliquots should not be thawed more than twice; however, used aliquots can be re-boiled.

2.3. Yeast GPCR Assay

1. FDGlu: Fluorescein-D-glucopyranoside (Invitrogen; Molecular Probes) (*see* **Note 2**). Stocks of 20 m*M* FDGlu in 100% DMSO are stored at –20°C.
2. FDG: Fluorescein di-β-D-galactopyranoside (Invitrogen, Paisley, UK; Molecular Probes) (*see* **Note 3**). Stocks of 20 m*M* FDG in 100% DMSO are stored at –20°C.
3. CPRG: Chlorophenol red-β-D-galactopyranoside (Sigma). Stocks of 1 mg/mL CPRG in H_2O are filter sterilized and stored at 4°C.
4. 3-AT: 3-amino-1,2,4-triazole (Sigma, *see* **Note 4**). 1 *M* stock in MilliQ water, filter sterilized. The solution is stored in the dark at 4°C (wrap bottle in foil). 3-AT is heat labile and will be destroyed if added to medium hotter than 55°C. Make fresh every month. Handle this product with care, the solid is carcinogenic.

5. 10× BU salts: 70 g $Na_2HP0_4.7H_2O$, 30 g NaH_2PO_4, made up to 1 L in MilliQ water and adjusted to pH 7.0. The solution is autoclaved at 121°C for 15 min and stored at room temperature.
6. FDGlu assay medium (200 mL): 20 mL 10 × YNB, 10 mL 40% glucose, 20 mL 10× BU salts, 100 μL 20 m*M* FDGlu (giving final concentration of 10 μ*M*), 400 μL 1 *M* 3-AT (giving default final concentration of 2 m*M*; *see* **Note 4**). Make up to 200 mL with WHAUL medium (pH 7.0).
7. FDG assay medium: 20 mL 10× YNB, 10 mL 40% glucose, 20 mL 10× BU salts, 100 μL 20 m*M* FDG (giving final concentration of 10 μ*M*), 400 μL 1 *M* 3-AT (giving default final concentration of 2 m*M*; *see* **Note 4**). Make up to 200 mL with WHAUL medium (pH 7.0).
8. CPRG assay medium: 20 mL 10× YNB, 10 mL 40% glucose, 20 mL 10× BU salts, 20 mL 1 mg/mL CPRG, 400μL 1 *M* 3-AT (giving default final concentration of 2 m*M*; *see* **Note 4**). Make up to 200 mL with WHAUL medium (pH 7.0).

3. Methods

Yeast host strains are stored at –80°C. Working stocks are maintained on YPD agar plates and can be stored at 4°C for several weeks. GPCR genes are cloned into a yeast expression vector, and the highest expression level is attempted initially (*see* **Note 5**). p426GPD *(10)*, a high copy episomal plasmid, with a strong constitutive promoter, is recommended.

Previously untested GPCRs are usually transformed into a panel of engineered yeast strains expressing different Gpa1p/G_α chimeras (*(1)*; *see* **Note 6**). The GlaxoSmithKline system consists of 11 isogenic host yeast strains, with the prefix MMY, containing different integrated Gpa1p/G_α chimeras (**Table 1**) in which the C-terminal five amino acids of Gpa1p are replaced with the equivalent sequence from mammalian G_α proteins *(7, 8)*.

The MMY strains have two chromosomally integrated reporter genes, *FUS1-HIS3* and *FUS1-lacZ*. The preferred assay is to measure His3p-mediated cell growth, induced by agonism of the GPCR, which can be quantified using a fluorometric indicator of cell number (**Fig. 1A**; *see* **Note 2**). Alternatively, assays may be configured measuring the β-galactosidase reporter (**Fig. 1B**; *see* **Note 3**) for which various fluorogenic and chromogenic substrates are available.

Table 1
Genotypes of yeast strains used for GPCR research at GlaxoSmithKline

Strain	Genotype
W303-1A	*MATa his3 ade2 leu2 trp1 ura3 can1*
MMY9	W303-1A *fus1::FUS1-HIS3 FUS1-lacZ::LEU2 far1Δ::ura3Δ gpa1Δ::ADE2Δ sst2Δ::ura3Δ*
MMY11	MMY9 *ste2Δ::G418*^{R}
MMY12	MMY11 *TRP1::GPA1*
MMY14	MMY11 *TRP1::Gpa1/*$G_{\alpha q(5)}$
MMY16	MMY11 *TRP1::Gpa1/*$G_{\alpha 16(5)}$
MMY19	MMY11 *TRP1::Gpa1/*$G_{\alpha 12(5)}$
MMY20	MMY11 *TRP1::Gpa1/*$G_{\alpha 13(5)}$
MMY21	MMY11 *TRP1::Gpa1/*$G_{\alpha 14(5)}$
MMY22	MMY11 *TRP1::Gpa1/*$G_{\alpha o(5)}$
MMY23	MMY11 *TRP1::Gpa1/*$G_{\alpha i1(5)}$
MMY24	MMY11 *TRP1::Gpa1/*$G_{\alpha i3(5)}$
MMY25	MMY11 *TRP1::Gpa1/*$G_{\alpha z(5)}$
MMY28	MMY11 *TRP1::Gpa1/*$G_{\alpha s(5)}$
YIG28	MMY23 *URA3::pRS306GPD-hCB*$_1$
YIG6	MMY23 *URA3::pRS306GPD-hCB*$_2$

Strains are derived from the parent host W303-1A with several modifications to the pheromone-response pathway, enabling assays to be configured for heterologous GPCRs in MMY9 and MMY11. Chimeric G proteins were chromosomally integrated at the *trp1* locus of MMY11 as described by Olesnicky et al. *(7)* to generate the MMY12-28 panel of coupling strains. Gpa1/$G_{\alpha x(5)}$ denotes derivatives of Gpa1p in which the five C-terminal residues are replaced by corresponding sequence from the mammalian G_α subunit indicated. The CNR1_V0 and CNR2_V0 genes encoding human cannabinoid receptors hCB$_1$ and hCB$_2$, respectively, were chromosomally integrated at the *ura3* locus of MMY23 to generate YIG28 and YIG6.

To set up an assay, cells are grown to saturation selecting for the transformed plasmid, then seeded at low cell density into assay medium lacking histidine and dispensed into assay plates containing ligands or compounds. Plates are incubated at 30°C for approximately 24 h and then read in a plate reader. Once the best coupling strain is identified, corresponding to the optimal G_α chimera/GPCR combination, a number of optimization steps may be carried out. 3-AT is a competitive inhibitor of the *HIS3* protein (His3p) which can be titrated into the assay to regulate background activity caused by leakiness of the reporter or

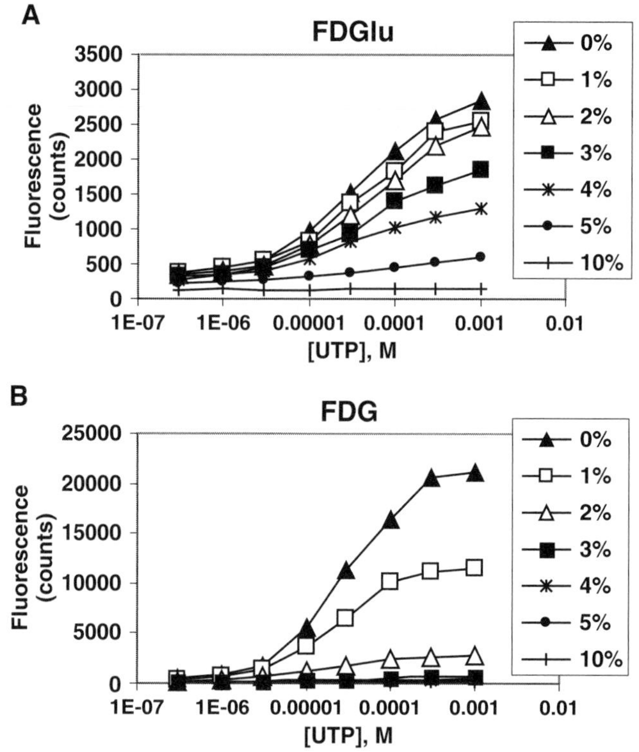

Fig. 1. Comparison of (**A**) FDGlu (growth) and (**B**) FDG (β-galactosidase) readouts for the human $P2Y_2$ receptor expressed in the MMY14 yeast strain. P2RY2_V0 was expressed in MMY14 and tested for activation of the pheromone-response pathway with the agonist UTP in the presence of a range of DMSO concentrations (0, 1, 2, 3, 4, 5, and 10% as indicated). The results illustrate a much larger fluorescein signal obtained using FDG but also a greater sensitivity to DMSO compared with the FDGlu readout. FDG exhibits similarly increased sensitivity to other solvents including methanol, ethanol, and DMF compared with FDGlu (data not shown).

constitutive activity of GPCRs (*see* **Note 4**). This is a key tool for optimizing the assay and generating a good signal window. Other factors influencing assay quality are seeding density, incubation time, and receptor expression level (*see* **Note 5**).

3.1. Yeast Transformation

1. Working stocks of the yeast host strains are generated by streaking from –80°C stocks onto YPD agar plates and grown for approximately 3 days at 30°C or until the colonies are 2–3 mm in diameter. These plates can then be maintained at 4°C for a number of weeks.
2. A single colony of each yeast strain is picked into 5 mL YPD medium and the culture shaken at 220 oscillations per minute and 30°C overnight (12–24 h). The flask capacity should be at least 5 times the volume of the yeast culture to ensure good aeration.

3. The following day, the cells should have grown to a dense culture (approximately 5 OD_{600}) approaching saturation. A 1/100 dilution is made into 100 mL YPD and grown for 4–8 h (approximately 2–3 generations). Cells should be in the mid-logarithmic growth phase.
4. Cells are harvested by centrifugation at 600 $\times g$ for 1 min using a bench-top centrifuge, resuspended in 1 mL sterile distilled water, transferred to a 1.5 mL microfuge tube, and then harvested by centrifugation for 10 s using a microfuge.
5. An adaptation of the lithium acetate method is used for the DNA transformation *(11)*. Each cell pellet is resuspended in 1 mL LiAc-TE (giving a 100-fold concentration of the original culture). 50 µL cells are used per transformation and 5 µL ssDNA added per 50 µL cells. If large numbers of transformations are to be done, this step can be scaled appropriately.
6. 1 µg of plasmid DNA is added, followed by 300 µL LiAc/PEG/TE, and the cell suspension mixed using a micropipette. If chromosomal integration is being attempted, larger amounts of DNA can be used (*see* **Note** 7). The transformation mixtures are incubated at room temperature for 10 min.
7. The transformations are heat shocked in a 42°C water bath for 20 min and then transferred to room temperature. 50 µL of the mixture is plated directly onto WHAUL+His plates (*see* **Note 8**). These are incubated at 30°C for 3 days or until well-defined colonies are visible.
8. Single colonies are picked with a sterile inoculation loop or blunt-end toothpick, patched onto a fresh WHAUL+His plate, and incubated a further 24 h at 30°C. This should generate enough cells as working stocks to be tested in several GPCR assays. The plates may be stored at 4°C.

3.2. Yeast GPCR Assay to Identify Active Transformants

1. A loop scraping of a single colony (or patch or streaked plate derived from a single colony) is inoculated into an appropriate volume of WHAUL+His (*see* **Note 9**). The yeast cultures are incubated overnight (18–24 h) shaking at 30°C.
2. FDGlu assay medium is prepared as described in **Section 3**. It is important to use WHAUL medium buffered at pH 7.0 using BU salts, as this is optimal for most GPCR-ligand interactions and for the activity of the reporter enzymes. A key variable is 3-amino triazole, which needs to be optimized for each GPCR/assay. A recommended default concentration for initial experiments is 2 m*M* in the final assay mixture. This can be varied (typically 0–20 m*M*) in subsequent experiments (*see* **Note 4**).

3. Typically four transformants of the GPCR construct are tested for each yeast strain (*see* **Note 10**). If the cells have been grown in a 96-well plate (*see* **Note 9**) it can be assumed they have reached saturation overnight (approximately 5 OD_{600}). A 1:250 dilution of each mini-culture into FDGlu assay medium is carried out. This can be achieved by transferring 6 μL of the saturated resuspended yeast cultures into 1.5 mL assay mix in a deep well 96-well block.
4. Assay plates should be prepared containing test compounds dispensed such that solvent concentrations are equal in every well. 96-well or 384-well plates may be used (*see* **Note 11**). It is recommended that final concentrations of solvents do not exceed 2% for FDGlu assays (**Fig. 1A**) and 1% for FDG assays (**Fig. 1B**).
5. When testing large numbers of transformants, a multi-channel, multi-dispensing micro-pipette may be used to distribute the yeast/assay mixture into the appropriate wells of the assay plate. The yeast/assay mixtures in the deep well block are agitated (by pipetting up and down) to ensure yeast are in suspension and dispensed at 100μL per well into the assay plate.
6. Plates are lidded, wrapped with cling film, and incubated at 30°C without shaking for 24 h.
7. Positive fluorescein signals become measurable between 16 and 24 h depending on the receptor, with signal window increasing over time. Plates are read at ex 485/em 535 nm in a fluorescence plate reader, for example, Tecan Spectrafluor Plus, Wallac Victor, or PerkinElmer Viewlux.

3.3. Assay Optimization

1. Assays are optimized to achieve the highest pEC_{50} value of a reference agonist, often the endogenous ligand, and/or the highest ratio between signal output in the presence and absence of a reference agonist (signal window). Parameters for achieving a preferred strain are receptor expression level (plasmid copy number, promoter strength, and chromosomal integration) and Gpa1/G_{α} chimera (*see* **Notes 5–7**). The preferred yeast strain is stored at –80°C (*see* **Note 12**).
2. Once the best strain is identified, assay parameters routinely optimized are: 3-AT concentration, initial seeding density, incubation time, substrate concentration, and DMSO concentration. Other parameters (e.g., incubation temperature and concentrations of media components) could conceivably affect characteristics of the assay but are not routinely varied during the optimization phase.

3. When optimizing assay conditions the protocol is largely the same as in 3.2 except that larger overnight cultures are grown (*see* **Note 9**) and optical density readings taken to enable accurate determinations of seeding density.
4. The non-invasive nature of the assay means that assay plates may be read at multiple time points (i.e., 16, 24, 40 h) to monitor development of the fluorescent signal, which can continue over at least 48 h. This can allow the activity of poorly expressed receptors to be detected. However, strains/assays are optimized to generate acceptable data over a maximum of 24 h, for convenience in later routine screening activities.

3.4. Compound Profiling Assays

1. For compound dilution, Greiner 384-well V-bottom polypropylene plates are supplied with test compounds (3 m*M* in DMSO) in columns 1 and 13. Eleven-point serial dilutions are prepared in 100% DMSO across the plate, at a dilution factor of three- or fourfold, and skipping columns 6 and 18. These plates are stored at –20°C for 1 month to allow re-stamping in the event of assay failure.
2. Assay ready compound plates are prepared for 384-well compound profiling assays as follows: 0.5 μL is transferred from compound dilution plates to Greiner 384-well black compound plates using the Biomek FX (Beckman Coulter, High Wycombe, Bucks, UK). Columns 6 and 18 are controls for the normalization of data and calculation of Z'. Column 6 (low control/minimum effect) wells receive 0.5 μL of DMSO. Column 18 (high control/maximum effect) wells receive 0.5 μL of an appropriate standard agonist or antagonist compound of the test receptor. These plates are sealed and stored at 4°C for up to 1 week and thereafter at –20°C for up to 2 months.
3. Each month, the GPCR assay strains are streaked from –80°C frozen stocks on to WHAUL+His agar plates, grown for 3 days at 30°C, and stored for up to 6 weeks at 4°C. These plates are used as the source for inoculum of appropriate volumes of WHAUL+His medium (*see* **Note 9**). After 18–24 h incubation with shaking (this parameter may be optimized and standardized for each assay), OD_{600} is measured (*see* **Note 13**). Overnight culture is diluted into FDGlu assay medium to achieve 0.02 OD_{600}. For agonist assays, 50 μL/well of this yeast/assay mix is dispensed into assay ready compound plates using a Multidrop384 or Matrix Wellmate (both ThermoScientific, Waltham, MA) (*see* **Note 14**). For antagonist assays, this mixture is supplemented with an appropriate concentration (EC_{80}) of a standard agonist. Plate seals are applied and plates incubated without shaking at 30°C in a humid atmosphere.

4. Plates are read after 24 h (±20 min) using stacking plate readers (LJL Analyst or Tecan Spectrafluor Plus with integrated Zymark Twister). Plate seals are removed before reading. A two-stage quality control process is applied to the data. Robust statistics *(12)* are calculated from n=16 low and n=16 high controls (columns 6 and 18, respectively), and Z′ derived, as a measure of well to well variability *(13)*. Plates falling below preset Z′ limits (typically Z′=0) are not analyzed further. Next, data for test compounds are normalized to high and low pharmacological effect (mean of columns 18 and , respectively) and analyzed using a four-parameter logistic fit *(14)* to derive pXC_{50} values (i.e., pIC_{50} or pEC_{50}). In each assay occasion, three or more known pharmacological standards (where available) are included among the set of test compounds. On assay occasions where less than two-thirds of pharmacological standard pXC_{50} values fall within preset limits (e.g., 3-month rolling mean ± 3S.D.), all data are discarded.
5. pXC_{50} values from assays passing QC are used to define structure–activity relationships (SAR) and inform lead optimization chemistry. For agonist assays, intrinsic activity data (fitted maximum for test compound as a proportion of fitted maximum for pharmacological standard) may also be captured.
6. SAR optimization efforts during drug discovery are often sustained over several years, and their success depends on the relevance and stability of the assays which support them. To illustrate the long-term stability of the yeast assay format, pEC_{50} values for the standard cannabinoid agonist HU-210 at yeast strains YIG28 and YIG6, which contain chromosomally integrated cannabinoid CB_1 and CB_2 receptors, respectively, are shown in **Fig. 2**.

3.5. Hit Identification Assays

1. The protocols described above can be readily applied to identify novel receptor ligands in diversity screening (high-throughput screening, HTS) campaigns. During HTS, large collections of compounds are tested at a single high concentration for their ability to activate (in the case of agonists) or block the effect of a reference agonist (in the case of antagonists) in the yeast assay. The general processes of plate preparation and assay validation for HTS utilized in GlaxoSmithKline are common to different assay formats and have been described elsewhere in this edition (*see* **Note 15**).
2. To ensure plates are read at 24 h (or other optimized time) and for ease of handling, assay plates are processed in batches. Batch size is determined by speed of the plate reader: for a

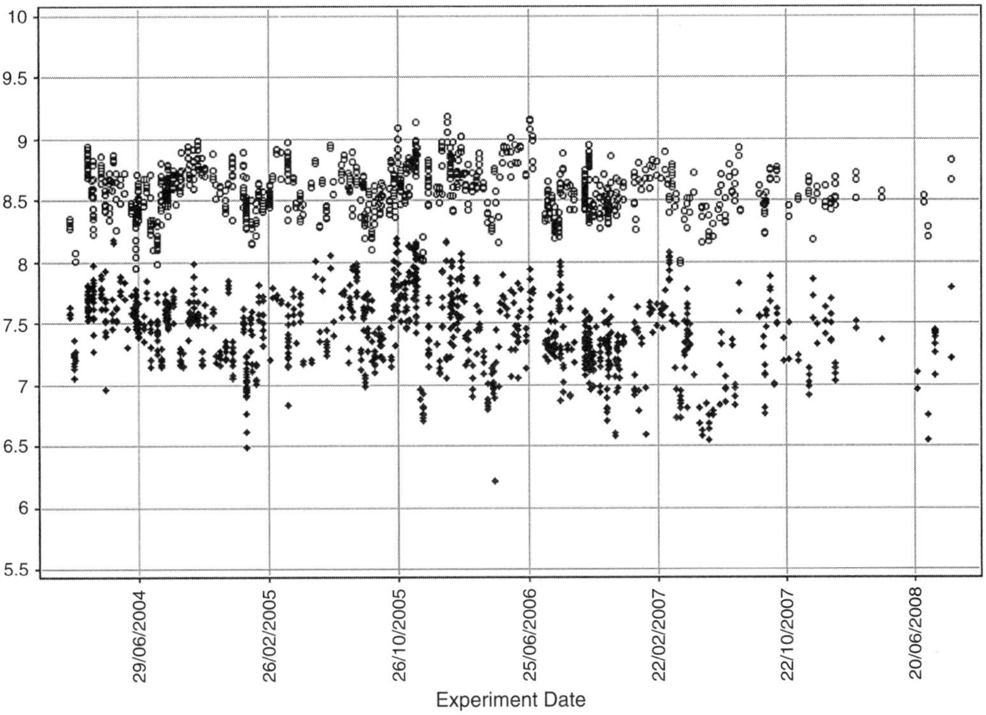

Fig. 2. Stability of yeast-based compound profiling assays over time. pEC_{50} values for the standard agonist HU-210 at the cannabinoid CB_1 (closed circles) and CB_2 (open circles) receptors, over the course of more than 4 years, are shown. A total of 1177 determinations made using yeast strain YIG28, which expresses the human cannabinoid CB_1 receptor from a chromosomally integrated expression cassette, yielded pEC_{50} 7.45 ± 0.3 (mean ± S.D.). Similarly, 1074 determinations made using yeast strain YIG6, which expresses the human cannabinoid CB_2 receptor from a chromosomally integrated expression cassette, yielded pEC_{50} 8.6 ± 0.2 (mean ± S.D.). Data were collected from March 2004 to August 2008.

384-well assay read on a Tecan Spectrafluor Plus, up to eight batches of 30 plates are processed per assay day (i.e., 4 × 240 plates = 368000 wells per week).

3. Yeast cultures may be grown over a longer time course by inoculating into WHAUL+His medium as described in **Section 3.4.3** and maintaining at 4°C without shaking for 24 or 48 h, then incubating at 30°C with shaking for 16–24 h, using an Innova 4230 refrigerated programmable incubator. This can extend the number of assay days per working week (i.e., four assay days per five-day working week).

4. Yeast assays may be scaled to 1536-well high-density plates. 50 nL test compound in DMSO is dispensed into assay plates (*see* **Note 11**) using an Echo550 liquid handler (Labcyte, Sunnyvale, CA, USA). 5 μL FDGlu assay medium containing yeast cells is added using MultidropCombi nanoliter (ThermoScientific, Waltham, MA, USA). After 24 h incubation, plates are read on Viewlux (PerkinElmer, Waltham, MA, USA).

5. The critical limitation in conversion of 384- to 1536-well assays is plate patterning or edge effects owing to evaporation from the small assay volume (5 μL) over the relatively long time course of assay (24 h). Optimization of both plate seals and incubation conditions are required to address this. We have recently completed a successful HTS campaign in 1536-well format using Breathseal (Greiner Bio-one) plate seals and rotating carousel-type humidified incubators (*see* **Note 16**).

4. Notes

1. Laboratory yeast strains grow in media containing trace elements plus sources of carbon and nitrogen. The media utilized here are supplemented with glucose (dextrose) as the carbon source and yeast nitrogen base (YNB) which provides trace elements and a source of nitrogen. Omission of either precludes cell growth. WHAUL is a synthetic-complete "drop out" mixture of amino acids that are not essential for growth but are an important component of GPCR assays because they enhance growth rates. The GlaxoSmithKline yeast strains are derived from W303-1A *(15)* which has *trp1, his3, ade2, ura3*, and *leu2* auxotrophies, and WHAUL lacks tryptophan, histidine, adenine, uracil, and leucine to enable use of these auxotrophic selectable marker genes encoded on transforming plasmids. The *TRP1*, *ADE2*, and *LEU2* markers were utilized during construction of the MMY strains, and *HIS3* is the reporter gene. Therefore, tryptophan, adenine, and leucine are not required as nutrient supplements but histidine is required for growth of cultures in the absence of GPCR agonism. The only marker that can be used to select for GPCR constructs is *URA3*. Expression constructs derived from pRS306 *(16)*, p416, and p426 *(10)* are suitable.
2. The cell growth readout has been found to minimize bell-shaped agonist concentration-response curves and to be less sensitive to non-specific inhibitory effects of solvents and compounds seen in β-galactosidase assays (**Fig. 1**). This minimizes false positives during hit identification campaigns for antagonists. His3p is recommended because of the ability to moderate background activity using 3-AT (*see* **Note 4**). FDGlu is a substrate for the yeast exoglucanase, Exg1p, that is constitutively expressed and secreted *(17)*. Exg1p converts FDGlu to fluorescein providing a quantitative measure of cell growth without the requirement to lyse cells. This may be used in conjunction with growth readouts such as *FUS1-HIS3*.

3. β-Galactosidase activity may be measured in a variation of the standard assay. β-Galactosidase assays are most successful when used in conjunction with the *HIS3* reporter in histidine-free, 3-AT containing media. In the absence of this selection, yeast growth appears to "quench" β-galactosidase reporter products. A variety of β-galactosidase substrates exists. FDG is converted to fluorescein and read in a fluorescence plate reader. The amplification obtained with the β-galactosidase reporter used in conjunction with the growth reporter can lead to larger fluorescein signals and signal-to-background ratios than the FDGlu assay. However, β-galactosidase is also more sensitive to solvents and toxic compound effects. DMSO must not exceed 1% (**Fig. 1**). CPRG (a yellow substrate) is converted by β-galactosidase into chlorophenol red (a red product) providing a visual readout for GPCR agonism, which may be quantified (for 96-well plates) by reading at 570 nm. The dynamic range of CPRG and other absorbance readouts is less than for the fluorescence (FDGlu, FDG) readouts, and optical scattering because of yeast cells settling to the bottom of assay wells can interfere with photometric measurement, especially in 384-well format.
4. His3p (imidazoleglycerol-phosphate dehydratase), an enzyme catalyzing the sixth step in histidine biosynthesis, is modulated by the competitive inhibitor 3-amino triazole (3-AT) *(18)*. The MMY strains exhibit low levels of *HIS3* expression in the absence of transformed GPCRs, which vary from strain to strain and reflect slight differences in affinities between chimeric G_α subunits with the yeast $G_{\beta\gamma}$. MMY28 has a significantly higher background than other strains in the series. GPCRs may also exhibit constitutive activity in the absence of agonist, ranging from barely measurable to full activation depending on the GPCR. 10 m*M* 3-AT is usually sufficient to eliminate all background response. If detection of constitutive activity is important (for instance to identify coupling of an orphan GPCR in the absence of ligand), the assay may be "sensitized" by using a very low level of 3-AT and a higher seeding density of cells. Increasing [3-AT] generally causes agonist response curves to shift to the right. It can also reveal partial agonism of compounds that appear as full agonists at low [3-AT].
5. Failure to obtain functional coupling is often due to poor expression of the heterologous GPCR. A high copy plasmid with a strong constitutive promoter (e.g., p426GPD; *(10)*) provides the best chance of obtaining good expression levels. If necessary, high constitutive activity can be reduced through the use of weaker promoters (CYC, ADH, TEF; *(10)*), low copy plasmids (e.g., p416GPD), or chromosomal integration

(*see* **Note 7**). In situations where no functional coupling is obtained, codon optimization, fusion to N-terminal secretory leader sequences (such as that from alpha factor pheromone), or construction of receptor chimeras may remedy low expression or incorrect trafficking.

6. Chimeric G proteins can enable coupling of diverse GPCR coupling classes to a common signaling pathway. The C terminus of the G_α subunit contains important determinants for GPCR interactions and Gpa1p derivatives incorporating the C-terminal five amino acids of mammalian G_α subunits are used in the GlaxoSmithKline yeast strains. GPCRs exhibit strong coupling preferences for different G_α chimeras which can reflect their mammalian G_α coupling *(8)*. However, accumulated experience has found that this is a crude approximation and the optimal strain needs to be identified empirically. For instance, G_α chimeras using the C-terminal five amino acids of $G_{\alpha s}$ tend to couple inefficiently, and $G_{\alpha s}$-coupled GPCRs often couple better to a Gpa1p/$G_{\alpha i}$ chimera in yeast. Many GPCRs also couple in several of the strains, with differences in coupling efficiency reflected in the pEC_{50} of a reference agonist. MMY24 is considered the most generic strain for coupling a wide range of GPCRs with moderate efficiency.
7. Chromosomal integration is used to generate a stable GPCR-expressing strain that will ensure reproducible data over long-term use and may also be maintained on non-selective medium (e.g., YPD). The promoter-GPCR expression cassette should be transferred from episomal plasmids such as p426GPD, into an integrating vector (e.g., pRS306; *(16)*) that lacks a yeast DNA replication origin. For p426GPD, restriction sites such as PvuII, PvuI, or BglI are convenient for transfer of this cassette. The integrating construct must be linearized within the selectable marker to ensure efficient integration. Suitable sites in *URA3* are *Nsi*I, *Stu*I, or *Nde*I. The linearized DNA is transformed into the yeast using the same method as described for episomal plasmids. Transformation of higher amounts of DNA (5–10 μg) can lead to multiple integration events and larger GPCR responses, therefore numerous colonies should be tested to identify the preferred integrant strain.
8. The transformation efficiency of LiAc-competent yeast can be very high for episomal plasmids. Different quantities of the transformation mixture can be plated on multiple agar plates to obtain single colonies. Transformation of episomal plasmids should yield colonies of uniform size. A range of different sized or sectored colonies is indicative that the GPCR expression is toxic. In this case, a range of colonies should be picked for assays, and if results are inconsistent, chromosomal

integration should be attempted. In a chromosomal integrative transformation, integrants will emerge as large colonies from a lawn of smaller non-viable colonies. These arise from non-integrative transformation of the linearized construct, which is able to support a few generations of yeast growth in the absence of chromosomal integration.

9. Culture volumes can be adjusted according to the experiment. For testing large numbers of independent colonies in single concentration–response curves, colonies can be picked into 100 μL WHAUL+His in the wells of a 96-well plate. To optimize conditions for a single yeast clone, 5 mL cultures grown in a shake flask are appropriate. For large-scale compound profiling HTS, larger volume cultures (e.g., 15–100 mL) can be grown to mid-logarithmic phase to ensure accurate cell density calculations. For larger volume cultures, correspondingly greater quantities of inoculum are transferred to the sterile loop.
10. Yeast strains derived from W303 exhibit a low level of reversion to URA^+ meaning that some colonies on the transformation plate may be revertants not transformants. The level of reversion can be assessed using a "no DNA" control transformation. Otherwise, the reproducibility between individual colonies is typically extremely high.
11. For compound profiling assays, a wide variety of plasticware has been tested and is suitable, including black- and optical bottom plates. The main criterion for plasticware is for opaque well walls to avoid crossover of fluorescent signals. For top-read plate readers, Greiner 384-well black-bottomed plates are recommended. For bottom-read plate readers, Greiner 384-well black optical-bottomed plates are recommended. For 1536-well assays, Greiner black HiBase 1536-well plates are recommended.
12. For frozen stocks of yeast strains, 750 μL of saturated yeast in YPD are mixed with 250 μL of a 60% solution of sterile glycerol in distilled water (final glycerol concentration 15%) in cryovials and stored at –80°C.
13. Expression of some GPCRs can have toxic effects resulting in slower growth rates of the yeast strains. In these situations, a QC check is introduced and overnight cultures are not used when their density falls outside set limits, for example, 1–3 OD_{600}.
14. When handling larger volumes of assay mixture for dispensing to multiple assay plates, cells are maintained in suspension by gentle stirring using a magnetic stirrer. Rarely, flocculation of cells in the pre-prepared assay mixture has been observed, occurring over a 1–3 h time course. This effect may be strain-dependent and can be overcome by processing smaller batches of assay mix/cells.

15. We have observed empirically that in yeast agonist assays, the rate of false positives (compounds giving concentration-dependent and reproducible fluorescence signals not specific to the expressed receptor) is low, generally less than 0.1%. Moreover, we commonly observe the majority of chemotypes identified in yeast agonist HTS also to be active in assays of the same receptor expressed in mammalian cells, for example, GTPγS binding. In contrast, yeast antagonist assays are consistently observed to have higher primary hit rates and are more liable to false-positive hits. Consequently, it is important to include both a specificity assay (yeast cells functionally expressing an unrelated GPCR) and a confirmation assay (usually the same receptor in a mammalian-based assay format such as intracellular calcium, cAMP, or GTPγS-binding assays) to validate hits from yeast antagonist HTS before progression. Decreasing the final concentration of test compounds in HTS (normal range is 3–30 μ*M*) can also reduce false-positive rates in antagonist HTS.
16. Assay conversion from 384- to 1536-well format can necessitate re-optimization of numerous assay parameters, in particular concentrations of 3-AT and FDGlu. Even after optimization, some negative impact on assay quality parameters such as Z' and false-negative and false-positive hit rates, concomitant with assay conversion from 384- to 1536-well format, is observed. As a result, 1536-well conversion is only attempted for high-quality 384 assays.

Acknowledgments

The authors thank all GlaxoSmithKline and visiting scientists who have contributed to the development of the yeast assay over the last 13 years. The authors are grateful in particular to Kalpana Patel (BR&AD) for providing data for **Fig. 1** and Carl Haslam for **Fig. 2**. Adaptation of the yeast assay to 1536-well format is largely the work of Carl Haslam, Victoria Holland, Kerri Hildick, and Parita Shah (all S&CP).

References

1. Dowell, S.J. and Brown, A.J. (2002) Yeast assays for G protein-coupled receptors. *Receptors Channels* **8**, 343–352.
2. Bardwell, L. (2004) A walk-through of the yeast mating pheromone response pathway. *Peptides* **25**, 1465–1476.
3. Price, L.A., Kajkowski, E.M., Hadcock, J.R., Ozenberger, B.A., and Pausch, M.H. (1995) Functional coupling of a mammalian somatostatin receptor to the yeast pheromone response pathway. *Mol. Cell Biol.* **15**, 6188–6195.

4. Price, L.A., Strnad, J., Pausch, M.H., and Hadcock, J.R. (1996) Pharmacological characterization of the rat A2a adenosine receptor functionally coupled to the yeast pheromone response pathway. *Mol. Pharmacol.* **50**, 829–837.
5. Erickson, J.R., Wu, J.J., Goddard, J.G., Tigyi, G., Kawanishi, K., Tomei, L.D., and Kiefer, M.C. (1998) Edg-2/Vzg-1 couples to the yeast pheromone response pathway selectively in response to lysophosphatidic acid. *J. Biol. Chem.* **273**, 1506–1510.
6. Ishii, J., Tanaka, T., Matsumura, S., Tatematsu, K., Kuroda, S., Ogino, C., Fukuda, H., and Kondo, A. (2008) Yeast-based fluorescence reporter assay of G protein-coupled receptor signalling for flow cytometric screening: FAR1-disruption recovers loss of episomal plasmid caused by signalling in yeast. *J. Biochem.* **143**, 667–674.
7. Olesnicky, N.S., Brown, A.J., Dowell, S.J., and Casselton, L.A. (1999) A constitutively active G protein-coupled receptor causes mating self-compatibility in the mushroom Coprinus. *EMBO J.* **18**, 2756–2763.
8. Brown, A.J., Dyos, S.L., Whiteway, M.S., White, J.H., Watson, M.A., Marzioch, M., Clare, J.J., Cousens, D.J., Paddon, C., Plumpton, C., Romanos, M.A., and Dowell, S.J. (2000) Functional coupling of mammalian receptors to the yeast mating pathway using novel yeast/mammalian G protein alpha-subunit chimeras. *Yeast* **16**, 11–22.
9. Sherman, F. (2002) Getting started with yeast. *Methods Enzymol.* **350**, 3–41.
10. Mumberg, D., Muller, R., and Funk, M. (1995) Yeast vectors for the controlled expression of heterologous proteins in different genetic backgrounds. *Gene* **156**, 119–122.
11. Gietz, R.D., Schiestl, R.H., Willems, A.R., and Woods, R.A. (1995) Studies on the transformation of intact yeast cells by the LiAc/SS-DNA/PEG procedure. *Yeast* **11**, 355–360.
12. Royal Society of Chemistry – Analytical Methods Committee (1989) Robust statistics – how not to reject outliers. *Analyst* **114**, 1693–1697.
13. Zhang, J.H., Chung, T.D., and Oldenburg, K.R. (1999) A simple statistical parameter for use in evaluation and validation of high throughput screening assays. *J. Biomol. Screen.* **4**, 67–73.
14. Bowen, W.P. and Jerman, J.C. (1995) Nonlinear regression using spreadsheets. *Trends Pharmacol. Sci.* **16**, 413–417.
15. Rothstein, R. (1991) Targeting, disruption, replacement, and allele rescue: integrative DNA transformation in yeast. *Methods Enzymol.* **194**, 281–301.
16. Sikorski, R.S. and Hieter, P. (1989). A system of shuttle vectors and yeast host strains designed for efficient manipulation of DNA in *Saccharomyces cerevisiae. Genetics* **122**, 19–27.
17. Cid, V.J., Alvarez, A.M., Santos, A.I., Nombela, C., and Sanchez, M. (1994) Yeast exo-beta-glucanases can be used as efficient and readily detectable reporter genes in *Saccharomyces cerevisiae. Yeast* **10**, 747–756.
18. Fields, S. (1993) The two-hybrid system to detect protein–protein interactions. *Methods Companion Methods Enzymol.* **5**, 116–124.

Chapter 16

GPCR Microspot Assays on Solid Substrates

Ye Fang and Joydeep Lahiri

Summary

Multiplexing and miniaturization make microarrays an attractive tool for biomolecular interaction analysis. Adequate shelf life, mechanical stability through multiple assay steps, and amenability to a microplate format for screening are core requirements for the practical large-scale implementation of microarray technology. G protein-coupled receptor (GPCR) microarrays require the co-immobilization of the receptors and their associated lipid membranes. The vulnerability of solid-supported membranes to desorption and the unique surface requirements for GPCR function provide formidable challenges for the fabrication of GPCR microarrays. The chapter describes air-stable GPCR microarrays and their utility for selectivity profiling of GPCR drugs with high fidelity.

Key words: G protein-coupled receptor, Microarray, Selectivity profiling, Multiplexing, Fluorescence.

1. Introduction

Air-stable G protein-coupled receptor (GPCR) microarrays consist of an indexed series of microscopic spots of GPCR membranes *(1–4)*. GPCRs and other membrane proteins (e.g., ion channels, receptor tyrosine kinases) make up around a third of the proteome of a cell *(5)* and are key targets for therapeutic intervention *(6)*. Relative to assaying a single receptor at a time, microarrays not only enable analysis of many receptor–ligand interactions in a single assay but also limit the consumption of precious receptors.

Unique to GPCR microarrays is the co-immobilization of a receptor and its associated membranes in each microspot. This is because the functions of membrane proteins often demand association with lipid molecules and are strongly dependent on the

Wayne R. Leifert (ed.), *G Protein-Coupled Receptors in Drug Discovery, vol. 552*

Book doi: 10.1007/978-1-60327-317-6_16

biophysical characteristics (e.g., long-range fluidity) of the membrane. Long-range lateral fluidity of the host membrane precludes covalent immobilization of the bulk lipid; however, physisorbed membranes on solid supports are unstable due to their propensity to desorption upon exposure to air. The solid support should also enable the correct folding of the transmembrane and extramembrane domains of the GPCR (and associated G proteins). Taken together, these demanding requirements made the practical realization of GPCR microarrays an elusive goal. We first reported air-stable GPCR microarrays *(1)* and their utility for selectivity profiling of drug candidate molecules against multiple receptors *(7–9)*. Here, using a five-element GPCR microarray as a model system, we describe a three-step protocol for GPCR microspot-based assays: (i) microarray fabrication, (ii) selection and characterization of fluorescent ligands in both simplexed and multiplexed formats, and (iii) multiplexed binding assays for selectivity profiling.

2. Materials

2.1. GPCR Membranes, Fluorescent Probes

1. Human muscarinic receptor subtype-1 (M1) (Euroscreen, Brussels, Belgium).
2. Human muscarinic receptor subtype-2 (M2) (Euroscreen).
3. Human motilin receptor (MOTR) (Euroscreen).
4. Human $\delta 2$ opioid receptor (OP1) (Euroscreen).
5. Human neurotensin receptor subtype-1 (NTS1) membrane preparation (Perkim Elmer Life Sciences, Boston, MA, USA).
6. Human β_1-adrenergic receptor (β_1-AR) membrane preparation (Perkim Elmer Life Sciences).
7. Cy3B-telenzepine (Cy3B-TEL) (GE Healthcare, Rutgers, NJ, USA).
8. Bodipy-tetramethylrhodamine (TMR)-CGP12177 (BT-CGP) (Invitrogen, Carlsbad, CA, USA).
9. Cy5-neurotensin 2-13 (Cy5-NT) (Corning Inc., Corning, NY, USA).
10. Bodipy-TMR-motilin 1-16 (BT-MOT) (Corning Inc.)
11. Cy5-naltrexone (Cy5-NAL) (Corning Inc.)
12. Neurotensin (Sigma, St. Louis, MO, USA).
13. Protease-free bovine serum albumin (BSA) (Sigma Chemical Inc., St. Louis, MO, USA).
14. Deionized water (>18 Ω; MilliQ-UV, Millipore, Bedford, MA, USA).

15. Ligand-binding buffer: 10 mM $MgCl_2$, 0.1% BSA, 50 mM Hepes–KOH (pH 7.4), and 1 mM EDTA (ethylenediaminetetraacetic acid) in deionized water.
16. GPCR membrane reformulation buffer: 10% sucrose, 0.5% BSA, 10% glycerol, 50 mM Tris–HCl, 2.5 mM $MgCl_2$, pH 7.4 in deionized water.

2.2. Instruments and Consumables

1. Genipix 4000B scanner (Axon Instruments, Union City, CA, USA).
2. Quill-pin printer (Cartesian Technologies Model PS 5000, Irvine, CA, USA).
3. Quill pin CMP3 (Telechem, Atlanta, GA, USA).
4. White low volume 384-well microplate (Corning Inc.).
5. γ-Aminopropylsilane-coated glass slide (GAPS II) (Corning Inc.)
6. FlexiPERM micro 12 chambers (Sigma).
7. Prism Software (Graph Pad Software Inc., La Jolla, CA, USA).

3. Methods

3.1. Preparation of Air-Stable GPCR Microarrays

Air-stable GPCR microarrays can be fabricated using standard contact pin printing technologies *(1–4)*. The air stability is achieved by (i) choosing appropriate surface chemistry that enables both long-range fluidity and stable association with the substrate surface of lipid bilayers *(1, 10)* and (ii) protecting the membrane microspots through closely packed soluble proteins surrounding the microspots and through disaccharide molecules associated with the lipid headgroups *(7)*.

1. The quality of GAPS-coated glass slides is first assessed using a typical water contact angle measurement based on 2-μL water droplets. Only slides with water contact angles within the range of 25–35° should be used (*see* **Note 1**) to ensure optimal performance.
2. The GPCR membrane reformulation buffer is prepared fresh using deionized water. The water-soluble protein BSA molecules will effectively form packed layer(s) surrounding the GPCR-membrane microspots during the array fabrication and post-printing processes *(7)*. The disaccharides sucrose or trehalose also protects the integrity and functionality of GPCR membranes from the typical deterioration of the membranes when fabricated and stored under dry conditions *(7, 11)*.

3. GPCR membranes obtained from commercial sources are reformulated (*see* **Note 2**). The receptor fragments are centrifuged down to the bottom of a centrifuge tube at approximately 5000 × *g*. After careful removal of the supernatant, the GPCR membrane reformulation buffer is added to resuspend the receptor fragments such that the total concentration of membrane proteins is about 1–2 mg/mL. When necessary, the membrane suspensions are further sonicated on an icy water bath for 5 min or are homogenized again using a homogenizer to improve the homogeneity of membrane fragments.
4. CMP3 model quill-pins are used to produce GPCR microspots with a spot diameter of approximately 130 μm. Different quill pins can be used, depending on the desired shape and diameter of the microspots.
5. Microarray printing is performed using the Cartesian quill-pin printer under controlled humidity (relative humidity of approximately 60%). Briefly, a receptor suspension of 7 μL is added to a well of the low-volume 384-well microplate. Replicate microspots are obtained after 20 pre-prints using a single sample loading of the pin. Typically, a total of 16 grids of sub-microarrays, each with four replicates for each receptor, are printed onto a single GAPS slide. Each grid of the sub-microarray is separated with a pitch corresponding to the footprint of a conventional 96-well microplate. The onboard sonicator is used to clean the pin during each sample loading step (*see* **Note 3**).
6. The printed microarrays are further processed by 1-h incubation within a controlled humidity chamber (relative humidity of 80–90%) to ensure the stable association of GPCR membranes with the surface. Afterwards, the microarrays are dried and the slides are packed in a nitrogen-filled polypropylene mailer and sealed in an alumina pouch. The microarrays stored at 4°C are functional up to at least 3 months.

3.2. Characterization and Selection of Fluorescent Ligands Using GPCR Microspot Assays

Fluorescence detection is the most popular technology for microspot-based assays because of its high sensitivity and multi-color capability. Because of the complexity of GPCR–ligand interactions *(12, 13)*, selecting appropriate fluorescent ligands is crucial to successful GPCR microspot assays. The binding of labeled ligands can be characterized by both the equilibrium saturation assay and the kinetic assays. The saturation experiments measure the specific binding of labeled ligand at equilibrium at various concentrations of the labeled ligand, resulting in an equilibrium binding constant. The kinetic experiments measure the time course of binding and dissociation to determine the rate constants for labeled ligand binding and dissociation, which permit a calculation of the equilibrium dissociation constant. These kinetic measurements can be diffusion limited; true kinetic constants may be evaluated by adapting the experiments to flow cell formats with flow rates that overcome mass transport limitations. Assays can be performed in simplex or multiplexed formats. For multiplexed assays, the microarrays are incubated with a cocktail of labeled ligands in the absence and presence of a cocktail containing excess unlabeled counterparts. Following is a protocol for simplex binding assays. **Figure 1** shows the characteristics of Cy5-NT binding to NTS1 in a five-element microarray using simplex assays.

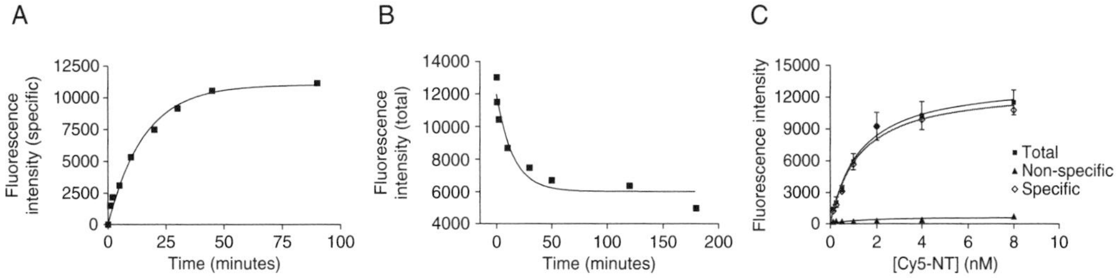

Fig. 1. Binding characteristics of Cy5-NT to NTS1 in the five-element GPCR microarrays. (**A**) The binding association curve of 2 nM Cy5-NT. (**B**) The dissociation curve of bound Cy5-NT at 2 nM. The Cy5-NT pre-bound NTS1 microarrays were subject to exposure to the binding buffer solution only for different period of time to determine the remaining bound Cy5-NT. (**C**) The saturation curve of Cy5-NT. The microarrays were incubated with various concentrations of Cy5-NT in the absence (total) and presence (non-specific) of 2 μM neurotensin. Results showed that (i) the binding of Cy5-NT proceeds to equilibrium within 30 min when its concentrations used are close to the K_d; (ii) the binding of Cy5-NT is specific to the receptor; and (iii) the binding of Cy5-NT follows the law of mass and is reversible. The binding constants of Cy5-NT are $1.0 \pm 0.1 \times 10^6\ M^{-1}\ s^{-1}$ (the apparent association rate constant at 2 n*M*), $1.0 \pm 0.1 \times 10^{-3}\ s^{-1}$ (the apparent dissociation rate constant), and 1.4 ± 0.3 nM (the binding affinity constant) ($n = 3$).

1. The stored microarrays are first brought back to room temperature and quickly rehydrated in a humid chamber (relative humidity of ~85%). The FlexiPERM micro-12 chamber is assembled on the slide such that each well contains a sub-microarray.
2. The binding affinity of a labeled ligand is first determined using an equilibrium saturation assay. Here a concentration series of the labeled ligand in the absence and presence of excess unlabeled counterpart is used to titrate its cognate receptor(s). The specific binding signal, obtained by subtracting the non-specific signal obtained in the presence of the counterpart from the total binding signal, is plotted as a function of labeled ligand concentration. Non-linear regression is used to determine the binding affinity of the labeled ligand. An ideal labeled ligand should have a binding affinity lower than 20 nM to its cognate receptor(s).
3. The binding kinetics of a labeled ligand can also be determined. Here the microarray is first incubated with the labeled ligand in the absence and presence of its unlabeled

counterpart in excess (1000 ×). After a certain period of incubation, the arrays are directly blow dried using air and examined with a fluorescence scanner. The amount of specific binding is plotted as a function of time. Conversely, to measure the dissociation rate constant, after a 1-h incubation period with the labeled ligand, the microarray is quickly dried and covered with 100 μL of the binding buffer without any ligands. At certain time points, the array is dried and examined using a fluorescence scanner. The total binding signal is plotted as a function of time. Both apparent association and dissociation rate constants are calculated using non-linear regression methods with the Prism (or similar) software. The association rate constants determine the optimal assay time (typically 30–60 min), whereas the dissociation rate constants dictate the limits for the washing protocol used for multiplexed binding assays.

4. Once its binding affinity is determined, the labeled ligand at a concentration of EC_{50} or EC_{80} is used to determine its specificity to its cognate receptor(s) as well as its cross-activity to other receptors in the microarray. An ideal labeled ligand should have a binding specificity of greater than 70% to its cognate receptor(s) and have minimal cross-activity (<15%) to other receptors (*see* **Note 4**).
5. The parent ligand can be tagged with a different color when the initial label results in cross-talk issues with other receptors in a specific channel. The newly labeled ligand also needs to be validated experimentally. For example, for the five-element GPCR microarray consisting of the M1, M2, NTS1, MOTR, and OP1 receptors, an acceptable set of fluorescently labeled ligands are Cy3B-TEL (M1 and M2), Cy5-NT (NTS1), BT-MOT (MOTR), and Cy5-NAL (OP1) (*see* **Note 5**).

3.3. Multiplexed Binding Assays Using GPCR Microarrays

1. The ligand binding buffer for the five-element GPCR microarrays is used initially; however, the assay buffer composition, its ionic strength, the cations present, and the pH buffering reagents are first optimized (*see* **Note 6**).
2. A cocktail of labeled ligands, each at $\sim EC_{50}$ or EC_{80}, is prepared using the optimized ligand binding buffer.
3. The microarray is incubated with the cocktail-labeled ligands in the absence and the presence of a drug compound for 1 h. After washing twice with the binding buffer alone, the microarrays are dried and imaged with a fluorescence scanner. The binding of labeled ligands is quantified by measuring the fluorescence intensities of each microspot. Four replicates in an array are typically used for accurate statistical analysis of each receptor. The difference between the signals in the absence and the presence of the drug

compound is a direct indicator of the binding of the drug compound to the receptor(s). The binding profile across the receptors in the microarray is an indicator of selectivity of the drug compound.

4. Notes

1. The GAPS coating is susceptible to environmental modification because of reactive primary amines and undergoes a slow evolution over time even under optimal packaging conditions.
2. GPCR membranes can be liposomes containing reconstituted receptors or membrane fragments containing over-expressed receptors made from the standard cell membrane preparation approach. Many commercially available GPCR preparations can be used for fabricating GPCR microarrays after reformulation. These preparations differ greatly in homogeneity, active receptor concentration (so-called B_{max}), concentration of total membrane proteins, and buffer compositions. Therefore, reformulation and normalization are necessary.
3. Printing GPCR membranes is tricky because biological membranes are susceptible to environmental changes and often significantly alter the wetting and dewetting properties of pins during the printing.
4. The cross-activity is mostly non-specific in nature. For the five-element microarrays, both CyB-TEL and BT-MOT exhibit non-specific binding to both NTS1 and OP1 receptors in the microarrays *(7)*.
5. Labeled ligands are synthesized using standard amine coupling chemistry and characterized using microspot-based assays *(7)*. Motilin (Phe–Val–Pro–Ile–Phe–Thr–Tyr–Gly–Glu–Leu–Gln–Arg–Met–Gln–Glu–Lys–Glu–Arg–Asn–Lys–Gly–Gln–OH) is a natural ligand of MOTR. Bodipy-TMR-motilin 1-16 (BT-MOT) is synthesized through amine coupling of the N-terminal lysine residue of motilin 1–16 with an amine-reactive bodipy-TMR dye, and purified and confirmed with mass spectroscopy. Neurotensin (Pyr–Leu–Tyr–Glu–Asn–Lys–Pro–Arg–Arg–Pro–Tyr–Ile–Leu–OH) is a 13 amino acid peptide neurotransmitter for NTS1. Cy5-NT is synthesized through amine coupling of the N-terminal amine of neurotensin 2–13 with an amine reactive Cy5 dye, and purified and confirmed using mass spectroscopy. Naltrexone is a non-addictive antagonist of OP1. Compared to fluorescein-naltrexone, Cy5-naltrexone (Cy5-NAL) is a more hydrophilic

derivative of naltrexone and exhibits better binding characteristics (high specificity to OP1 and low cross-activity to other receptors).

6. The assay buffer composition could have significant impact on the pharmacological properties of the ligands. For example, certain cations such as Zn^{2+}, Mg^{2+}, and Na^{+} act as positive or negative allosteric modulators for several GPCRs *(14)*. The binding of the Cy5-NT to NTS1 was found to be significantly reduced by the presence of Na^{+} *(7)*. Both Zn^{2+} and Co^{2+} dose dependently inhibit the binding of the BT-CGP to the β_1-AR in microarrays *(7)*. The inhibitory effect of the cations is primarily observed as an increase in the dissociation constant rather than as a change in the association constant. In addition, the buffer reagents themselves can also impact the binding characteristics of labeled ligands.

References

1. Fang, Y., Frutos, A.G., and Lahiri, J. (2002) Membrane protein microarrays. *J. Am. Chem. Soc.* **124**, 2394–2395.
2. Fang, Y., Frutos, A.G., and Lahiri, J. (2002) G protein-coupled receptor microarrays. *ChemBiochem* **3**, 987–991.
3. Fang, Y., Lahiri, J., and Picard, L. (2003) G protein-coupled receptor microarrays for drug discovery. *Drug Discov. Today* **8**, 755–761.
4. Fang, Y., Hong, Y., Webb, B.L., and Lahiri, J. (2006) Applications of biomembranes for drug discovery. *MRS Bulletin* **31**, 541–545.
5. Hopkins, A.L., and Groom, C.R. (2002) The druggable genome. *Nature Rev. Drug Discov.* **1**, 727–730.
6. Drews, J. (2000) Drug discovery: A historical perspective. *Science* **287**, 1960–1963.
7. Fang, Y., Peng, J., Ferrie, A.M., and Burkhalter, R.S. (2006) Air-stable G protein-coupled receptor microarrays and ligand binding characteristics. *Anal. Chem.* **78**, 149–155.
8. Hong, Y., Webb, B.L., Pai, S., Ferrie, A., Peng, J., Lai, F., Lahiri, J., Biddlecome, G., Rasnow, B., Johnson, M., Min, H., Fang, Y., and Salon, J. (2006) Multiplexed compound screening using GPCR microarrays and ligand cocktails. *J. Biomol. Screen.* **11**, 435–438.
9. Posner, B., Hong, Y., Benvenuti, E., Potchoiba, M., Nettleton, D., Lui, L., Ferrie, A., Lai, F., Fang, Y., Miret, J., Wielis, C., and Webb, B. (2007) Multiplexing G protein-coupled receptors in microarrays: A radioligand-binding assay. *Anal. Biochem.* **365**, 266–273.
10. Fang, Y. (2006) Spreading and segregation of lipids in air-stable lipid microarrays. *J. Am. Chem. Soc.* **128**, 3158–3159.
11. Luzardo, M.C., Amalfa, F., Nunez, A.M., Diaz, S., Lopez, A.C.B., and Disalvo, E.A. (2000) Effect of trehalose and sucrose on the hydration and dipole potential of lipid bilayers. *Biophys. J.* **78**, 2452–2458.
12. Gurwitz, D., and Haring, R. (2003) Ligand-selective signaling and high content for GPCR drugs. *Drug Discov. Today* **8**, 1108–1109.
13. Kobilka, B. (2004) Agonist binding: A multistep process. *Mol. Pharmacol.* **65**, 1060–1062.
14. Swaminath, G., Lee, T.W., and Kobilka, B. (2003) Identification of an allosteric binding site for Zn^{2+} on the β_2-adrenergic receptor. *J. Biol. Chem.* **278**, 352–356.

Chapter 17

Resonant Waveguide Grating Biosensor for Whole-Cell GPCR Assays

Ye Fang, Ann M. Ferrie, and Elizabeth Tran

Summary

Current drug discovery campaigns for G protein-coupled receptors (GPCRs) heavily rely on assay technologies that use artificial cell systems tailored to a point-of-contact readout and as a consequence are mostly pathway biased. Recently, we have developed label-free optical biosensor cellular assays that are capable of examining systems cell biology of endogenous receptors and systems cell pharmacology of GPCR ligands in both physiologically and disease relevant environments. We have shown that these biosensor assays enable high-throughput screening of pathway-biased ligands acting on endogenous β_2-adrenergic receptor in cells. These biosensor cellular assays hold the potential to reduce attrition rates in drug discovery and development process.

Key words: G protein-coupled receptor, Optical biosensor, Resonant waveguide grating biosensor, Dynamic mass redistribution, Ligand-directed functional selectivity.

1. Introduction

Resonant waveguide grating (RWG) biosensor is an optical biosensor that is capable of detecting minute changes in local index of refraction near the sensor surface *(1)*. Since local index of refraction within a cell is a function of density and its distribution of biomass (e.g., proteins, molecular complexes) *(2)*, RWG biosensor non-invasively detects stimulus-induced dynamic mass redistribution (DMR) in native cells without the need for any labels and cellular manipulations *(3–6)*. Common to current cell-based assays is the use of labels and cellular manipulations, which could require significant assay development efforts and often lead to many complications in receptor

Wayne R. Leifert (ed.), *G Protein-Coupled Receptors in Drug Discovery, vol. 552*

Book doi: 10.1007/978-1-60327-317-6_17

biology and ligand pharmacology *(7, 8)*. Instead of measuring single point of contacts within complex signaling pathways, RWG biosensor can follow the evolution of receptor signaling in time and space, leading to a kinetic and integrative response, termed DMR. The DMR measure is mostly pathway unbiased but pathway sensitive *(9–13)*. With the recent advancements in biosensor design and instrumentation *(5, 9)*, these biosensors are easily scalable and enable high-throughput screening of drug compounds for endogenous G protein-coupled receptors (GPCRs) in native cells *(14)*.

For whole-cell sensing, a RWG biosensor is considered as a three-layer waveguide configuration: a substrate with an optical grating, a high index of refraction waveguide coating, and a cell layer (**Fig. 1a**). The biosensor employs the resonant coupling of light into the waveguide by means of a diffraction grating. When illuminated with broadband light at a fixed and nominally normal angle of incidence, these sensors reflect only a narrow band of wavelengths that is a sensitive function of the index of refraction of the biosensor and is governed by *(1)*:

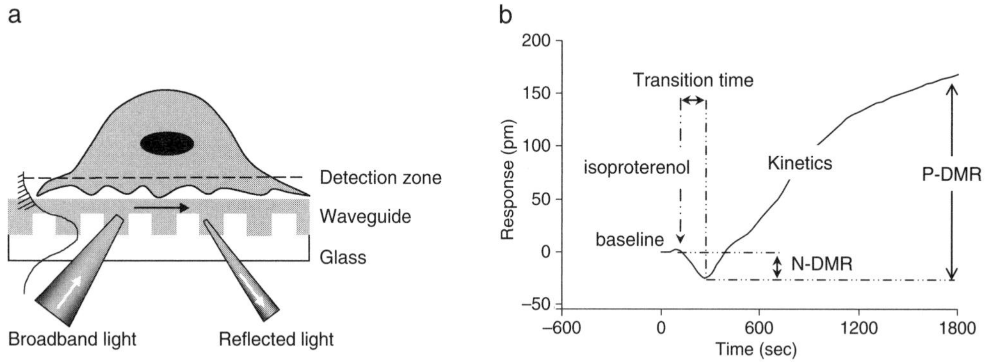

Fig. 1. RWG biosensor for whole-cell GPCR sensing. (**a**) A three-layer waveguide system for detecting ligand-induced DMR signals in living cells using RWG biosensor. Cells are cultured on the sensor surface. (**b**) The DMR signal of quiescent A431 cells induced by 0.1 n*M* isoproterenol. Isoproterenol is a full agonist of β_2AR.

$$\sin(\theta) = n_{eff} - l\frac{\lambda}{\Lambda}$$

where θ is the maximum efficiency coupling angle, n_{eff} the effective index of refraction of the waveguide, ℓ the diffraction order, λ the resonant wavelength, and Λ the grating period.

RWG biosensor utilizes the evanescent wave to characterize ligand-induced alterations in the cells. The evanescent wave is an electromagnetic field created by the total internal reflection of resonant light in the waveguide thin film, whose intensity exponentially decays away from the sensor surface. The distance from the sensor surface at which the electric field strength has decreased to $1/e$ of its initial value is the penetration depth or detection zone or sensing volume (typically ~150 nm). This feature indicates that the biosensor only samples the bottom portion of the cells contacting with the sensor surface (**Fig. 1a**).

Using a three-layer waveguide system, we have found that a ligand-induced change in effective refractive index (i.e., the detected signal) is governed by *(3)*:

$$\Delta N = S(C)\alpha d \sum_i \Delta C_i(t)\left[e^{\frac{-z_i}{\Delta Z_C}} - e^{\frac{-z_{+1i}}{\Delta Z_C}}\right]$$

where $S(C)$ is the sensitivity of the biosensor to the cell layer, ΔZ_c the penetration depth into the cell layer, α the specific refraction increment (about 0.18/mL/g for proteins), $\Delta C_i(t)$ the change in local concentration of biomolecules at the given location at a specific time, z_i the distance where the mass redistribution occurs, and d an imaginary thickness of a slice within the cell layer. This theory predicates, as confirmed by experimental studies *(3–6, 9–13)*, that the biosensor is able to monitor cell signaling in real time, a stimulus-induced optical response is dominated by the vertical DMR, and the resultant DMR signal is an integrated cellular response containing contributions from many cellular events mediated through a receptor. The DMR signals are often manifested by a shift in resonant wavelength of the biosensor (**Fig. 1b**).

The full activation of endogenous β_2-adrenergic receptor (β_2AR) in human epidermoid carcinoma A431 cells leads to a prototypical G_s-mediated signaling *(13)*. The DMR signal mediated through the activation of β_2AR offers multiple parameters to differentiate pathway-biased activity of many ligands acting on the receptor *(13)*. Assays using a subset of Library of Pharmaceutically Active Compounds (Sigma Chemical Co.) show the ability of the biosensor cellular assay for screening pathway-biased ligands. Here using the endogenous β_2AR in A431 cells as a model system we describe a three-step protocol for whole-cell GPCR sensing using RWG biosensors: (i) preparation of cells, (ii) detecting cellular responses upon stimulation using the biosensor, and (iii) extracting DMR parameters for analysis of ligand pharmacology and receptor biology.

2. Materials

2.1. Tissue Culture Medium and Cell Line

1. Dulbecco's modified Eagle's medium (DMEM; Invitrogen, Carlsbad, CA, USA).
2. Heat-inactivated fetal bovine serum (FBS; Invitrogen).

3. Penicillin-streptomycin liquid (100 ×; Invitrogen).
4. Complete cell culture medium: DMEM supplemented to a final concentration of 10% with heat-inactivated FBS, 4.5 g/L of glucose, 2 m*M* of glutamine, 50 U/mL of penicillin, and 50 μg/mL of streptomycin.
5. Serum-free starvation medium: DMEM supplemented to a final concentration of 4.5 g/L of glucose, 2 m*M* of glutamine, 50 U/mL of penicillin, and 50 μg/mL of streptomycin.
6. Trypsin-EDTA: 0.25% Trypsin with EDTA.4Na$^+$ (Invitrogen).
7. Human epidermoid carcinoma A431 cells (American Type Cell Culture, Manassas, VA, USA).

2.2. Microplates and Instruments

1. Corning 75 cm^2 tissue culture-treated polystyrene flask with vented cap (T-75) (Corning Inc., Corning, NY, USA).
2. Corning 384-well polypropylene compound storage plate (Corning Inc.).
3. Epic® 384-well microplate tissue culture treated (Corning Inc.) (*see* **Note 1**).
4. Matrix 16-channel electronic pipettor (Thermo Fisher Scientific, Hudson, NH, USA).
5. Epic® system (Corning Inc.; *see* **Note 2**).
6. BioTek cell plate washer ELx405 (BioTek Instruments Inc., Winooski, VT, USA).

2.3. The RWG Biosensor Cellular Assays

1. Betaxolol, dopamine, ICI118551, (−)-isoproterenol, norepinephrine, pindolol, propranolol, and salbutamol (Tocris Chemical Co., St. Louis, MO).
2. Catechol, halostachine, and S(−)-epinephrine (Sigma Chemical Co., St. Louis, MO, USA).
3. Hank's balanced salt solution (HBSS), 1 × with calcium and magnesium, but no phenol red (Invitrogen).
4. 1 *M* HEPES buffer solution, pH7.1 (Invitrogen).
5. Assay buffered solution (1 × HBSS, 10 m*M* HEPES, pH 7.1).
6. Library of Pharmaceutically Active Compounds (Sigma Chemical Co.).

2.4. Data Analysis Software

1. Epic® Offline Viewer (Corning Inc.).
2. Microsoft Excel (Microsoft Inc., Seattle, WA, USA).
3. Prism Software (GraphPad Software Inc., La Jolla, CA, USA).

3. Methods

3.1. Preparations of Cells for Assaying Endogenous β_2 AR by RWG Biosensor

This protocol employs standard cell culture and starvation techniques to prepare cells for assaying the endogenous β_2AR in A431 cells (*see* **Note 3**). Simple modifications of this protocol can be used for assaying receptors in different types of native or engineered cells, including suspension cells (*see* **Note 4**). These modifications include the cell culture medium and time, initial seeding numbers of cells, cell synchronization, and types of biosensor surfaces.

1. The wild-type human epidermoid carcinoma A431 cells received from ATCC are passed in T-75 flasks using the recommended protocol. The cells up to at least 25 passages after received from ATCC are appropriated for the biosensor cellular assays in our laboratory. The native A431 cells are passed when approaching confluence with trypsin/EDTA to provide new maintenance cultures on T-75 flasks and experimental cultures on the Epic 384-well tissue culture-treated microplate. A 1:10 split of the native cells will provide maintenance cultures on T-75 flasks that are approaching confluence after 5 days. Cells on a T-75 flask are sufficient for experimental cultures on at least one biosensor microplate.
2. Once the cells reach confluence in the T-75 flask, the cells are harvested using 1 × trypsin-EDTA solution. After centrifuging the cells down, the supernatant is removed and the cell pallet is resuspended in freshly prepared complete cell culture medium.
3. Approximately 1.8×10^4 cells at passages 3–25 suspended in 50 μL of the complete medium are added into each well of an Epic 384-well biosensor microplate (*see* **Note 5**). The cell plating is carried out using a 16-channel electronic pipettor. Air bubbles trapped in the bottoms of the wells at this stage, if any, are manually removed by the pipettor.
4. After incubation in the laminar flow hood for ~20 min, the cells are then cultured for 24 h at 37°C under air/5% CO_2. At this point the cells usually reach approximately 80–90% confluency. After rinsing twice with the serum-free starvation medium, the cells are incubated for a further 24 h in the serum-free DMEM at 37°C under air/5% CO_2. During the starvation, the cells continue to grow until approaching 100% confluence and reaching a quiescent state through serum withdrawal and contact inhibition *(15)* (*see* **Note 6**).

3.2. Biosensor Cellular Assays for Kinetic Measurements of Receptor Signaling and Ligand Pharmacology

This protocol describes both one-step and sequential two-step kinetic assays. The one-step assay is useful for determining agonism of individual ligands, determining competitive antagonism of a ligand against an agonist under non-equilibrium condition, and examining cellular responses upon costimulation. The two-step assay is useful for assaying antagonism of ligands, determining competitive antagonism of a ligand against an agonist under equilibrium condition, and analyzing systems cell biology of an agonist-induced signaling. The systems cell biology analysis is assessed based on the impact of chemical and biochemical (e.g., interference RNA) intervention of specific cellular signaling cascades on the agonist-induced DMR signal *(4–6, 9, 10)*. For the two-step assays, the separation time between the two stimulations are typically within tens of minutes.

1. The assay-buffered solution is made ready and stored at room temperature. Compounds are generally dissolved in dimethyl sulfoxide (DMSO) and stored at high concentrations (10–100 m*M*) at –20°C.
2. Compound solutions are made by diluting the stored concentrated solutions with the assay-buffered solution at room temperature and transferred into a 384-well polypropylene compound storage plate using a pipettor to prepare a compound source plate. Two separate compound source plates are applied when a two-step assay is performed.
3. The starved cells are washed twice with the assay-buffered solution using the BioTek washer and maintained in 30 μL of the assay-buffered solution to prepare a cell assay plate.
4. Both the cell assay plate and the compound source plate(s) are incubated in the hotel of the Epic system for at least 1 h (*see* **Note 7**). When a compound solution contains greater than 0.1% DMSO, the DMSO in the corresponding well of the cell assay plate is carefully matched (*see* **Note 8**).
5. After approximately 1 h of incubation in the reader system, the baseline wavelengths of all biosensors in the cell assay microplate are recorded and normalized to zero. Afterwards, a 2–10 min continuous recording is carried out to establish a baseline. At this point, the baseline should reach a steady state, leading to a net-zero response (**Fig. 1b**) (*see* **Note 9**).
6. Cellular responses are triggered by transferring 10 μL of the compound solutions from the compound source plate into the cell assay plate using the on-board liquid handler. Afterwards, the cellular responses are continuously monitored for a period of time (typically 1 h for GPCR signaling) (*see* **Note 10**).
7. For studying the influence of chemical or biochemical interventions, a second stimulation with an agonist at a fixed dose (typically a dose at EC_{80} or EC_{100}) is applied. The cellular

responses are continuously recorded. The resonant wavelengths of all biosensors in the microplate can be normalized again to establish a second baseline, right before the second stimulation.

3.3. Biosensor Cellular Assays for High-Throughput Screening

Once the DMR signal is known for a receptor–agonist pair in a cell type, a two or multiple end-point assay can be developed in order to screen compounds in high-throughput manner. Since the biosensor cellular assays are non-invasive in nature, both agonism and antagonism screening modes can be incorporated in a single screening campaign. The following is an example of high-throughput screening of agonists for endogenous G_s-coupled receptors in A431 cells using a subset of LOPAC library of compounds.

1. The Sigma-Aldrich LOPAC 1280™ library of compounds includes 1280 bioactive small organic molecules against many target classes including several GPCRs. The compounds received are stored in barcoded 96-well microplates as 10 m*M* solution in neat DMSO. Four of these compound microplates are aliquoted and reconfigured into a single 384-well compound source microplate. After appropriate dilution with the assay-buffered solution, a 384-well compound source plate having 320 compounds in wells from columns 3–2 is made ready, such that the final concentration of each ligand is 4 μ*M*. The DMSO concentration is 0.4%. The wells in the columns 1 and 2 only contain the assay-buffered solution having 0.4% DMSO and are used as a negative control. The wells in the columns 23 and 24 only contain 2 n*M* epinephrine in 0.4% DMSO and are used as a positive control.
2. The starved A431 cells in the biosensor microplate are washed with the assay-buffered solution twice and maintained in 30 μL of the buffered solution containing 0.4% DMSO.
3. Both the compound source plate and the cell assay plate are incubated in the hotel of the reader system for 1 h. After a baseline read, 10 μL 4 × compound solutions are transferred into the cell assay plate. After 50 min of stimulation, a second end-point read is recorded. The shift in resonant wavelength in each well is calculated and plotted as a function of compounds.

3.4. Data Analysis

The practical applications of these biosensor cellular assays are numerous. This section presents a brief description of some of these assays to study receptor signaling and ligand pharmacology.

3.4.1. Extracting Kinetic Information from Ligand-Induced DMR Signals

RWG biosensors measure ligand-induced DMR signals in living cells. The resultant DMR signal is a real-time kinetic response and contains high information contents. As exampled in the isoproterenol response in quiescent A431 cells, following the steady baseline is an initial decrease in signal (termed negative-DMR, N-DMR) and a subsequent increase in signal (positive-DMR, P-DMR) (**Fig. 1b**). Multiple parameters can be extracted from the DMR signal, each of which can be used to analyze ligand pharmacology and receptor biology. These parameters include overall dynamics, number of phases, the transition time from one phase to another, and amplitudes, duration, and kinetics of each phase.

1. After a 2 min baseline recording, the quiescent A431 cells are stimulated with isoproterenol at different doses. The cellular response is continuously monitored for 1 h until reaching an elevated plateau.
2. The amplitudes of both N-DMR and P-DMR events are calculated using the Epic offline viewer. The transition time for the P-DMR event to occur is calculated using Microsoft Excel, whereas the kinetics of the P-DMR event is determined by fitting it with a one-phase association non-linear regression process using the Prism software.

3.4.2. Determining Agonist Potency and Efficacy

To determine the efficacy and potency of an agonist, the cells are stimulated with a concentration series of the agonist. The kinetic responses of cells are recorded and subsequently analyzed for the dose dependency of the cellular responses. **Figure 2a** shows the dose-dependent DMR signals of quiescent A431 cells induced by isoproterenol. **Figure 2b** shows the time-dependent amplitudes of isoproterenol-induced DMR signals in A431 cells. The isoproterenol response displays classical dose dependency, that is, both the amplitudes and kinetics increase until reaching a maximal level at saturating concentrations. The potency and efficacy of the agonist can be determined in many different ways. Typically the amplitude of a DMR event (e.g., the P-DMR event for the isoproterenol response) at a specific time point is plotted as a function of agonist doses to determine the potency and efficacy of the agonists (**Fig. 2b**).

3.4.3. Determining Relative Potency of Antagonists

To determine relative potency of antagonists, the potency of a β_2AR agonist such as epinephrine is determined first using the above-mentioned method (**Section 3.4.2**). Epinephrine at EC_{80} is chosen to determine the relative potency of β_2AR antagonists, such as betaxolol, ICI 118551, and propranolol. The quiescent A431 cells are pretreated with each antagonist at different doses for about 5 min to 1 h. Afterward a baseline read, and the agonist responses are triggered by transferring 10 μL of the 5 × solution of the agonist into the cell assay plates. Later, the amplitudes of the agonist P-DMR event in the presence of an antagonist at different doses are calculated based on the shift in resonant wavelength before and 50 min after stimulation. Non-linear regression analysis

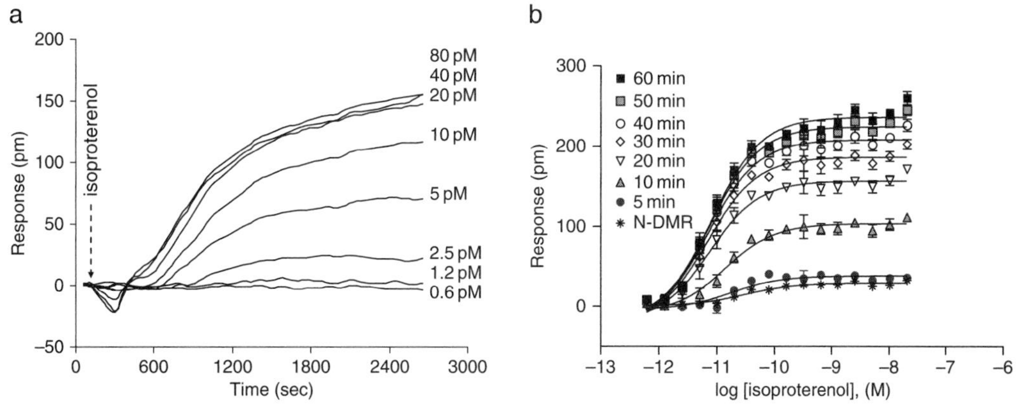

Fig. 2. The dose-dependent isoproterenol responses of quiescent A431 cells. (**a**) Real-time kinetic responses. (**b**) The time-dependent amplitudes. A431 cells were cultured on the Epic 384-well tissue culture-treated microplate and grown to confluence. After starvation, the cells were stimulated with isoproterenol at different doses as indicated. The amplitudes were calculated based on the difference of resonant wavelength between before and a specific time after stimulation. The broken arrow indicated the time when isoproterenol is introduced.

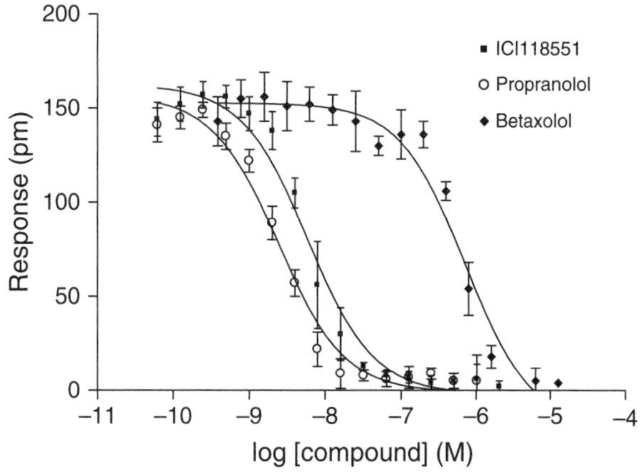

Fig. 3. The dose-dependent inhibition of the 2 n*M* (–)-epinephrine response of quiescent A431 cells by three β_2AR antagonists, ICI118551, propranolol, and betaxolol. The amplitudes of the P-DMR event of the epinephrine DMR signals were plotted as a function of antagonist concentration. The P-DMR amplitudes were calculated based on the shift in resonant wavelength before and 50 min after the epinephrine stimulation.

is used to determine the relative potency of the antagonists against the agonist. **Figure 3** shows the dose-dependent inhibition of the epinephrine response by the three β_2AR antagonists.

3.4.4. Determining Ligand-Directed Functional Selectivity

GPCRs display rich behaviors in cells and many ligands can induce operative bias to favor specific portions of the cell machinery and exhibit pathway-biased efficacies *(16, 17)*. To determine ligand-directed functional selectivity with the biosensor cellular assays, panels of structurally similar β_2AR ligands that have a wide spectrum of efficacies are chosen and used to stimulate the quiescent A431 cells. The DMR signals are recorded, and multiparameter analysis is carried out to determine the correlation between the structures of ligands and the characteristics of their optical signals *(13)*. **Figure 4** graphically depicts the chemical structures of agonists examined and their corresponding DMR signals in quiescent A431cells.

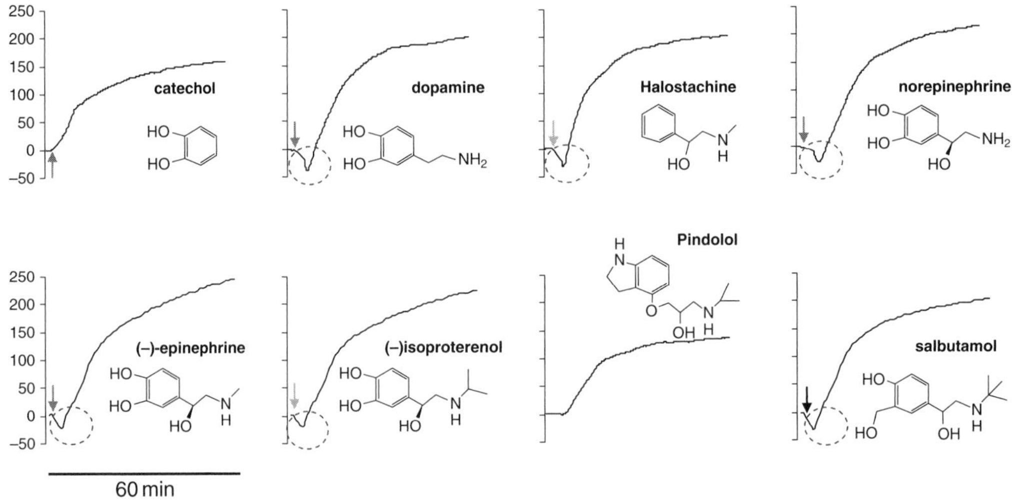

Fig. 4. The structures of β_2AR ligands and their DMR in quiescent A431 cells. The ligands included (–)epinephrine (8 n*M*), (–)isoproterenol (10 n*M*), norepinephrine (100 n*M*), dopamine (32 μ*M*), halostachine (500 μ*M*), catechol (500 μ*M*), salbutamol (164 n*M*), and pindolol (8 μ*M*). The gray arrows indicated the time when the agonist is introduced. The *y*-axis is the response in picometer (pm). The inhibition profiles by propranolol suggest that these ligand-induced DMR signals are specific to the β_2AR *(13)*. (Reproduced with permission from *(13)*).

3.4.5. Determining Competitive Antagonism

The competitive antagonism can be assessed under two distinct experimental conditions: equilibrium and non-equilibrium conditions. The equilibrium competitive assay is performed using a two-step stimulation procedure, wherein the cells are pretreated with an antagonist at a fixed dose, followed by stimulation with an agonist at different doses. The non-equilibrium assay is performed using costimulation of cells with an agonist in several independent dose series, each series in the presence of an antagonist at a fixed dose. The Schild analysis is then carried out. **Figure 5** shows an example of the non-equilibrium assay to determine the competitive antagonism of propranolol against epinephrine acting on the β_2AR in A431 cells.

3.4.6. Screening Pathway-Biased Agonists

The pathway-biased agonists can be assessed using two different types of assays: kinetic and end-point assays. The quiescent A431 cells are stimulated with a subset of the LOPAC compounds at a fixed dose (each at 1 μ*M*). The cellular response of each biosensor

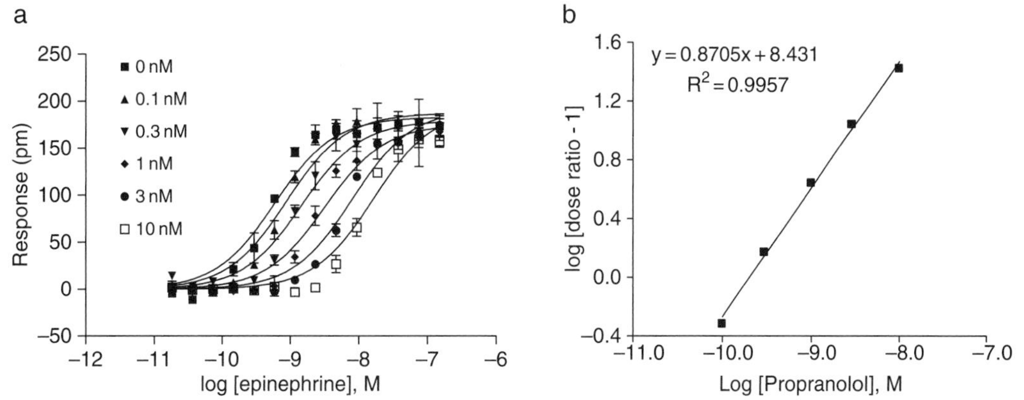

Fig. 5. Schild analysis for the competitive antagonism of propranolol against epinephrine under non-equilibrium condition. (**a**) The amplitudes of the epinephrine responses in the presence of propranolol were plotted as a function of epinephrine concentration. The amplitudes were calculated based on the shift in resonant wavelength before and 50 min after stimulation. The cells were stimulated with epinephrine at different doses. Propranolol at different fixed doses was added into each epinephrine dose series. (**b**) The Schild plot analysis. The results indicate that propranolol is a competitive antagonist against epinephrine under the non-equilibrium condition.

well is calculated based on the shift in resonant wavelength before and 50 min after stimulation. The difference between the positive and negative controls is used to calculate assay robustness. The relative ratio of an agonist response to the positive control is an

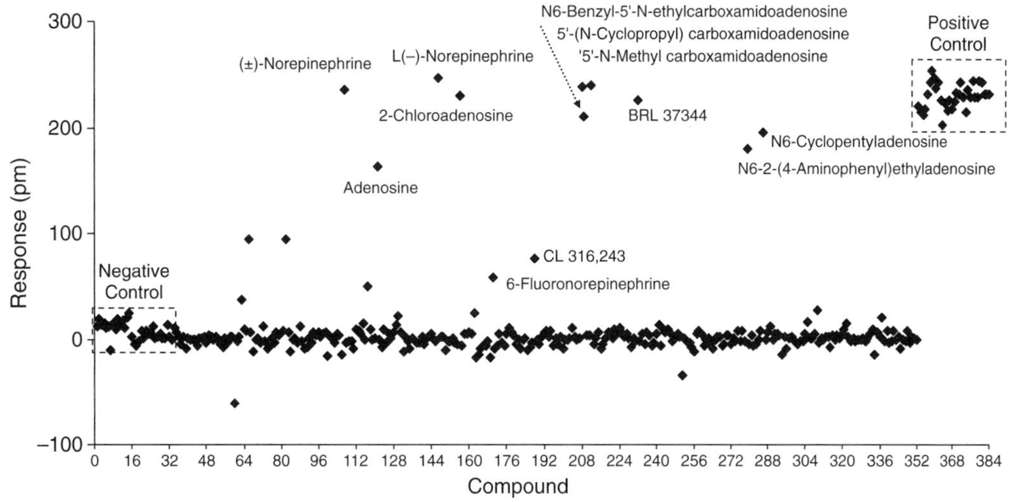

Fig. 6. The response of quiescent A431 cells as a function of compound. The quiescent A431 cells were stimulated with a subset of LOPAC library of compounds. The shift in resonant wavelength before and 50 min after stimulation was calculated for each well. The negative controls (the vehicle only) led to a response of 8 ± 7 pm (n=32), whereas the positive controls (2 nM (−)-epinephrine) led to a response of 230 ± 12 pm (n=32), indicating a robust assay with a Z' factor of 0.74. This end-point screening identified all agonists in this subset of compounds for both the endogenous β_2AR and adenosine receptors in A431. Several other compounds whose mechanisms to trigger the DMR responses are unknown were also identified.

indicator of the ability of the agonist to trigger the receptor signaling; a ratio of less than 1 indicates that the agonist is a partial agonist. **Figure 6** shows an example of screening pathway-biased agonists using the end-point assays.

4. Notes

1. Two types of biosensor microplates are commercially available and are ready to culture. They are Epic 384-well tissue culture treated and Epic 384-well fibronectin coated. Within each well of either type of microplates, there is an RWG biosensor.
2. The Epic system is the first high-throughput screening biosensor system for both biochemical and cell-based assays *(4–6, 14)*. The system consists of two components: a disposable SBS (Society for Biomolecular Sciences) standard 384-well biosensor microplate in which each well contains an RWG biosensor and an optical reader that utilizes a linear array of fiber optic heads for recording cellular responses in the biosensor microplate. The commercially available Epic system is a standalone optical reader. An external liquid handling accessory can be directly attached to the reader system. This system is capable of measuring as many as 40,000 wells in an 8 h period, based on end-point measurements. For kinetic assays, the temporal resolution is approximately 7 or 15 s, depending on the scanning mode selected. Here a beta version of the Epic system is used, in which an on-board liquid handler is available for onsite compound addition. The entire reader system is maintained at 26°C.
3. A431 cell line is chosen because it endogenously expresses a large number of the β_2AR but no β_1AR or β_3AR *(18)*. The endogenous β_2AR is a prototypical G_s-coupled receptor and has served as a model system for studying GPCR signaling cycle, including receptor trafficking *(19, 20)*.
4. The biosensor cellular assays are applicable to both adherent and suspension cells. For adherent cells such as A431, the cells are directly cultured on the surfaces of the 384-well Epic microplate tissue culture treated. For weakly adherent cells such as human embryonic kidney 293, the cells are directly cultured on the surfaces of the 384-well Epic microplate fibronectin coated. For suspension cells, the cells are brought to contact with the surface of a biosensor microplate through either gravity or chemical interactions (e.g., covalent coupling or specific biomolecular interactions of the cell surface molecules).

5. The seeding number of cells on the biosensor microplates is usually optimized first. Since the biosensor measures an averaged response of a population of cells located in the area illuminated by the incident light, a cell layer of high confluency is usually used to achieve optimal results.
6. Synchronizing cells into a specific state is not necessary. However, it can be, in some cases, beneficial to receptor biology analysis, assay reproducibility, and robustness. This is because the biosensor assays are sensitive to cellular context (e.g., passages, proliferating and quiescent states, and confluency) due to the integrative nature of the DMR signals measured with the biosensor. The cellular environment is known to modulate receptor pharmacology, rendering many GPCR ligands to often display cellular context-dependent pharmacological profiles *(21)*.
7. Preincubation (~ tens of minutes) of both the cell assay plates and the compound source plates can significantly reduce the environmental effects on cellular response. A temperature-controlling unit is built in the reader system to minimize any temperature fluctuation.
8. DMSO is a high index of refraction solvent. Also, DMSO is often considered a cytotoxic agent and has significant impact on cell biology.
9. Although cells are dynamic and constantly undergo micromotion (i.e., a dynamic movement and remodeling of cellular structure under unstimulated conditions), the cells generally give rise to an almost net-zero DMR response, following the cell preparation and assay protocol described in **Sections 3.2** and **3.3**. This is partly because of the low spatial resolution of the biosensors, also partly due to highly ordered structure of intracellular macromolecules in cells, most of which have just completed a single cycle of division at the time of assay.
10. GPCR agonist-induced optical responses in living cells typically last for about 1 h until they reach a plateau.

References

1. Tiefenthaler, K., and Lukosz, W. (1989) Sensitivity of grating couplers as integrated-optical chemical sensors. *J. Opt. Soc. Am. B* **6**, 209–220.
2. Barer, R., and Joseph, S. (1954) Refractometry of living cells. Part I. basic principles. *Quart. J. Microsc. Science* **95**, 399–423.
3. Fang, Y., Ferrie, A.M., Fontaine, N.H., Mauro, J., and Balakrishnan, J. (2006) Resonant waveguide grating biosensor for living cell sensing. *Biophys. J.* **91**, 1925–1940.
4. Fang, Y. (2006) Label-free cell-based assays with optical biosensors in drug discovery. *Assay Drug Dev. Technol.* **4**, 583–595.
5. Fang, Y. (2007) Non-invasive optical biosensor for probing cell signaling. *Sensors* 7, 2316–2329.
6. Fang, Y., Frutos, A.G., and Verkleeren R. (2008) Label-free cell-based assays for GPCR screening. *Comb. Chem. High Throughput Screen.* **11**, 357–369.

7. Cooper, M.A. (2006) Optical biosensors: where next and how soon. *Drug Discov. Today* **11**, 1061–1067.
8. Milligan, G. (2003) High-content assays for ligand regulation of G protein-coupled receptors. *Drug Discov. Today* **8**, 579–585.
9. Fang, Y., Ferrie, A.M., Fontaine, N.H., and Yuen, P.K. (2005) Characteristics of dynamic mass redistribution of EGF receptor signaling in living cells measured with label free optical biosensors. *Anal. Chem.* **77**, 5720–5725.
10. Fang, Y., Li, G., and Peng, J. (2005) Optical biosensor provides insights for bradykinin B2 receptor signaling in A431 cells. *FEBS Lett.* **579**, 6365–6374.
11. Fang, Y., Li, G., and Ferrie, A.M. (2007) Non-invasive optical biosensor for assaying endogenous G protein-coupled receptors in adherent cells. *J. Pharmacol. Toxicol. Methods* **55**, 314–322.
12. Fang, Y., and Ferrie, A.M. (2007) Optical biosensor differentiates signaling of endogenous PAR_1 and PAR_2 in A431 cells. *BMC Cell Biol.* **8**, e24.
13. Fang, Y., and Ferrie, A.M. (2008) Label-free optical biosensor for ligand-directed functional selectivity acting on β_2 adrenoceptor in living cells. *FEBS Lett.* **582**, 558–564.
14. Li, G., Ferrie, A.M., and Fang, Y. (2006) Label-free profiling of endogenous G protein-coupled receptors using a cell-based high throughput screening technology. *J. Assoc. Lab. Automat.* **11**, 181–187.
15. Coller, H.A., Sang, L., and Roberts, J.M. (2006) A new description of cellular quiescence. *PLoS Biol.* **4**, e83.
16. Kenakin, T. (2005) New concepts in drug discovery: collateral efficacy and permissive antagonism. *Nat. Rev. Drug Discov.* **4**, 919–927.
17. Perez, D.M., and Karnik, S.S. (2005) Multiple signaling states of G protein-coupled receptors. *Pharmacol. Rev.* **57**, 147–161.
18. Delavier-Klutchko, C., Hoebeke, J., and Strosberg, A.D. (1984) The human carcinoma cell line A431 possesses large numbers of functional β_2-adrenergic receptors. *FEBS Lett.* **169**, 151–155.
19. Morris, A.J., and Malbon, C.C. (1999) Physiological regulation of G protein-linked signaling. *Physiol. Rev.* **79**, 1373–1430.
20. Shih, M., and Malbon, C.C. (1994) Oligodeoxynucleotides antisense to mRNA encoding protein kinase A, protein kinase C, and β_2-adrenergic receptor kinase reveal distinctive cell-type-specific roles in agonist-induced desensitization. *Proc. Natl. Acad. Sci. USA* **91**, 12193–12197.
21. Nelson, C.P., and Challiss, R.A.J. (2007) "Phenotypic" pharmacology: the influence of cellular environment on G protein-coupled receptor antagonist and inverse agonist pharmacology. *Biochem. Pharmacol.* **73**, 737–751.

Chapter 18

FRET-Based Measurement of GPCR Conformational Changes

Sébastien Granier, Samuel Kim, Juan José Fung, Michael P. Bokoch, and Charles Parnot

Summary

The C-termini of G protein-coupled receptors (GPCRs) interact with specific kinases and arrestins in an agonist-dependent manner suggesting that conformational changes induced by ligand binding within the transmembrane domains are transmitted to the C-terminus. Förster resonance energy transfer (FRET) can be used to monitor changes in distance between two protein domains if each site can be specifically and efficiently labeled with a donor or acceptor fluorophore. In order to probe GPCR conformational changes, we have developed a FRET technique that uses site-specific donor and acceptor fluorophores introduced by two orthogonal labeling chemistries. Using this strategy, we examined ligand-induced changes in the distance between two labeled sites in the β_2 adrenoceptor (β_2-AR), a well-characterized GPCR model system. The donor fluorophore, Lumio™Green, is chelated by a CCPGCC motif [*Fl*uorescein *As*enical *H*elix or *H*airpin binder (FlAsH) site] introduced through mutagenesis. The acceptor fluorophore, Alexa Fluor 568, is attached to a single reactive cysteine (C265). FRET analyses revealed that the average distance between the intracellular end of transmembrane helix (TM) six and the C-terminus of the β_2-AR is 62 Å. This relatively large distance suggests that the C-terminus is extended and unstructured. Nevertheless, ligand-specific conformational changes were observed *(1)*. The results provide new insight into the structure of the β_2-AR C-terminus and ligand-induced conformational changes that may be relevant to arrestin interactions. The FRET labeling technique described herein can be applied to many GPCRs (and other membrane proteins) and is suitable for conformational studies of domains other than the C-terminus.

Key words: GPCR, Conformational Changes, Fluorescence Spectroscopy, FRET, Orthogonal Labeling Method, Membrane protein expression and purification.

1. Introduction

G protein-coupled receptors (GPCRs) are versatile membrane proteins that regulate a wide variety of physiological functions. They respond to a large array of structurally diverse ligands and are the largest group of targets for drug discovery. Structure/function

Wayne R. Leifert (ed.), *G Protein-Coupled Receptors in Drug Discovery, vol. 552*

Book doi: 10.1007/978-1-60327-317-6_18

analysis has identified amino acids important for G protein coupling and ligand binding for several well-characterized GPCRs *(2)*. Few studies have directly addressed the mechanism by which diffusible ligands activate GPCRs. We have developed a number of fluorescence methods to characterize the structure of the β_2 adrenoceptor (β_2-AR) and monitor ligand-induced conformational changes in real time *(3–5)*. Our previous studies primarily focused on ligand-induced conformational changes in transmembrane (TM) segments, which are directly involved in ligand binding and G protein coupling. However, agonists also induce structural changes that promote phosphorylation of the carboxyl terminus by GPCR kinases and subsequent binding of arrestins *(6, 7)*. These processes are important for receptor desensitization and agonist-induced internalization. Recent studies demonstrate that arrestin is also a signaling molecule *(7, 8)*. Of interest, arrestin-dependent activation of ERK has been observed in response to both agonists and inverse agonists *(9, 10)*, suggesting that a given ligand may have differential efficacy for the stimulatory G protein (Gs) and arrestin signaling pathways. The β_2-AR is activated by a broad spectrum of diffusible ligands and therefore makes an ideal GPCR model system to study ligand-induced conformational changes and the structural basis of ligand efficacy. Moreover, the three-dimensional structure of the β_2-AR in the inactive state has been recently solved *(11, 12)*.

We have developed a Förster resonance energy transfer (FRET)-based approach to monitor ligand-induced movement of the carboxyl terminus relative to the cytoplasmic end of transmembrane 6 (TM6). FRET refers to the transfer of energy between two fluorophores through a non-radiative dipole–dipole interaction. The efficiency of energy transfer is dependent upon the distance between two probes and thus is useful for extracting structural information. The FRET efficiency (E) can be expressed in terms of the distance (R) between the donor and the acceptor fluorophores and the characteristic Förster distance (R_0) for a given pair of fluorophores (based on their spectral characteristics, see *Methods* below). Donor fluorophores were attached to a CCPGCC motif [*Fl*uorescein *A*r*s*enical *H*elix or *H*airpin binder (FlAsH)] introduced at position 351–356 in the proximal C-terminus (10 residues after the palmitoylation site) or at the distal C-terminus (after residue 413). Acceptor fluorophores are introduced at a single reactive cysteine (C265) at the cytoplasmic end of TM6. FRET analyses provided evidence that the C-terminus is in an extended conformation; nevertheless we observed ligand-specific effects on FRET between C265 and both the proximal and the distal FlAsH sites *(1)*. The results provide insights into structural features that may be relevant to the interactions between the C-terminus of the β_2-AR and regulatory proteins such as GPCR kinase and arrestins.

2. Materials

2.1. Receptor Expression and Purification from Sf9 Insect Cells

1. Bac-to-Bac® Baculovirus Expression System (Invitrogen, Carlsbad, CA, USA).
2. MAX Efficiency® DH10Bac™ Chemically Competent Cells (Invitrogen).
3. SOC (Super Optimal Catabolite) medium (Invitrogen).
4. LB agar: isopropyl-β-D-thiogalactopyranoside (IPTG) 40 μg/mL, kanamycin 50 μg/mL, tetracycline 10 μg/mL, gentamycin 7 μg/mL, BLUO-GAL (dissolved in dimethylsulfoxide, DMSO) 300 μg/mL (Invitrogen).
5. ESF-921 medium (Expression Systems, Woodland, CA, USA) (store at 4°C, light sensitive).
6. *Sf* 9 cells SFM adapted (Invitrogen).
7. Cellfectin® Transfection Reagent and Grace's medium without serum (Invitrogen).
8. M1 anti-Flag antibody (Sigma, St.-Louis, MO, USA).
9. Alexa Fluor® 488 protein labeling kit (Invitrogen).
10. Lysis buffer: 10 mM Tris–HCl, pH 7.5, with 1 mM EDTA, 1 μM alprenolol, 160 μg/mL benzamidine, and 2.5 μg/mL leupeptin.
11. Solubilization buffer: 20 mM Tris–HCl, pH 7.5, with 1.0% (w/v) *n*-dodecyl-β-D-maltopyranoside (DDM) (Anatrace, Maumee, Ohio, USA), 100 mM NaCl, 160 μg/mL benzamidine, 2.5 μg/mL leupeptin, and 1 μM alprenolol.
12. Dounce tissue grinder (Wheaton Science Products, Millville, NJ, USA).
13. ANTI-FLAG® M1 Agarose Affinity Gel (Sigma).
14. Glass Econo-column (internal diameter 1.5 cm, length 10 cm) (Bio-Rad, Hercules, CA, USA).
15. Binding buffer: 75 mM Tris–HCl, pH 7.4.
16. Washing solution: 10 mM Tris–HCl (pH 7.4), 3 m*M* $MgCl_2$.
17. [^{3}H]-dihydroalprenolol ([^{3}H]-DHA, Perkin-Elmer, Waltham, MA, USA).
18. Sephadex® G50 Medium and Superfine gel filtration media (GE Healthcare, Chicago, IL, USA).
19. Poly-prep® chromatography columns (0.8 cm × 4 cm) (Bio-Rad).

2.2. Fluorescence Labeling of Purified Receptors

1. Lumio™Green In-cell labeling kit (Invitrogen, store at –20°C, light sensitive, stable for at least 12 months). Safety concern – Lumio™Green contains small amounts

of an organic arsenic compound. Wear protective gear and handle according to institutional chemical hygiene plan.

2. Tris(2-carboxyethyl) phosphine hydrochloride (TCEP).
3. Alexa Fluor® 568 C5 maleimide (Invitrogen): Resuspend the powder in DMSO, make 10 μL aliquots at 10 mM, and store at –80°C with dessication. Stable for at least 2 months.
4. Econo-column Bio-Rad (ID 0.7 cm, length 10 cm).
5. HEPES Low Salt (HLS) buffer (20 mM HEPES, pH 7.5, 100 m*M* NaCl, and 0.1% (w/v) DDM) (make fresh as required).

2.3. Fluorescence Spectroscopy

1. Experiments are performed on a SPEX FluoroMax-3 spectrofluorometer (Horiba Jobin Yvon, or similar equipment) with photon counting mode using an excitation and emission bandpass width of 2 nm in S/R (signal over reference) acquisition mode. Unless otherwise indicated, all experiments were performed at 25°C.
2. Micro Fluorometer Cell 5 × 5 mm (NSG Precision Cells, Inc., Farmingale, NY, USA).

3. Methods

3.1. Receptor Expression and Purification from Sf9 Insect Cells

3.1.1. Preparation of the cDNA Template

1. Use classical molecular biology methods to modify the cDNA template. It needs to be epitope-tagged at the amino-terminus with the cleavable influenza-hemagglutinin signal sequence followed by the FLAG epitope, and at the carboxyl-terminus with six histidines.
2. Digest the mutated cDNA with appropriate enzymes and clone into pFastBac1 vector (Invitrogen).
3. Confirm the constructs by restriction enzyme analysis and DNA sequencing.

3.1.2. Bacterial Transformation

1. Transform the DH10Bac competent cells with 50 ng of the cDNA of interest.
2. Spread the transformation on LB agar Bacmid plate (*see* **Note 1** for details on plate preparation).
3. Incubate the plate for at least 48 h at 37°C.
4. Amplify a white colony (in which the cDNA has been transposed) in 3 mL of SOC medium containing 25 μg/mL kanamycin, 5 μg/mL tetracycline, and 3.5 μg/mL gentamycin (shake for at least 20 h at 37°C before making the miniprep).

3.1.3. Isolation of Bacmid DNA by Miniprep

1. Isolate the Bacmid DNA by a classic isopropanol precipitation method.
2. Dry the Bacmid DNA pellet for 5 min under sterile conditions.
3. Resuspend in 40 μL of a sterile Tris buffer (10 mM, pH 8.0) and allow to dissolve for 20 min (*see* **Note 2**).
4. Sequence the Bacmid DNA using primers designed to cover the entire open reading frame.

3.1.4. Transfection of Sf9 Cells and Baculovirus Production

1. Dilute 15 μL of CellFectin into 1 mL Grace's medium without serum (day 0).
2. Add 5 μL of Bacmid DNA to the solution and incubate at RT for 15–30 min. During this incubation, pellet 10×10^6 *Sf*9 cells in log-phase (*see* **Note 3**) in a 50-mL Corning tube at $100 \times g$ (the cells should be actively dividing and greater than 90% viable). Aspirate off the supernatant and gently resuspend the cells in the transfection mix by tapping the tube. Incubate in the shaker at 27°C for 4–5 h (loosen the cap for ventilation).
3. At 5 h, add 4 mL of cell media and put back the cells in the incubator (shake at 200 rpm to keep in suspension).
4. At 48 h (day 2), add an equal volume of media (5 mL). The cells should have divided at least once since the transfection. Transfer the cells into a 125-mL autoclaved pyrex flask and turn down the shaker's speed from 200 to 130 rpm.
5. At 72 h, the cells should not have divided again and need to be checked for cell surface staining to detect the viral production (*see* **Note 4**). Often the cell surface staining will be >50% at this time point. If this is the case, the virus can be harvested by pelleting the cells at $500 \times g$ for 10 min and keeping the supernatant (store the virus at –80°C, add serum to 5% final to make 1 mL aliquots). If the staining is <50%, then feed the cells 2–3 mL/day until 50% staining is reached. Most P1 Bacmid viruses are harvested between 72 and 96 h.

3.1.5. Amplification of the P1 Viruses

1. Pellet 3×10^8 cells (100 mL at 3×10^6 cells/mL) at $100 \times g$ for 10 min using two 50-mL sterile centrifuge tubes.
2. Resuspend the cells in 100 mL of *Sf*9 media using a 300-mL flask.
3. Add 1 mL of the P1 virus into the resuspended cells (1/100 dilution).
4. At 24 h, feed the cells with 50 mL of RT *Sf*9 media (the cells should have divided).
5. At 48 h, stain the cells as described for the P1 virus. Staining should show that >50% of all cells are staining (the cells should look large and infected and likely have not divided). If the cells have divided and the staining is <<50%, then feed the cells another 50 mL and check again at 72 h.

6. Harvest the P2 virus by centrifugation by spinning the cells at 500 × *g* for 10 min.
7. Store the virus as described for the P1 in 10 mL aliquots.
8. To determine the optimal amount of P2 virus needed for protein expression, infect 10 mL of *Sf*9 cells with 1/100 (i.e., 100 μL of P2 virus in 10 mL of *Sf*9 cells at a density of 3×10^6 cells/mL), 1/200, 1/500, 1/1000 dilutions.
9. At 52 h, determine the amount of receptor in each condition by binding experiments on *Sf*9 cells.

3.1.6. Binding Experiments on Sf9 Cells

1. Dilute the infected cells 100 times into a mix containing the binding buffer and saturating amount of the radioligand (10 nM [^{3}H]-DHA is used for the β_2-AR) (final volume of 500 μL).
2. Incubate at 24°C for 1 h under constant shaking (200 rpm).
3. Separate free radioligand from bound by filtering onto a Whatman glass fiber filter (0.8–1.2 μm). Rinse the filters three times with 4 mL of cold washing solution.
4. Measure the remaining radioactivity by liquid scintillation spectrometry. Non-specific binding is determined in the presence of 1 μM of non-radiactive ligand (alprenolol is used for the β_2-AR).

3.1.7. Cells Infection and Receptor Expression

1. Infect *Sf*9 cell cultures at a density of $\sim 3 \times 10^6$ cells/mL with appropriate viruses.
2. Harvest after 52 h by centrifugation (10 min at 5000 × *g*). The cell pellets can be kept at –80°C until their use for purification.

3.1.8. Lysis and Solubilization of Cell Pellets

1. Lyse the cell pellets (~20 mL for 1 liter of cell culture) in 100 mL of lysis buffer for 10 min at 4°C.
2. Following centrifugation (20 min at 30,000 × *g*), resuspend the lysed cells in 100 mL of solubilization buffer.
3. Homogenize with 30 strokes of tight dounces using Wheaton dounce tissue grinder.
4. Stir for 1 h at 4°C.

3.1.9. M1 Flag Purification

1. Following centrifugation (20 min at 30,000 × *g*), supplement the supernatant with 2 mM $CaCl_2$ (*see* **Note 5**).
2. Load the supernatant onto 1 mL of M1 Flag resin at a rate of 1 mL/min. Wash the resin extensively with HLS buffer supplemented with 2 mM $CaCl_2$.
3. Elute the Flag-tagged receptors by adding HLS buffer containing 2 mM EDTA and 200 μg/mL of Flag peptide. Collect

1 mL fraction and probe for the presence of protein using OD at 280 nm or Bradford reagent (5 μL in 50 μL of Bradford reagent diluted five times in water).

3.1.10. Ligand-Affinity Purification

1. If applicable, purify the eluate from the M1 anti-Flag column on a ligand-sepharose affinity column and finally through a second M1 Flag antibody affinity resin purification step.
2. Store the purified detergent-soluble receptor in HLS buffer at 4°C.

3.1.11. Determination of the Concentration of Functional, Purified Receptor by Binding Experiments

1. Incubate the purified receptor in triplicate in HLS buffer with a saturating concentration of radioligand (10 nM [^{3}H]-DHA for the β_2-AR) in a total volume of 100 μL for 1 h at room temperature.
2. Separate free [^{3}H]-DHA from bound by passing through a Sephadex G50 Medium column (4 cm × 0.8 cm; 2 mL of gel bed, elution with 1 mL of HLS buffer). Non-specific binding is determined in the presence of 1 μM alprenolol. Routinely, the final receptor concentration of functional receptor reaches 3 μM for a total volume of 1 mL.

3.2. Fluorescence Labeling of Purified Receptors

The biarsenical FlAsH compound Lumio^{TM}Green binds to a tetracysteine motif (CCPGCC) that can be introduced into specific sites within the protein of interest, thus providing a labeling chemistry orthogonal to single-cysteine labeling (*see* **Note 6**). For site-specific labeling of the β_2-AR with Lumio^{TM}Green and Alexa 568 to monitor the distance between TM6 and the C-terminus by FRET, we generated a modified β_2-AR with a single FRET acceptor site at the cytoplasmic end of TM6 and two different FRET donor sites in the carboxyl terminus (**Fig. 1**). We started with a modified version of the β_2-AR where 4 of the 13 endogenous cysteines (C77, C327, C378, and C406) were mutated to alanine, valine, or serine (β_2-AR-Δ4). Five of the nine remaining cysteines are not available for derivatization because of palmitoylation (C341) or disulfide bond formation (C106, C184, C190, and C191). The three remaining cysteines, C116, C125, and C285, are poorly labeled with maleimide reagents. This leaves C265 at the cytoplasmic end of TM6 as the only remaining maleimide-reactive cysteine. This site was used for attachment of the FRET acceptor Alexa568 maleimide. For the C-terminal FRET donor sites, we used the fluorophore 4′,5′-bis(1,2,3-dithioarsolan-2-yl)-fluorescein, also called Fluorescein Arsenical Helix or Hairpin binder (FlAsH), commercially known as Lumio^{TM}Green labeling reagent (**Fig. 1**). This fluorophore binds specifically to a CCPGCC motif (FlAsH site). The first FlAsH site was introduced by

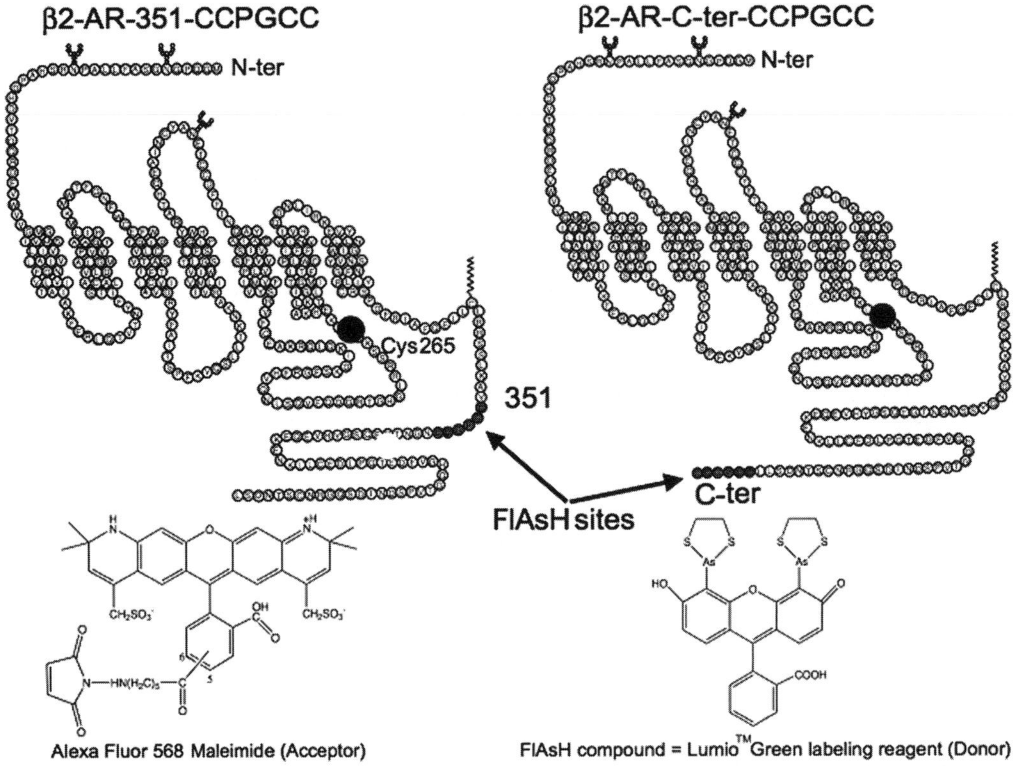

Fig. 1. Engineered β_2-ARs and fluorophores used in this study. The FlAsH site (CCPGCC) was introduced in two alternate regions of the C-terminal domain of β_2-ARs. One starts at position 351 and is named β_2-AR-351-CCPGCC (*left*). The other was added to the C-terminus of the receptor (β_2-AR-C-ter-CCPGCC, *right*). Fluorophores used in this study are FlAsH (the donor which reacts with CCPGCC) and Alexa Fluor 568 maleimide (the acceptor which reacts with Cysteine 265).

replacing residues G351–S356, located 10 residues after the palmitoylation site (β_2-AR-351-CCPGCC), and the other was introduced following the last amino acid at the C-terminus (β_2-AR-C-ter-CCPGCC) (**Fig. 1**).

3.2.1. Double Labeling of the Receptor for FRET

1. Purified receptors (100 μL) are first reacted overnight at 16°C in the dark with three equivalents of Lumio™Green labeling reagent and tris(2-carboxyethyl)phosphine (TCEP) (100 μM).
2. Alexa Fluor 568 maleimide (1.1 equivalents) is then added to the mixture for 10 min at 4°C. For acceptor-only labeling, purified receptors (100 μL) are first incubated overnight at 16°C in the dark in the exact same conditions as for the doubly labeled receptor but without Lumio™Green and TCEP. Then, 1.1 equivalents of Alexa Fluor 568 maleimide are added to the mixture for 10 min at 4°C.
3. The 100 μL fluorophore-labeled receptors are then separated from the free dye by gel filtration on a Sephadex G50

Superfine column (ID 0.7 cm, length 10 cm, gel bed of about 4.5 mL) equilibrated with a HLS buffer containing 0.01% cholesterolhemisuccinate (*see* **Note 7**).

4. The donor/receptor and acceptor/donor ratio is determined by dividing the bound dye concentration (calculated by using the maximum absorbance of the donor or acceptor-labeled receptor) by the donor or receptor concentration (determined by absorbance or ligand binding, respectively). The ratio of donor to receptor ranged from 0.8 to 1 dye per receptor. The typical acceptor/donor labeling ratios ranged from 1 to 1.3 (extinction coefficients : $\varepsilon_{FlAsH,528}$ = 70,000 $cm^{-1}M^{-1}$ and $\varepsilon_{Alexa568,578}$ = 91,300 $cm^{-1}M^{-1}$).

3.3. Fluorescence Spectroscopy

3.3.1. Drug-Induced Changes in FRET Efficiency for β2-AR-351-CCPGCC and β2-AR-C-ter-CCPGCC Constructs

For each FRET experiment, fluorescence spectra are taken for both the doubly labeled receptor and the acceptor-only labeled receptor. For each type of receptor, two types of emission scans are acquired.

1. The first emission scan (donor scan) uses the excitation maximum for the donor fluorophore.
2. The second emission scan (acceptor scan) uses the excitation maximum for the acceptor fluorophore. The donor/acceptor pair uses 508 nm excitation for the donor and 578 nm excitation for the acceptor.
3. For testing the effects of β_2-AR specific drugs, samples with or without drugs are gently mixed and incubated for 15 min at 24°C. Three separate samples are used for testing each type of drug and individual spectra are acquired and averaged.
4. Emission spectra of the solutions containing the drugs only are also obtained at both the donor and acceptor excitation wavelengths and subtracted from the spectra obtained from the samples containing both the receptor and drug (see below).
5. Background fluorescence of the buffer is subtracted from spectra derived from the sample containing only the receptor.
6. Removal of acceptor bleedthrough and correction of drug-induced acceptor fluorescence intensity changes are carried out as described in detail under the analysis section.

3.3.2. Analysis of FRET Data

1. In this section, we use the following symbols to refer to the experimental emission spectra used for analysis, determined using the receptor with donor on CCPGCC motif (Lumio^{TM}-Green) and acceptor (Alexa 568) on C265, or the receptor labeled only with acceptor on C265, after excitation at the

donor wavelength (ExcD) or at the acceptor wavelength (ExcA):

$$\begin{cases} A & = \text{receptor labeled with donor and acceptor, ExcD} \\ A' & = \text{receptor labeled with donor and acceptor, ExcA} \\ B & = \text{receptor labeled with acceptor, ExcD} \\ B' & = \text{receptor labeled with acceptor, ExcA} \\ \mathrm{A_{drug}} & = \text{same as } A\text{, with drug, ExcD} \\ \mathrm{A'_{drug}} & = \text{same as } A'\text{, with drug, ExcA} \\ \mathrm{S_{buff}} & = \text{buffer, ExcD} \\ \mathrm{S'_{buff}} & = \text{buffer, ExcA} \\ \mathrm{S_{drug}} & = \text{drug alone, in buffer, ExcD} \\ \mathrm{S'_{drug}} & = \text{drug alone, in buffer, ExcA} \end{cases}$$

Background fluorescence from either buffer or drug is removed as follows:

$$C = A - S_{buff}$$

$$C' = A' - S'_{buff}$$

$$D = A_{drug} - S_{drug}$$

$$D' = A'_{drug} - S'_{drug}$$

$$E = B - S_{buff}$$

$$E' = B' - S_{buff}$$

In spectrum E, the only signal is from direct excitation of the acceptor at ExcD. In spectra C and D, the signal from direct excitation of the acceptor is mixed with donor and FRET signals. However, the contribution from direct excitation of the acceptor in spectrum *C* and *D* is proportional to spectrum *E*, with a scaling factor that depends on the amount of acceptor fluorophores in the different samples. Importantly, the amount of acceptor is directly proportional to the intensities in spectra *C'*, *D'*, and *E'*, where the donor and the FRET signals do not contribute at all. Thus, the contribution from direct excitation of acceptor in spectra C and D can be subtracted as follows:

$$\begin{cases} \mathrm{F} = & C - E \times \frac{C'_{\mathrm{max}}}{E'_{\mathrm{max}}} \\ \mathrm{G} = & D - E \times \frac{D'_{\mathrm{max}}}{E'_{\mathrm{max}}} \end{cases}$$

where "max" is defined as the intensity at the acceptor emission peak. The wavelength used to determine this value is 603 nm. If the intensity of the acceptor changes in response to the drug, the emission peaks for spectra *C'* and *D'* will be different:

$$\text{Drug response} = \frac{D'_{\text{max}}}{C'_{\text{max}}}$$

This change in intensity will also modify the signal obtained when using ExcD, in spectrum G. For instance, if the drug response is 2 in spectrum *D'*, then the acceptor signal in spectrum *G* should actually be divided by 2 to have only the changes due to FRET (note that in our experiments, the responses were actually in the order of 1–3%). More generally, the acceptor signal in spectrum *G* should be corrected for FRET-independent drug response using the following correction factor:

$$\text{Correction factor} = 1 - \frac{C'_{\text{max}}}{D'_{\text{max}}}$$

Because only the acceptor signal is affected, this correction factor should only be applied to the contribution of the acceptor in the total spectrum, which is a mix of donor and acceptor signals. The acceptor signal can be extracted using spectrum *E*, and properly scaling it as was done above to obtain spectra *F* and *G*:

$$\text{Acceptor signal in spectrum } G = E \times \frac{G_{\text{max}}}{E_{\text{max}}}$$

Thus, the final corrected spectrum where the FRET-independent response to drug has been subtracted is

$$H = G - E \times \frac{G_{max}}{E_{max}} \times 1 - \frac{C'_{max}}{D'_{max}}$$

Finally, spectra are normalized to keep the area under the curve constant, which also removed the contribution from any drug-induced fluorescence intensity change of the donor. The proximity ratio is then

$$\text{Proximity ratio} = \frac{I_{\text{A}}}{I_{\text{A}} + I_{\text{D}}}$$

where I_{D} and I_{A} are the peak intensities of the donor and the acceptor, respectively.

When comparing the responses to drugs, we used the proximity ratio. The drug response is calculated as the change in proximity ratio between spectrum *F* and spectrum *H*.

To be able to accurately calculate the distances between the fluorescent probes using the Förster theory, the proximity ratio needs to be corrected to give the true FRET efficiency *(13)* as follows:

$$\text{FRET efficiency} = \frac{\mathrm{I_A}}{\mathrm{I_A} + \gamma \mathrm{I_D}}$$

$$\text{FRET efficiency} = \frac{I_\mathrm{A}}{I_\mathrm{A} + \gamma I_\mathrm{D}}$$

$$\gamma = \frac{\eta_\mathrm{A}\Phi_\mathrm{A}}{\eta_\mathrm{D}\Phi_\mathrm{D}}$$

The correction factor γ is defined as

$$\gamma = \frac{\eta_\mathrm{A}\Phi_\mathrm{A}}{\eta_\mathrm{D}\Phi_\mathrm{D}}$$

where η_D and η_A are the collection efficiencies of the donor and the acceptor signals, and Φ_D and Φ_A are the fluorescence quantum yields of the donor and the acceptor, respectively. We assume $\eta_\mathrm{A}/\eta_\mathrm{D}$ to be 1 to obtain the following equation:

$$\text{FRET efficiency} = \frac{\mathrm{I_A}}{\mathrm{I_A} + (\Phi_\mathrm{A}/\Phi_\mathrm{D})\mathrm{I_D}}$$

Φ_D and Φ_A were measured by using the following relation *(14)*:

$$\Phi_\mathrm{x} = \Phi_\mathrm{st} \times \frac{\mathrm{F_x}}{\mathrm{F_{st}}} \times \frac{\mathrm{OD_{st}}}{\mathrm{OD_x}}$$

$$\Phi_\mathrm{x} = \Phi_\mathrm{x} \times \frac{F_\mathrm{x}}{F_\mathrm{st}} \times \frac{OD_\mathrm{st}}{OD_\mathrm{x}}$$

where subscripts st and x refer to the standard and unknown solutions, respectively. *F* is the relative integrated fluorescence intensity and *OD* is the optical density at the exciting wavelength. Rhodamine 6G was chosen as the standard (quantum yield equal to 0.90 in water *(15)*). Emission spectra were obtained at 25°C using 490 nm excitation while collecting fluorescence from 496 to 800 nm. The signal from buffer solution was subtracted from each sample and from the standard before integration.

2. Steps taken for data analysis of FRET levels in the double-labeled (DL) receptors are illustrated in **Fig. 2A**.

   The proximity ratios are calculated for both constructs (**Fig. 2B**, bar graph). The FlAsH/Alexa 568 proximity ratio is significantly higher for β_2-AR-351-CCPGCC than for β_2-AR-C-ter-CCPGCC (54.11 ± 0.57 vs. 45.64 ± 0.09 in %).

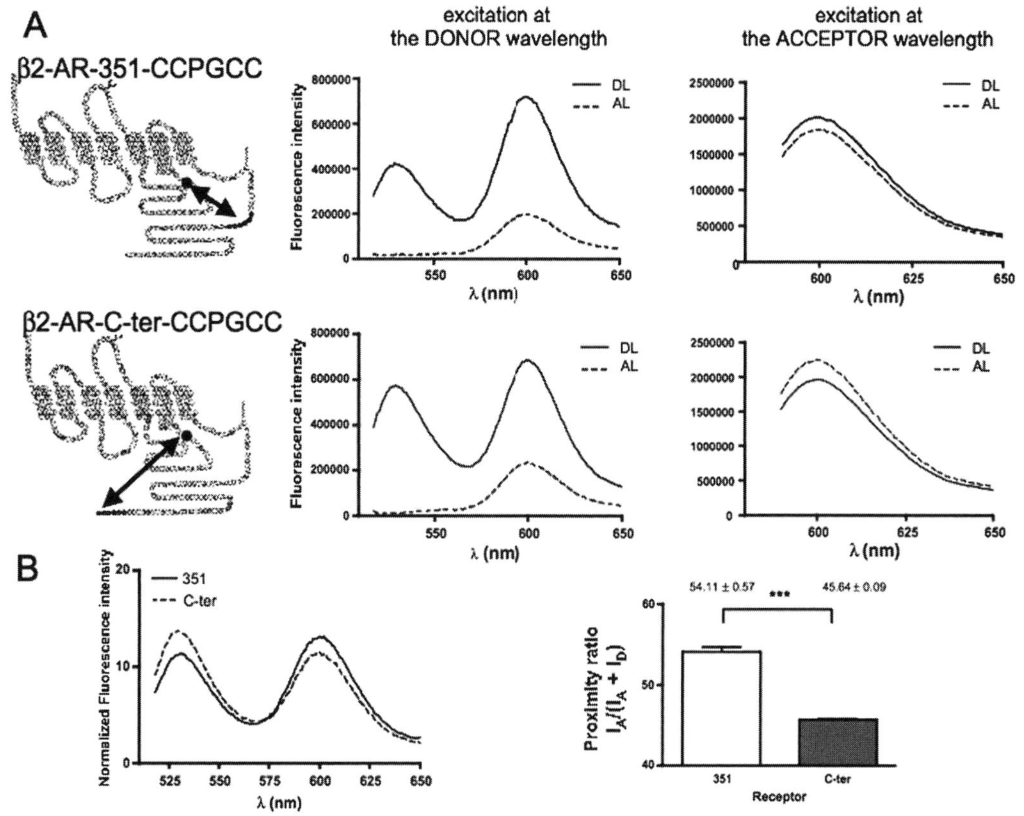

Fig. 2. Proximity ratio between FlAsH and Alexa Fluor 568 for β_2-AR-351-CCPGCC and β_2-AR-C-ter-CCPGCC receptors. (**A**) Characteristic spectra used for FRET calculations: Both constructs were labeled as described under experimental procedures. Emission scans were acquired using 15 nM of desalted double-labeled (DL, *solid line*) receptor or receptor labeled only with the Alexa Fluor 568 (AL, *dotted line*). Emission scans were obtained for excitation at the donor wavelength (FlAsH, 508 nm) and at the acceptor wavelength (Alexa Fluor 568, 578 nm). The spectra represent the average of triplicate determinations and are representative of three independent sets of labeling reactions made on the same receptor preparation. (**B**) Normalized spectra from panel A and proximity ratios. Averaged spectra from triplicate determinations for β_2-AR-351-CCPGCC (351, *solid line*) and β_2-AR-C-ter-CCPGCC (C-ter, *dotted line*) were normalized as described under experimental procedures. Proximity ratios (*right*) were calculated and plotted as the mean ± SEM of three independent experiments performed in triplicate.

3. To measure conformational changes in the receptor, we measured the FRET efficiency before and after treatment with the full agonist, isoproterenol. The result is illustrated in **Fig. 3**.
4. To calculate FRET efficiencies, we determined the fluorescence quantum yield of FlAsH and Alexa 568 bound to the receptor as described above. We found that the FlAsH quantum yields were similar when conjugated to either β_2-AR-351-CCPGCC or β_2-AR-C-ter-CCPGCC (0.42 ± 0.03 vs. 0.44 ± 0.05). The Alexa 568 quantum yields are also similar for both constructs (0.121 ± 0.016 vs. 0.114 ± 0.013).

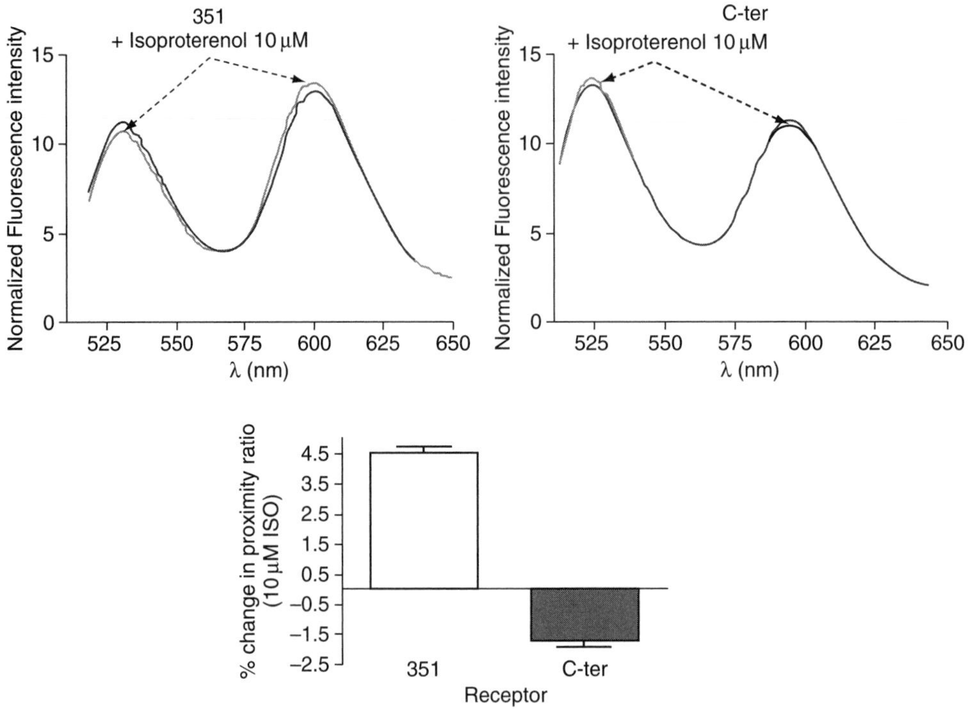

Fig. 3. Effects of isoproterenol on proximity ratio of labeled β_2-AR receptors. β_2-AR-351-CCPGCC (left panel) or β_2-AR-C-ter-CCPGCC (right panel) were incubated 15 min with or without 10 μM isoproterenol. Spectra represent the average of triplicate determinations. The bottom panel represents the percentage change in proximity ratio induced by 10 μM isoproterenol for both constructs calculated from three independent experiments performed in triplicate with two different receptor preparations.

Using these values we determined the basal FRET efficiency to be 83.35% for β2-AR-351-CCPGCC and 77.02% for β_2-AR-C-ter-CCPGCC.

3.3.3. Determination of R_0

The R_0 values for the FlAsH-Alexa568 FRET pair were calculated using the relationship:

$$R_0 = (9.765 \times 10^3)(J(\lambda) \times k^2 \times \Phi_D \times n^{-4})^{1/6} \quad \text{(in A)}$$

where κ^2 is the orientation factor (assumed to be equal to 2/3), n is the refractive index (equal to 1.3), Φ_D is the quantum yield of the donor, and $J(\lambda)$ is the spectral overlap integral between the emission spectrum of β_2-AR-FlAsH and the absorption spectrum of β_2-AR-Alexa568 (in $cm^3\ M^{-1}$). The R_0 value for the FRET pair used in this study (FlAsH-Alexa568) was found to be 75 Å. From FRET efficiencies and R_0, we used the Förster theory ($R^6 = R_0{}^6(1-E)/E$) to calculate $R_{Proximal}$ (56.96 ± 0.17 Å) and R_{Distal} (62.05 ± 0.04 Å).

4. Notes

1. Preparation of Bacmid plates: all the components used must be sterile otherwise the plate would not be storable for months at 4°C. Heat 500 mL of LB agar 25 min using microwaves and let it cool for 20 min. Add the appropriate antibiotic, IPTG, and bluo Gal and pour the mix under sterile conditions. Plates are stable for at least 6 months at 4°C.
2. No pipetting, just flick the tube a couple of times. Check the purity and quantity of your DNA by absorption spectroscopy by checking the A260 and the A260/A280 ratio. Expect ~1 mg/mL DNA and a A260/A280 ratio of ~1.9.
3. Insect cells needs to be incubated at 27–28°C and cultured in suspension by using a shaker with a constant speed (~130 rpm). The cell density for maintenance needs to be kept under 9×10^6 cells per mL of culture.
4. The viral production is detected through the monitoring of cell surface Flag-tagged receptor. Use M1 anti-Flag antibody labeled with the Alexa 488 dye (the protocol is given in great details in the labeling kit). Dilute 100 μL of the cell culture in 400 μL of cell media in a 12-well cell culture plate, add 1 μL of fluorescent M1 and incubate for 15 min (protect from light). Check the fluorescence under a fluorescence microscope (GFP filter, removed the media just before checking). Expect a bright membrane fluorescence.
5. The addition of $CaCl_2$ is of major importance because the M1 binding to the Flag epitope is Ca^{2+}-dependent.
6. This orthogonal labeling scheme (single cysteine + CCPGCC motif) can be applied to other systems provided the single cysteine labeling reaction is well controlled and characterized. For the β_2-AR, this has been accomplished through the monitoring of the reactivity of each cysteine in the receptor.
7. You can check the gel filtration assay by using a fluorescent receptor visible by eye or after illumination with a portable UV lamp. Usually, 700 μL is necessary before the receptor is eluted (in ~300 μL).
8. To obtain FRET-based kinetic data for the conformational change, the ratio of the fluorescence intensities at two fixed wavelengths (λ_{max}'s for the donor and the acceptor), that is, the proximity ratio, can be monitored continuously instead of recording the full emission spectrum. Usually, the control software for the spectrofluorometer provides this ratiometric acquisition mode.

Acknowledgment

S.G. thanks Brian Kobilka for his constant support and for the supervision of this project.

References

1. Granier, S., Kim, S., Shafer, A. M., Ratnala, V. R., Fung, J. J., Zare, R. N., and Kobilka, B. (2007) Structure and conformational changes in the C-terminal domain of the beta2-adrenoceptor: Insights from fluorescence resonance energy transfer studies. *J. Biol. Chem.* **282**, 13895–13905.
2. Ji, T. H., Grossmann, M., and Ji, I. (1998) G protein-coupled receptors. I. Diversity of receptor-ligand interactions. *J. Biol. Chem.* **273**, 17299–17302.
3. Swaminath, G., Xiang, Y., Lee, T. W., Steenhuis, J., Parnot, C., and Kobilka, B. K. (2004) Sequential binding of agonists to the beta2 adrenoceptor. Kinetic evidence for intermediate conformational states. *J. Biol. Chem.* **279**, 686–691.
4. Ghanouni, P., Gryczynski, Z., Steenhuis, J. J., Lee, T. W., Farrens, D. L., Lakowicz, J. R., and Kobilka, B. K. (2001) Functionally different agonists induce distinct conformations in the G protein coupling domain of the beta2 adrenergic receptor. *J. Biol. Chem.* **276**, 24433–24436.
5. Ghanouni, P., Steenhuis, J. J., Farrens, D. L., and Kobilka, B. K. (2001) Agonist-induced conformational changes in the G protein-coupling domain of the beta2 adrenergic receptor. *Proc. Natl. Acad. Sci. USA* **98**, 5997–6002.
6. Benovic, J. L. (2002) Novel beta2-adrenergic receptor signaling pathways. *J. Allergy Clin. Immunol.* **110**, S229–S235.
7. Reiter, E., and Lefkowitz, R. J. (2006) GRKs and beta-arrestins: roles in receptor silencing, trafficking and signaling. *Trends Endocrinol. Metab.* **17**, 159–165.
8. Lefkowitz, R. J., and Shenoy, S. K. (2005) Transduction of receptor signals by beta-arrestins. *Science* **308**, 512–517.
9. Ren, X. R., Reiter, E., Ahn, S., Kim, J., Chen, W., and Lefkowitz, R. J. (2005) Different G protein-coupled receptor kinases govern G protein and beta-arrestin-mediated signaling of V2 vasopressin receptor. *Proc. Natl. Acad. Sci. USA* **102**, 1448–1453.
10. Azzi, M., Charest, P. G., Angers, S., Rousseau, G., Kohout, T., Bouvier, M., and Pineyro, G. (2003) Beta-arrestin-mediated activation of MAPK by inverse agonists reveals distinct active conformations for G protein-coupled receptors. *Proc. Natl. Acad. Sci. USA* **100**, 11406–11411.
11. Rasmussen, S. G., Choi, H. J., Rosenbaum, D. M., Kobilka, T. S., Thian, F. S., Edwards, P. C., Burghammer, M., Ratnala, V. R., Sanishvili, R., Fischetti, R. F., Schertler, G. F., Weis, W. I., and Kobilka, B. K. (2007) Crystal structure of the human beta2 adrenergic G protein-coupled receptor. *Nature* **450**, 383–387.
12. Rosenbaum, D. M., Cherezov, V., Hanson, M. A., Rasmussen, S. G., Thian, F. S., Kobilka, T. S., Choi, H. J., Yao, X. J., Weis, W. I., Stevens, R. C., and Kobilka, B. K. (2007) GPCR engineering yields high-resolution structural insights into beta2-adrenergic receptor function. *Science* **318**, 1266–1273.
13. Ha, T., Ting, A. Y., Liang, J., Caldwell, W. B., Deniz, A. A., Chemla, D. S., Schultz, P. G., and Weiss, S. (1999) Single-molecule fluorescence spectroscopy of enzyme conformational dynamics and cleavage mechanism. *Proc. Natl. Acad. Sci. USA* **96**, 893–898.
14. Chen, R. F. (1965) Fluorescence quantum yield measurements: vitamin B6 compounds. *Science* **150**, 1593–1595.
15. Magde, D., Wong, R., and Seybold, P. G. (2002) Fluorescence quantum yields and their relation to lifetimes of rhodamine 6G and fluorescein in nine solvents: improved absolute standards for quantum yields. *Photochem. Photobiol.* **75**, 327–334.

Chapter 19

FLIPR® Assays of Intracellular Calcium in GPCR Drug Discovery

Kasper B. Hansen and Hans Bräuner-Osborne

Summary

Fluorescent dyes sensitive to changes in intracellular calcium have become increasingly popular in G protein-coupled receptor (GPCR) drug discovery for several reasons. First of all, the assays using the dyes are easy to perform and are of low cost compared to other assays. Second, most non-$G\alpha_q$-coupled GPCRs can be tweaked to modulate intracellular calcium by co-transfection with promiscuous or chimeric/mutated G proteins making the calcium assays broadly applicable in GPCR research. Third, the price of instruments capable of measuring fluorescent-based calcium indicators has become significantly less making them obtainable even for academic groups. Here, we present a protocol for measuring changes in intracellular calcium levels in living mammalian cells based on the fluorescent calcium binding dye, fluo-4.

Key words: Intracellular calcium measurement, G protein-coupled receptors, probenecid, FLIPR, FlexStation, NOVOstar.

1. Introduction

Since the development of the fluorescent calcium indicator, fluo-3, by Tsien and colleagues in 1989 *(1)*, fluorescence-based assays of intracellular calcium have become increasingly popular. Initially, fluorescence microplate readers were excessively expensive due to the use of argon laser to excite the fluorophores, but recently instruments based on, for example, xenon flash lamps or light-emitting diodes (LEDs) have decreased price and installation requirements and thus made the instrument accessible even for academic groups. Initially, assays were restricted to using the 488 nm emission line of the

Wayne R. Leifert (ed.), *G Protein-Coupled Receptors in Drug Discovery, vol. 552*

Book doi: 10.1007/978-1-60327-317-6_19

argon laser, which led to the development of fluo-4 – a fluo-3 analog with peak excitation at 494 nm (compared to 506 nm for fluo-3) – and thus increased emission upon binding of calcium *(2)*.

The ease of use and relatively low cost has been a main driver for the increased use of intracellular calcium assays in G protein-coupled receptor (GPCR) drug discovery. Another reason for the increased popularity is the possibility of directing the signal transduction pathway of most GPCRs to calcium signaling via use of chimeric, mutated, and/or promiscuous G proteins *(3)*. The initial breakthrough in this regard was the observation by Conklin and colleagues that substitution of the extreme end of the C-terminal of G proteins also switched the signaling pathway *(4)*. Soon thereafter, Offermanns and colleagues discovered that the G proteins, $G\alpha_{15}$ and $G\alpha_{16}$, were promiscuous and were able to couple non-$G\alpha_q$-coupled GPCRs to the calcium signaling pathway *(5)*. Most recently, Kostenis and colleagues have shown that mutation of a glycine at position 66 of $G\alpha_q$ to, for example, aspartate provides a promiscuous G protein coupling many different GPCRs to the calcium signaling pathway *(6)*. Many chimeric/mutated variations of the G proteins linking $G\alpha_i$-, $G\alpha_s$-, or $G\alpha_{12}$-coupled receptors to the $G\alpha_q$ pathway have been made, but as pointed out no "G protein queen" truly superior to the others have been identified *(3)*, and it is thus our experience that it is worthwhile testing a series of G proteins when optimizing a novel calcium assay for a non-$G\alpha_q$-coupled receptor *(7, 8)*.

The principle of the fluo-4 assay is shown in **Fig. 1**. Fluo-4 is administered to the cells as an acetoxymethyl (AM) ester, which is cell membrane permeable. Once inside the cells, fluo-4, AM is hydrolyzed by intracellular esterases, which lead to the cell membrane impermeable negatively charged form, fluo-4^{5-}. Fluo-4^{5-} is an ingenious compound consisting of a BAPTA-like Ca^{2+} chelator merged with a fluorescein analog. Fluo-4 binds Ca^{2+} with a K_d of 345 nM *(2)* which is in the physiological range of intracellular Ca^{2+} levels in most cells *(9)*. Once Ca^{2+} binds to the BAPTA-like chelator site, the electronic and thus spectroscopic properties of the fluorophore changes, which are easily measured. Unfortunately, some cells express the organic anion transporter, which leads to export of the negatively charged fluo-4^{5-} and thus decreased signal. However, by adding probenecid, an inhibitor of the transporter, to the cells this export can be prevented. Nowadays, several intracellular calcium dyes, and even commercial calcium assay kits, are available, but the fluo-4-based assays remain the most popular and will thus be presented here.

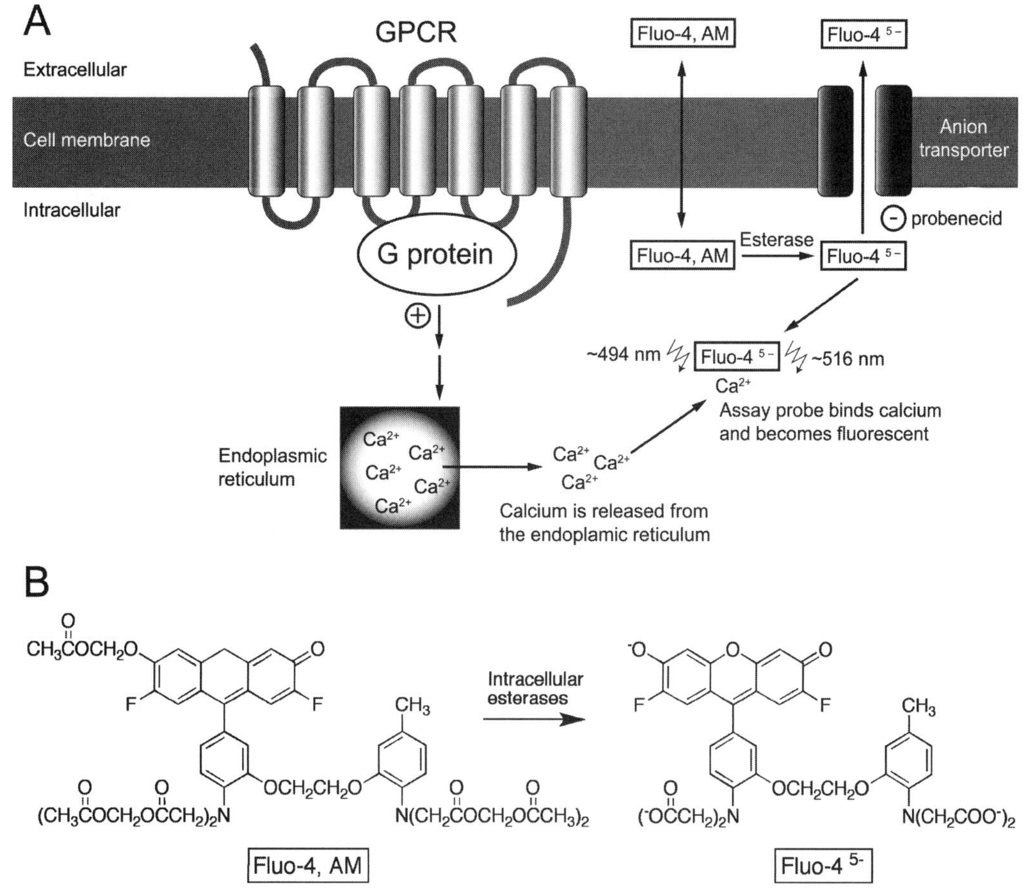

Fig. 1. Principle of the intracellular calcium assay in living mammalian cells based on the fluorescent calcium binding dye, fluo-4. (**A**) Fluo-4 is administered to the cells as a acetoxymethyl (AM) ester which is cell membrane permeable. Once inside the cells fluo-4, AM is hydrolyzed by intracellular esterases, which leads to the cell membrane impermeable negatively charged form, fluo-4^{5-}, capable of binding Ca^{2+}. Unfortunately, some cells express an organic anion transporter, which leads to export of the negatively charged fluo-4^{5-} and thus decreased signal. However, by adding probenecid, an inhibitor of the transporter, to the cells this export can be prevented. (**B**) The chemical structure of fluo-4, AM and fluo-4^{5-}. Note that fluo-4 consists of a BAPTA-like Ca^{2+} chelator merged with a fluorescein analog. Fluo-4 binds Ca^{2+} with a K_d of 345 nM which is in the physiological range of intracellular Ca^{2+} levels in most cells. Once Ca^{2+} binds to the BAPTA-like chelator site, the electronic and thus spectroscopic properties of the fluorophore are changed, which are easily measured.

2. Materials

2.1. Fluo-4-Based Intracellular Calcium Assay

1. HBSS–HEPES buffer: 10 mM HEPES in Hanks' Balanced Salt Solution without calcium, magnesium, or phenol red (5.33 mM KCl, 0.441 mM KH_2PO_4, 4.17 mM $NaHCO_3$, 137.93 mM NaCl, 0.338 mM Na_2HPO_4, 5.56 mM D-glucose). Adjust pH to 7.4 with 2 N NaOH. Store in refrigerator, but heat to room temperature before use.

2. $MgCl_2$ stock solution (1000 ×): 1 M $MgCl_2$ in double distilled water (ddH_2O). Store at room temperature.
3. $CaCl_2$ stock solution (1000 ×): 1 M $CaCl_2$ in ddH_2O. Store at room temperature.
4. HBSS–HEPES–Ca–Mg buffer: Add 50 μL $MgCl_2$ stock solution (1000 ×) and 50 μL $CaCl_2$ stock solution (1000 ×) to 50 mL HBSS–HEPES buffer. Make 50 mL buffer per 96-well plate. Use it the same day or else precipitate might form.
5. Probenecid solution (200 ×): 250 mM probenecid (Sigma-Aldrich, St. Louis, MO, USA) dissolved in 0.6 M NaOH. Use same day.
6. Wash buffer: Add 0.25 mL 200 × probenecid to 50 mL HBSS–HEPES–Ca–Mg buffer (*see* **Note 1**). Make 50 mL wash buffer per 96-well plate.
7. Fluo-4, AM solution (2 mM): Add 23 μL dimethyl-sulfoxide (DMSO) to a vial containing 50 μg fluo-4, AM (Invitrogen, Carlsbad, CA, USA), and vortex until dissolved.
8. Loading buffer: Mix 12 μL 2 mM fluo-4, AM solution with 12 μL pluronic acid (20% w/v in DMSO, Invitrogen, *see* **Note 2**), and vortex. Add 6 mL wash buffer and vortex again. This makes loading buffer containing 4 μM fluo-4, AM for one 96-well plate (*see* **Note 3**).

3. Methods

The method described below applies to mammalian cells adhered to the bottom of 96-well plates with clear bottom and black walls. For some cell types, it is necessary to coat the wells (e.g., with poly-D-lysine: *see* **Note 4**) prior to use in order to minimize dislodging of the cells during the washing steps. We have successfully used the protocol with Chinese hamster ovary (CHO), baby hamster kidney (BHK), and human embryonic kidney (HEK) cells, but in principle it should work with any mammalian cell line. Likewise, we have applied the protocol to cell lines either stably or transiently expressing the GPCR of interest. In general, we plate cells in 96-well plates the day before the assay and, for transient expression, transfect the cells 2 days before assay. However, these timelines should be optimized for each receptor/cell line combination as the time delay for optimal response might differ.

As the calcium response is time sensitive, you will need a fluorescence microplate reader with integrated automatic pipetting, which can dispense the ligand to the cells and immediately measure the fluorescence emission. Typically, the maximum read-out for a GPCR is reached 10–30 s after agonist application (*see*

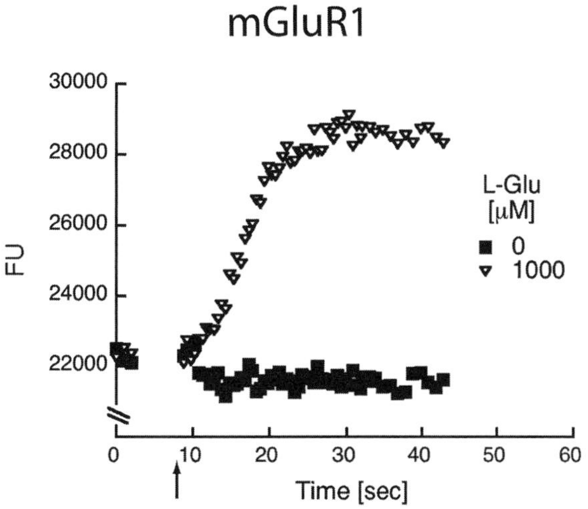

Fig. 2. Representative time-fluorescence curve of the metabotropic glutamate receptor subtype 1 (mGluR1) expressed in CHO cells *(12)*. Cells were loaded with fluo-4 as described in the present protocol, and fluorescence units (FU) were measured in a NOVOstar® microplate reader before and after addition of buffer (*closed squares*) or the endogenous agonist glutamate (L-Glu, added after 8 s as indicated by *arrow*) (*open triangles*).

Fig. 2). Furthermore, it is important that the fluorescence microplate reader excite and read from the bottom of the plate – close to the adhered cells. One of the first instruments was the FLIPR® (Molecular Devices, Sunnyvale, CA, USA), which has become synonymous with the name of the assay. The FLIPR® and other high-end plate fluorescence readers allow the user to apply ligands and read 96-, 384-, and even 1536-well plates simultaneously, which allow for very high throughput. More recently, less expensive instruments with lower throughput have been developed such as the FlexStation® (Molecular Devices, 8- or 16-well pipettor) and the NOVOstar® (BMG Labtechnologies, Offenburg, Germany, 1-well pipettor) (*see* **Note 5**).

It is well established that the cellular levels of receptor, G proteins, and effector proteins influence the potency and efficacy of agonists for GPCRs due to bottlenecks in the signaling cascade *(10)*. The use of a calcium-sensitive dye introduces another potential bottleneck as the maximally obtained intracellular calcium level might exceed the capacity of the fluo-4 probe. As with any GPCR assay, it is thus imperative to validate the calcium assay with a number of "standard" ligands with varying potency and efficacy and correlate the obtained potency and efficacy values with literature values before testing novel ligands. If large deviations for these standard ligands are observed, it might help to change the amount of DNA used for transfection, choose a stable cell line with higher/lower receptor expression level and/or change the concentration of fluo-4, AM used during the loading step (Step 2 below).

The protocol below relies on washing off the extracellular fluo-4 probe before the assay. This wash procedure can be harsh on some cell lines with low adherence such as HEK cells and thus introduce greater variability in the data. In that case, we normally use poly-D-lysine-coated 96-well plates (*see* **Note 4**) to prevent cell detachment during the washing steps. Also, having a full monolayer of cells in the wells helps the cells attach. Recently, several commercial vendors have developed no-wash assay kits such as Fluo-4 NW (Invitrogen) and Calcium Assay Kit (Molecular Devices), which, however, are significantly more expensive than the protocol described below. Also, some vendors do not fully disclose the content of their assay kits, which makes assay optimization more difficult.

3.1. Intracellular Calcium Assay in Living Mammalian Cells Using Fluo-4

1. Remove media from cells in the 96-well plate (*see* **Note 6**).
2. Add 50 μL loading buffer (room temperature) per well (*see* **Note 7**). Avoid light bleaching of the fluorescent probe (e.g., by wrapping the plate in aluminum foil).
3. Incubate the plate for 1 h at 37°C.
4. Prepare ligand solutions in wash buffer. Remember that the ligands will be diluted into 100 μL wash solution in the 96-well plate. Thus, if transferring 25 μL ligand solution to the cells, you should make a 5 × solution of the desired final ligand concentration. Place ligands in a 96-well plate. Always use negative (i.e., wash buffer) and positive (e.g., endogenous agonist) controls on each plate (*see* **Note 8**).
5. Following the incubation at 37°C, remove loading buffer, wash the wells twice with 100 μL wash buffer (room temperature), and finally add 100 μL wash buffer (room temperature) to each well (*see* **Notes 6** and 7 for advice on fluid removal and pipetting).
6. Transfer the plate to the fluorescence microplate reader and start the experiment (*see* **Note 9**). Choose wavelengths as close as possible to the fluo-4 excitation and emission maxima of 494 nm and 516 nm, respectively (we, e.g., use a 485 nm excitation filter and 520 nm emission filter on a NOVOstar® reader).

3.2. Data Analysis and Plate Design

All microplate readers measure fluorescence in arbitrary units (often referred to as fluorescence units, FU). Initially, the basal response of the cells is adjusted by setting the gain of the instrument, which is often set to ~25% of the maximum read-out of the instrument, making sure that the maximum responses obtained does not exceed the maximum read-out of the instrument. Usually, the microplate reader is programmed to make a series of fluorescence measurements prior to the addition of ligand, whereas the fluorescence is measured every second for 1–2 min – or at least until after the peak fluorescence response has been obtained (*see* **Fig. 2** for example of time–fluorescence curve).

All the previously mentioned microplate readers are controlled by sophisticated software which can be used to analyze the data. If the basal responses of the wells in a plate are very similar, it is often sufficient to use ΔFU (= peak FU – basal FU) as measure. However, if the basal response varies substantially over the plate, it might reduce the variability to adjust the data by dividing the peak FU or ΔFU with the basal FU. Also, intra- and/or inter-plate variability might decrease by normalizing the data to percent of peak response by the ionophore ionomycin (*see* **Note 8**).

It is our experience that some receptors/cell lines are affected by the so-called edge-effect, where cells in the outer rim of wells give substantially different responses than cells in the wells in the center of the plate, which could be due to thermal gradients across the plate or increased evaporation of media from the rim wells. One can try to reduce the edge-effect by pre-incubating newly seeded plates at room temperature for 1 h prior to incubation in the 37°C CO_2 incubator *(11)*, adding water between the rim wells or placing the microplate inside a large cell culture plate containing water, but often the best option is to *not* use the outer rim of wells. In any case, it is important to determine the magnitude of the edge-effect during implementation of a new assay and take appropriate action to reduce the intra-plate variability.

It is also our experience that some receptors/cell lines are sensitive to the addition of fluid by the microplate pipettor, which might be caused by dislodgement of cells from the plate bottom or mechanical force on the cell membrane/receptor. The effect is easily detected in control wells by comparison of the FU measurement before and after buffer addition. If there is a significant change in ΔFU, it might help to reduce the pipettor dispense speed and/or increase the pipettor height above the cells (note that this might affect mixing of the ligand solution with the buffer in the wells). If it is not possible to remove this fluid addition effect, one can use the negative controls (buffer addition) to adjust the read-outs of the test samples.

4. Notes

1. Some cells express the organic anion transporter, which exports the hydrolyzed negatively charged fluo-4^{5-} out of the cell, thus reducing the agonist-mediated signal (*see* **Fig. 1**).

Probenecid is an inhibitor of the transporter, but it is not necessary to add probenecid to cells not expressing the transporter, and in some cells probenecid might even decrease the agonist-mediated signal. Whether probenecid should be added or not, should thus be determined during implementation of a new assay.

2. Pluronic acid dissolved in DMSO can jellify upon storage at room temperature. Buy/make small amounts and inspect vial before use.
3. Often there is a linear relationship between concentration of fluo-4 in the loading buffer and obtained response. It might thus be necessary to use a higher concentration or possible to use a lower concentration of fluo-4 depending on the magnitude of the agonist-mediated response. Normal range of fluo-4 is 2–8 μM.
4. Prior to use, the 96-well plate is coated with poly-D-lysine (Sigma-Aldrich). Make a 4 mg/mL stock solution in sterile ddH_2O stored as frozen aliquots. Mix 50 μL of this stock solution with 6 mL Dulbecco's phosphate-buffered saline (PBS) without Ca^{2+} or Mg^{2+} (Invitrogen) and dispense 50 μL in each well. After 30–60 min, this solution is removed (invert plate on kitchen roll paper) and the wells are washed twice with 100 μL PBS. The plates are then ready for the cells.
5. The typical read-out time for a GPCR is 1 min/well, which translates to 1.5 h to perform a 96-well plate assay on a NOVOstar® plate reader. In spite of the ability to control the temperature in the cell plate chamber of the instruments, the fact that the last well has been incubated in assay buffer for 1.5 h longer than the first measured well can cause a drift in baseline and/or response values. In our experience, the drift varies quite substantially among receptors and cell lines and thus has to be established for each assay. However, usually it is possible to normalize drifts by strategic placement of negative and positive controls throughout the plate.
6. It is easy to dislodge cells in this step if using suction. Avoid this by inverting the plate and flinging the fluid into a bucket and then press the plate down on kitchen roll paper. Do not fling too hard as this can dislodge the cells, but not too soft either as this will leave too much fluid in the wells. Initially, inspect the cells in a microscope after flinging to see if cells have been detached.
7. It is easy to dislodge cells in this step. Avoid this by careful pipetting down the side of the well at slow dispense speed. Ideally, use an electronic 8- or 12-channel multistep pipette

(e.g., Matrix Multichannel Pipette; Thermo Scientific, Waltham, MA, USA) to quickly add buffer to the whole plate in a reproducible manner. Initially, inspect the cells in a microscope after pipetting to see if cells have been detached.

8. The ionophore ionomycin (Sigma-Aldrich, use 5 μM final concentration), which transports Ca^{2+} across the cell plasma membrane, can be used as positive control for proper loading of cells with fluo-4. Alternatively, many cell lines endogenously express adenosine receptors which elicit robust calcium responses in response to 10 μM adenosine-5′ -triphosphate (ATP, Sigma-Aldrich, make fresh from powder).
9. It is our experience that some receptors/cell lines display significant drift in basal and response fluorescence during the first minutes after insertion of the cell plate in the microplate reader due to auto luminescence and/or adjustment of the cells to the instrument temperature. This can be avoided by 5–10 min of incubation in the microplate reader prior to initiation of the experiment. It is also our experience that some receptors/cell lines are sensitive to the temperature in the plate chamber of the microplate reader. The temperature should thus be controlled by the microplate reader (usually set in the 25–37°C range). Note that the plate chamber might warm up significantly during a full day of experiments and that most microplate readers cannot cool the plate chamber.

Acknowledgments

Our work on FLIPR® assays of intracellular calcium has been supported by The Danish Medical Research Council, the Lundbeck Foundation, the Villum Kann Rasmussen Foundation, the Novo Nordisk Foundation, Fonden af 17-12-1981, the Augustinus Foundation, and the Direktør Ib Henriksen Foundation.

References

1. Minta, A., Kao, J. P. Y., and Tsien, R. Y. (1989) Fluorescent indicators for cytosolic calcium based on rhodamine and fluorescein chromophores. *J. Biol. Chem.* **264**, 8171–8178.
2. Gee, K. R., Brown, K. A., Chen, W. N. U., Bishop-Stewart, J., Gray, D., and Johnson, I. (2000) Chemical and physiological characterization of fluo-4 Ca^{2+}-indicator dyes. *Cell Calcium* **27**, 97–106.
3. Kostenis, E. (2006) G proteins in drug screening: From analysis of receptor-G protein specificity to manipulation of GPCR-mediated signalling pathways. *Curr. Pharm. Des.* **12**, 1703–1715.
4. Conklin, B. R., Farfel, Z., Lustig, K. D., Julius, D., and Bourne, H. R. (1993) Substitution of three amino acids switches receptor specificity of Gqα to that of Giα. *Nature* **363**, 274–276.

5. Offermanns, S., and Simon, M. I. (1995) G alpha 15 and G alpha 16 couple a wide variety of receptors to phospholipase C. *J. Biol. Chem.* **270**, 15175–15180.
6. Heydorn, A., Ward, R. J., Jorgensen, R., Rosenkilde, M. M., Frimurer, T. M., Milligan, G., and Kostenis, E. (2004) Identification of a novel site within G protein alpha subunits important for specificity of receptor-G protein interaction *Mol. Pharmacol.* **66**, 250–259.
7. Bräuner-Osborne, H., and Krogsgaard-Larsen, P. (1999) Functional pharmacology of cloned heterodimeric $GABA_B$ receptors expressed in mammalian cells. *Br. J. Pharmacol.* **128**, 1370–1374.
8. Christiansen, B., Hansen, K. B., Wellendorph, P., and Bräuner-Osborne, H. (2007) Pharmacological characterization of mouse GPRC6A, an L-α-amino acid receptor with ability to sense divalent cations. *Br. J. Pharmacol.* **150**, 798–807.
9. Takahashi, A., Camacho, P., Lechleiter, J. D., and Herman, B. (1999) Measurement of intracellular calcium. *Physiol. Rev.* **79**, 1089–1125.
10. Kenakin, T. P., and Morgan, P. H. (1989) Theoretical effects of single and multiple transducer receptor coupling proteins on estimates of the relative potency of agonists. *Mol. Pharmacol.* **35**, 214–222.
11. Lundholt, B. K., Scudder, K. M., and Pagliaro, L. (2003) A simple technique for reducing edge effect in cell-based assays. *J. Biomol. Screen.* **8**, 566–570.
12. Bjerrum, E. J., Kristensen, A. S., Pickering, D. S., Greenwood, J. R., Nielsen, B., Liljefors, T., Schousboe, A., Bräuner-Osborne, H., and Madsen, U. (2003) Design, synthesis, and pharmacology of a highly subtype-selective GluR1/2 agonist, (*RS*)-2-amino-3-(4-chloro-3-hydroxy-5-isoxazolyl)propionic acid (Cl-HIBO). *J. Med. Chem.* **46**, 2246–2249.

Chapter 20

Use of Fluorescence Indicators in Receptor Ligands

Kaleeckal G. Harikumar and Laurence J. Miller

Summary

Fluorescence techniques can provide insights into the environment of fluorescent indicators incorporated within a ligand as it is bound to its receptor. Fluorescent indicators of different sizes and chemical characteristics ranging from hydrophilic to hydrophobic that are incorporated into a receptor ligand can provide insights into the nature of the binding environment, the surrounding structures, and even into conformational changes associated with receptor activation. Methods for determining fluorescence spectral analysis, fluorescence quenching, fluorescence anisotropy, and fluorescence lifetimes of the ligand probes are described. The applications of these techniques to the CCK_1 receptor occupied by $Alexa^{488}$-CCK are utilized as examples. These methods represent powerful tools to expand our understanding of the structure and function of G protein-coupled receptors.

Key words: Cholecystokinin receptor, Collisional quenching, Emission spectra, Excitation spectra, Fluorescence anisotropy, Fluorescence lifetime, Fluorescent ligands.

1. Introduction

G protein-coupled receptors represent the largest group of membrane receptors, with several hundred members of this superfamily identified *(1)*. These receptors represent the most common target of drugs currently on the market *(2)*, yet we know relatively little about their structure, the molecular basis of their ligand binding, and the conformational states correlating with their activation and desensitization. We finally have high-resolution crystal structures for rhodopsin and for the β2-adrenergic receptor *(3, 4)*, but this represents only the beginning of what will be necessary to have substantial impact on the rational design and refinement of drugs acting at these targets. Novel methodologic approaches, such as those using fluorescence, can provide important new insights.

Wayne R. Leifert (ed.), *G Protein-Coupled Receptors in Drug Discovery, vol. 552*

Book doi: 10.1007/978-1-60327-317-6_20

Fluorescence has been applied to receptor characterization in two broad categories, involving the labeling of the receptor itself or the labeling of ligands for the receptor. While it is now relatively easy to build a recombinant receptor construct that includes a fluorescent tag, such as one of the analogues of green fluorescent protein (GFP), these fluorophores are quite large and can only be tolerated without substantial negative impact on function when attached to a few regions of the receptor. As such, they are most informative for localization of the tagged receptor to a cellular compartment or for the gross determination of protein–protein associations using resonance transfer techniques. Fluorescent analogues of natural ligands provide a very powerful experimental approach to provide information regarding the microenvironment of the receptor-bound ligand and insights into conformational changes that correlate with receptor activation. However, here too, fluorescent analogues of natural ligands are limited and require careful validation of their behaving like natural ligands in binding and stimulation of biological activity.

The latter approach is the focus of the current report. Fluorescent ligand spectroscopy has been used for the characterization of ligand binding domains and conformational changes that occur at multiple members of this superfamily, including rhodopsin *(5)*, the β2-adrenergic receptor *(6)*, the cholecystokinin (CCK) receptor *(7)*, the secretin receptor *(8)*, and the parathyroid hormone receptor *(9)*.

The major challenge for these studies is to develop fluorescent analogues of relevant ligands that preserve function, without modifying binding or biological activity. A wide variety of fluorophores that have very different chemical characteristics are available for incorporation into such ligands. These include aladan, nitrobenzoxadiazole, dansyl, acrylodan, various alexa moieties, fluorescein, rhodamine, and members of the Cye3/Cye5 series, each having distinct size and charge, affecting their hydrophobicity and hydrophilicity, as well as unique solvatochromatic characteristics *(7, 8, 10–12)*.

The fluorescence characteristics of the probe reflect its local environment. Fluorescence emission profiles are dependent on the polarity of the ligand-binding environment, with spectral shifts toward the blue region indicative of the probe binding to its receptor in a hydrophobic location, whereas shifts toward the red region are consistent with a more hydrophilic region of binding. The spectral characteristics of the fluorescence indicator are also affected by the viscosity and pH of the medium where it resides, and fluorescence quantum yields can be affected by local quenching. This refers to the decrease in the intensity of the fluorescence due to either static or dynamic interactions between quencher and indicator. Similarly, the fluorescence anisotropy refers to the rotational mobility of the fluorescence indicator within its excited state during the period of fluorescence decay. Time-resolved decay analysis can be used to determine the fluorescence lifetime of the fluorophore, another indication of its local environment.

2. Materials

2.1. Sample Preparation

1. CCK_1 receptor-bearing cell membranes (stored at –80°C in small aliquots). Quality of membrane preparation must be evaluated before these are utilized for fluorescence studies (*see* **Note 1**).
2. $Alexa^{488}$-CCK ($Alexa^{488}$-Gly-Asp-Tyr(SO_3)-Nle-Gly-Trp-Nle-Asp-Phe(NH_2)), a fully efficacious and high-affinity agonist ligand (*see* **Note 2**).
3. Krebs–Ringer–HEPES (KRH): 25 m*M* HEPES (pH 7.4), 104 m*M* NaCl, 5 m*M* KCl, 2 m*M* $CaCl_2$,1 m*M* KH_2PO_4, and 1.2 m*M* $MgSO_4$ (prepared freshly with protease inhibitors added) (*see* **Note 3**).
4. Bovine serum albumin (Sigma, St Louis, MO, USA) – 0.2% bovine serum albumin is added to the KRH medium before performing the assay.
5. Soybean trypsin inhibitor (Invitrogen, Carlsbad, CA, USA) – 0.01% soybean trypsin inhibitor is added to the KRH medium before performing the assay.
6. Low retention microfuge tubes (Fisher Scientific, Chino, CA, USA).
7. Refrigerated microcentrifuge.

2.2. Fluorescence Instrumentation

1. SPEX Fluoromax-3 spectrofluorophotometer (SPEX Industries, Edison, NJ, USA).
2. Datamax-3 software (SPEX Industries).
3. Quartz cuvette (Starna Cells Inc., Atascadero, CA, USA).

2.3. Spectral Profiles

1. $Alexa^{488}$-CCK bound to the CCK_1 receptor expressed in membranes that are studied in suspension (freshly bound).
2. $Alexa^{488}$-CCK ligand (synthesized in the laboratory using standard peptide chemical coupling reactions and purification) (*see* **Note 4**).
3. Non-fluorescent CCK peptide (Bachem, Torrance, CA, USA).
4. Solvents with different polarities (water, acetonitrile, methanol, isopropyl alcohol; Fisher Scientific).

2.4. Fluorescence Quenching Measurements

1. Alexa^{488}-CCK bound to the CCK_1 receptor in membranes that are studied in suspension (freshly bound).
2. Potassium iodide.
3. Potassium chloride.
4. Sodium thiosulfite ($Na_2S_2O_3$).
5. 2,2,6,6-tetramethyl piperidine *N*-oxyl (TEMPO).

2.5. Fluorescence Anisotropy Measurements

1. Alexa^{488}-CCK bound to the CCK_1 receptor in membranes that are in suspension (freshly bound).
2. Temperature-controlled cuvette holder (temperature of the cuvette is controlled by a external circulating water bath filled with 50%:50% water/antifreeze to maintain constant temperature (±0.5°C).
3. Automatic polarizer (attached to the spectrofluorophotometer; SPEX Industries).

2.6. Time-Resolved Fluorescence Spectroscopy

1. Alexa^{488}-CCK bound to the CCK_1 receptor in membranes that are in suspension (freshly bound).
2. Pulse-picked frequency-doubled titanium-sapphire picosecond laser source (Tsunami Spectra Physics Laser Division, Mountain View, CA, USA).
3. Interference filter systems with 6.8 nm path length.
4. Time-correlated single photon counter (Multi-channel plate photomultiplier – R1809U, Hamamatsu, Bridgewater, NJ, USA).
5. Ortec Maestro-32 software package (Ortec, Oak Ridge, TN, USA).
6. GLOBAL.EXE, windows version (Laboratory of Fluorescence Dynamics, University of California, Irvine, CA, USA).

3. Methods

A fluorescent ligand for the CCK receptor (Alexa^{488}-CCK utilized here) can be helpful to explore the molecular basis of ligand binding, providing insights into its microenvironment as it is bound to its receptor (**Fig. 1**). This can also be utilized to explore conformational changes that occur during agonist-stimulated activation. The complementary methods described below are meant to gather relevant information toward such insights.

Spectral emission profiles of the fluorescent ligand in various solvents are indicative of the influence of the environment on probe fluorescence. When the probe is bound to the receptor,

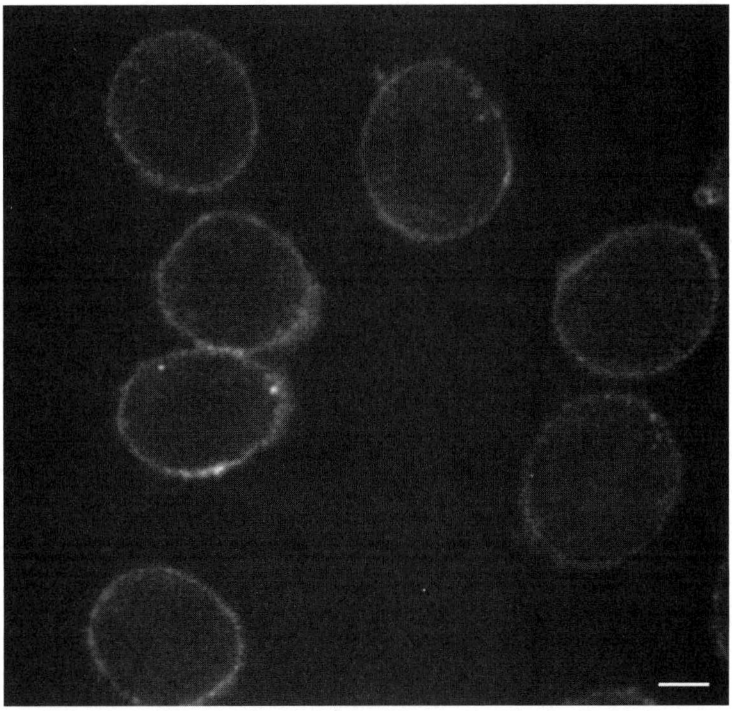

Fig. 1. Receptor localization. Shown are typical confocal microscopic images of Type 1 CCK receptors on CHO-CCKR cells occupied with Alexa^{488}-CCK. Scale bar: 25 μm.

changes in the position of the emission maximum along the spectrum and its quantum yield provide important information about the polarity of its microenvironment. Spectral shifts toward the blue region are indicative of a hydrophobic binding location, whereas shifts toward the red region are indicative of a more hydrophilic region of binding.

Collisional quenching of fluorescence provides complementary information about the microenvironment of the receptor-bound probe. Effective quenching with a hydrophilic quencher like potassium iodide is indicative of a hydrophilic environment, whereas effective quenching with TEMPO is more indicative of a hydrophobic environment. Collisional quenching is typically displayed using a Stern–Volmer plot, graphing the ratio of fluorescence intensity in the absence and presence of quencher versus quencher concentration. The slope of the line fitting these data determines the quenching constant, with a steeper slope indicative of greater quenching.

Fluorescence anisotropy provides an indication of the rotational freedom of the indicator within the ligand, as it is bound to the receptor. This, too, is dependent on the characteristics of the binding location. Greater exposure to aqueous solvent typically leads to greater anisotropy. Fluorescence lifetimes tend to vary inversely with anisotropy, such that greater rotational freedom, such as occurs in a hydrophilic environment, is often associated with a shorter lifetime.

3.1. Sample Preparation for Fluorescence Measurements

1. The CCK_1 receptor-bearing membranes (50 μg of membrane proteins) are incubated with 100 n*M* fluorescent CCK ligand (Alexa^{488}-CCK) for 20 min at room temperature in KRH medium (pH 7.4) (*see* **Note 5**). It is important to continuously mix the membrane suspension to allow uniform ligand binding and to protect the tubes from stray light to avoid bleaching.
2. After the incubation, the membrane suspension is cooled and the receptor-bound ligand fraction is separated from free ligand by centrifugation at 20,000 × g for 10 min at 4°C. Please note that the centrifuge should be cooled before starting the centrifugation, since ligand dissociation is often quite rapid at higher temperatures.
3. The membrane fraction is once again washed with ice-cold KRH medium, centrifuged, and resuspended in cold medium for fluorescence measurements. The fluorescent ligand-bound membrane suspension is kept cold to avoid dissociation of receptor-bound ligand. The membrane fraction should be carefully and completely resuspended to get a clear signal from the samples.

3.2. Fluorescence Spectroscopy (System Characteristics)

1. Steady-state fluorescence excitation and emission spectra are collected using a SPEX Fluoromax-3 spectrofluorometer. A standard fluorometer consists of a light source, excitation filter, emission filter, and an emission detector. Start the fluorometer and set up the excitation and emission wavelengths, slit width, and acquisition conditions using a constant increment. This should provide a stable and reliable signal.
2. The Alexa^{488}-CCK-bound CCK_1 receptor-bearing membrane suspension is transferred into a 1 mL quartz cuvette and the fluorescence is promptly recorded. The cuvette must be clean, since impurities can affect the fluorescence characteristics, including intensity and spectral patterns (*see* **Note 6**).
3. The excitation spectra are recorded by scanning from 400 to 500 nm at a constant emission of 521 nm.
4. The emission spectra are recorded from 500 to 650 nm by exciting samples at 482 nm (**Fig. 2A**) (*see* **Note 7**).
5. The spectra are collected using the Datamax-3 software attached to the Fluoromax-3 spectrofluorometer, with a band pass of 4.00 nm and 05 s integration time.

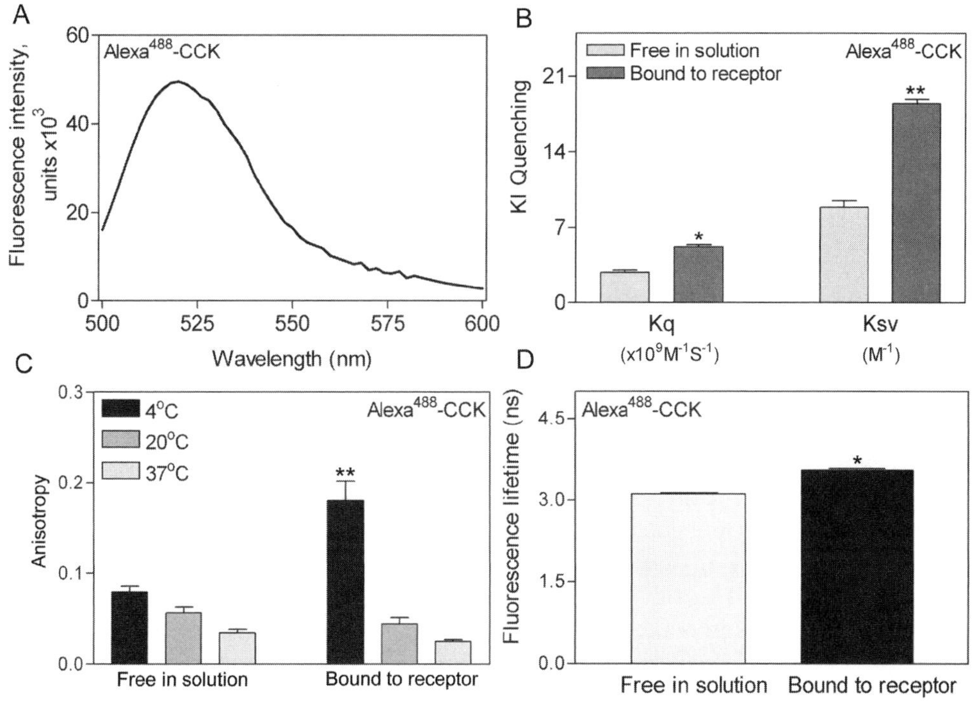

Fig. 2. Fluorescence properties. Some of the properties of Alexa^{488}-CCK bound to Type 1 CCK receptors on CHO-CCKR cells are shown. (**A**) Fluorescence emission spectrum of receptor-bound probe; (**B**) K_I collisional quenching constants – Stern–Volmer constant, K_{SV}, and bimolecular quenching constant, K_q, for probe when free in solution and when receptor bound; (**C**) steady-state fluorescence anisotropy values at three different temperatures for free and receptor-bound probe; (**D**) fluorescence lifetime values for free and receptor-bound probe. Data represent means ± S.E.M. of data from four different experiments. *$p<0.05$; **$p<0.01$ for receptor-bound probe characteristics relative to those of probe in solution.

6. Analogous emission and excitation spectra are collected with buffer as well as with cell membranes which were not exposed to fluorescent ligand, considered as background measurements. From this spectral analysis, the excitation and emission maxima can be established and recorded. Corrected spectra are acquired by subtracting the blank spectra from the sample spectra. This can be achieved by incorporating the blank spectral values in the correct application module.

3.3. Spectral Profiles

Fluorescence emission profiles of the probes containing the more solvatochromatic fluorophores, such as aladan, acrylodan and nitrobenzoxadiazole, can provide important information about the ligand binding environment *(7, 11)*.

1. Fluorescence emission spectra are recorded for Alexa^{488}-CCK while free in solution and while bound to membrane-associated CCK_1 receptor. The emission spectra of the receptor-bound Alexa^{488}-CCK in the absence or presence of

100-fold molar excess of non-fluorescent CCK peptide are recorded from 500 to 650 nm after excitation of the sample at 482 nm. The latter provides an important control.

2. Fluorescent probe emission profiles are collected in solvents with distinct dielectric constants. Approximately 1 n*M* fluorescent probe (Alexa^{488}-CCK) is mixed with solvents with decreased dielectric constants (water, buffer – 80; acetonitrile – 36.6; methanol – 33; ethanol – 24; isopropyl alcohol – 20.1) and emission spectra are recorded as discussed above (*see* **Note 8**). Corrected spectra are prepared by subtracting the emission spectrum from each sample with the corresponding solvent, and final emission peak values are recorded.

3.4. Fluorescence Quenching Measurements

Fluorescence quenching measurements refer to the reduction in the fluorescence intensity of the probe by molecular interactions or molecular rearrangements while in its excited state. To measure this, the fluorescence of Alexa^{488}-CCK bound to its receptor is quantified in the presence of various concentrations of the quenching reagent, such as potassium iodide.

1. Fluorescent ligand-bound CCK_1 receptor-bearing membranes in suspension are transferred into 1 mL quartz cuvette, where the sample is excited with 482 nm light and the steady-state fluorescence emission is measured at 521 nm. The Datamax-3 program is used for constant wavelength analysis. In constant wavelength emission acquisition mode, the fluorescence intensity is acquired by averaging two trial measurements at each point.
2. Fluorescence is recorded at optimal emission by fixing a constant excitation wavelength after sequential addition of freshly prepared potassium iodide solution to the Alexa^{488}-CCK-bound CCK_1 receptor preparation.
3. A stock solution (1 *M*) of potassium iodide in 10 m*M* $Na_2S_2O_3$, a reducing agent to avoid air-induced oxidation of iodide solution.
4. The potassium iodide solution is added sequentially to achieve the desired concentrations: 25–250 m*M* (*see* **Note 9**).
5. After each addition of potassium iodide, shake well and delay for 10 s before measuring the fluorescence intensity. The dilution effect and the effect of the ionic strength on the fluorescence are controlled by the addition of potassium chloride to the control samples.

3.4.1. Calculations

1. The blank-subtracted fluorescence intensity data are calculated using the Stern–Volmer equation, $F_o/F = 1 + K_{sv}\,[Q]$, where F_o/F is the ratio of the fluorescence intensities in the absence and the presence of potassium iodide.

2. The ratio of fluorescence intensities in the absence and presence of quencher are plotted relative to quencher concentrations, generating a linear fit. The Stern–Volmer quenching constant, $K_{sv,}$ is determined from the slope of this graph (**Fig. 2B**).
3. The bimolecular quenching constant (K_q) illustrates the efficiency of iodide quenching or the accessibility of quencher to the fluorescence indicator (**Fig. 2B**) (*see* **Note 10**). This is calculated utilizing the equation, $K_q = K_{sv}/(\tau)$, where τ represents the fluorescence lifetime of the probe.

3.5. Fluorescence Anisotropy Measurements

Fluorescence anisotropy refers to the rotational mobility of the fluorescence indicator. In practice, this refers to the correlation between polarization of fluorescence emission and excitation by the incident polarized light. If the molecules rotate significantly between excitation and emission, there is less correlation, consistent with a low level of fluorescence anisotropy.

1. Steady-state anisotropy measurements are performed using $Alexa^{488}$-CCK bound to receptor expressed in the membrane suspension (**Fig. 2C**). These measurements are carried out at various temperatures, as discussed below. The fluorescence intensities should be collected after 2 s, to allow the cuvette to achieve the temperature of the holder.
2. Measurements are carried out by using an L-format-based single-channel SPEX Fluromax-3 spectrofluorometer equipped with automatic polarizer and thermostatically controlled cuvette holder (*see* **Note 11**).
3. The excitation and emission polarizing filters are aligned to 0° and 55°, respectively.
4. The emission intensities are measured by setting up the excitation-side polarizer in the vertical position (V) and the emission-side polarizer in the horizontal (H) and vertical positions (V).
5. The emission intensities are collected by exciting the samples at 482 nm and the emission wavelength is fixed at 521 nm.
6. The polarization measurement is carried out by Constant Wavelength Analysis mode of 10 s integration time with a two trial measurement after a delay of 2 s. The polarization values are recorded at 4°C, 20°C, and 37°C.

3.5.1. Calculations

1. The anisotropy is calculated based on the polarization values using the following equation:

$$A = (I_{VV} - GI_{VH})/I_{VV} + 2GI_{VH})$$

where I_{VV} is the fluorescence intensity measured with both excitation and emission side polarizers aligned in the vertical positions and I_{VH} is the fluorescence intensity measured with the excitation side polarizer aligned in the vertical position and the emission side polarizer aligned in the horizontal position.

2. The values for G are calculated by the following equation:

$$G = I_{HH}/I_{HV}$$

where G represents the ratio of detection sensitivity of vertically and horizontally polarized light. G is dependent on the emission wavelength and expected to be 1 (*see* **Note 12**).

3.6. Time-resolved Fluorescence Spectroscopy

Time-resolved fluorescence spectroscopy is utilized to measure fluorescence lifetimes. Fluorescence lifetime is the period of time in nanoseconds that the fluorescent molecule is in the excited state before it returns to the ground state. This is determined by counting the number of photons emitted during the relevant time period. Once again, the fluorescence lifetime is dependent on the environment of the bound fluorescent ligand.

1. Time-correlated fluorescence spectroscopy is used to measure the fluorescence lifetimes of the probes when bound to the receptor (**Fig. 2D**). This is achieved by time-correlated single photon counting using a single photon counter.
2. The $Alexa^{488}$-CCK bound to its receptor in the membrane suspension is transferred into a cuvette of 1 cm path length.
3. Samples are excited using a pulse-picked frequency-doubled titanium-sapphire picosecond time scale laser source at room temperature.
4. The excitation wavelength based on the laser output is tuned with a pulse width of 1-2 picoseconds, yielding an approximate spectral bandwidth of 1 nm.
5. The fluorescence emission is passed through the interference filter centered at 521 nm with a 6.8 nm bandwidth and the single photons are detected by a microchannel plate photomultiplier R1809U (MCP, Hamamatsu).
5. The number of photons for a typical experiment should be more than 1000 photons to get meaningful data (*see* **Note 13**).
6. The photons are collected in 1080 channels with a width of 10.05 ps/channel.
7. A constant fraction discriminator (CFD; Tennelec TC455 Quad CFD) converts the photo arrival time to a pulse height, which is processed by a Multichannel Analyzer (MCA) (TRUMP-PCI-8 k) card and Mastero-32 software.

8. The fluorescence lifetime decay analysis is collected by using the modules for instrumental controls and analog/digital time amplitude conversion using Ortec Mastero-32 software package 9. The decay analysis is performed using the Windows version of GLOBALS.EXE *(13)*. The curve fitting utilized is based on the models of a single exponential and with two discrete exponential lifetime components. The quality of the exponential fit is based on the values of Chi square (χ^2) (close to 1) statistics.

3.6.1. Calculations

1. By assuming the fluorescence decay to be the sum of discrete exponentials, then the fluorescence intensity of decay is calculated based on this equation.

$$I(t) = \alpha_i e^{-t/\tau i}$$

where $I(t)$ is the intensity decay, τ_i is the decay time of the *i*th component, and α_i is a weighting factor (amplitude) representing the contribution of the particular lifetime component to the fluorescence decay.

2. The decay parameters are obtained using the non-linear least squares iterative fitting procedure based on the Marquardt algorithm and also using the PORT3 portable Fortran 3 program.
3. The fractional decay of the fluorescence for the *i*th component at wavelength $\lambda(f_i(\lambda))$ is calculated from the following equation:

$$f_i(\lambda) = (\alpha_i(\lambda)\tau_i / \Sigma\alpha_i(\lambda)\tau_i)$$

4. The mean average lifetime ($<\tau>$) for the bi-exponential decays of fluorescence are calculated with the following equation:

$$<\tau> = \Sigma f_i \tau_i$$

where $<\tau>$ is the average lifetime, f_i is the fraction of the *i*th decay component, and τ_i is the correspondent lifetime of the *i*th decay component.

4. Notes

1. Receptor-bearing membranes are prepared as described by Hadac et al. *(14)* and should be stored in small aliquots that are not allowed to be repeatedly thawed and refrozen. The quality of receptor in these membranes is measured by radioligand binding assays using ^{125}I-CCK ligand *(14)*.

2. Fluorescent Alexa^{488}-CCK is stored at –20°C in small aliquots wrapped in aluminum foil to protect them from light, also avoiding multiple cycles of thawing and refreezing. Alexa^{488}-CCK is able to bind saturably and specifically to the CCK_1 receptor with affinity not different from natural CCK *(7)*.
3. All the buffers and solvents used for fluorescence measurements are degassed and bubbled with nitrogen to prevent any quenching from dissolved oxygen.
4. Fluorescent Alexa^{488}-CCK is prepared by reacting the amino group of the CCK peptide with Alexa^{488}-succimidyl ester using a standard coupling reaction, followed by purification using reversed phase high-performance liquid chromatography *(15)*.
5. The membrane suspension should be incubated in low retention microcentrifuge tubes to avoid excessive loss of peptide due to adherence to the walls of the tubes.
6. The quartz cuvette is washed using concentrated nitric acid, water, and ethanol, followed by extensive washing with nanopure water to remove the impurities.
7. For acquiring the fluorescence excitation and the emission profiles, a fixed bandwidth, integration time, and wavelength increment are necessary to get reproducible signals. An average of three emission scans will give a spectral profile with adequate quality.
8. Spectral emission profiles for Alexa^{488}-CCK in each solvent are corrected for a blank emission spectrum for each corresponding solvent in the absence of fluorescent ligand.
9. The correct amount of potassium iodide solution was added to the fluorescent sample to yield the desired concentration.
10. Since quenching of the fluorophore is dependent on its fluorescence lifetime, the bimolecular quenching constant, an indication of the frequency of collisions between the diffusing molecules, provides insight into the environment in which the quenching molecules diffuse.
11. The L-format represents the method in which a single emission channel is used and the samples are excited using vertically polarized light with the emission intensities collected with vertical and horizontal channels.
12. Since the anisotropy measurement is carried out using an emission filter, and not a monochromator, and filters do not have any significant polarization, the value of G used is 1.
13. For the most meaningful data for analysis, it is recommended to collect 1000–2000 photons in the minimal period of time. This increases the signal-to-noise ratio.

Acknowledgments

This work was supported by a grant from the National Institutes of Health, DK32878, the Fiterman Foundation, and Mayo Clinic.

References

1. Lefkowitz, R.J. (2007) Seven transmembrane receptors: something old, something new. *Acta Physiol.* **190**, 9–19.
2. Lagerstrom, M.C. and Schioth, H.B. (2008) Structural diversity of G protein-coupled receptors and significance for drug discovery. *Nat. Rev. Drug Discov.* 7, 339–357.
3. Cherezov, V., Rosenbaum, D.M., Hanson, M.A., Rasmussen, S.G., Thian, F.S., Kobilka, T.S., et al. (2007) High-resolution crystal structure of an engineered human beta2-adrenergic G protein-coupled receptor. *Science* **318**, 1258–1265.
4. Rosenbaum, D.M., Cherezov, V., Hanson, M.A., Rasmussen, S.G., Thian, F.S., Kobilka, T.S., et al. (2007) GPCR engineering yields high-resolution structural insights into beta2-adrenergic receptor function. *Science* **318**, 1266–1273.
5. Farrens, D.L., Altenbach, C., Yang, K., Hubbell, W.L., and Khorana, H.G. (1996) Requirement of rigid-body motion of transmembrane helices for light activation of rhodopsin. *Science* **274**, 768–770.
6. Gether, U., Lin, S., and Kobilka, B.K. (1995) Fluorescent labeling of purified beta 2 adrenergic receptor. Evidence for ligand-specific conformational changes. *J. Biol. Chem.* **270**, 28268–28275.
7. Harikumar, K.G., Pinon, D.I., Wessels, W.S., Prendergast, F.G., and Miller, L.J. (2002) Environment and mobility of a series of fluorescent reporters at the amino terminus of structurally related peptide agonists and antagonists bound to the cholecystokinin receptor. *J. Biol. Chem.* **277**, 18552–18560.
8. Harikumar, K.G., Hosohata, K., Pinon, D.I., and Miller, L.J. (2006) Use of probes with fluorescence indicator distributed throughout the pharmacophore to examine the peptide agonist-binding environment of the family B G protein-coupled secretin receptor. *J. Biol. Chem.* **281**, 2543–2550.
9. Vilardaga, J.P., Bunemann, M., Krasel, C., Castro, M., and Lohse, M.J. (2003) Measurement of the millisecond activation switch of G protein-coupled receptors in living cells. *Nat. Biotechnol.* **21**, 807–812.
10. Cohen, B.E., McAnaney, T.B., Park, E.S., Jan, Y.N., Boxer, S.G., and Jan, L.Y. (2002) Probing protein electrostatics with a synthetic fluorescent amino acid. *Science* **296**, 1700–1703.
11. Harikumar, K.G., Pinon, D.I., and Miller, L.J. (2006) Fluorescent indicators distributed throughout the pharmacophore of cholecystokinin provide insights into distinct modes of binding and activation of type A and B cholecystokinin receptors. *J. Biol. Chem.* **281**, 27072–27080.
12. Vilardaga, J.P., De Neef, P., Di Paolo, E., Bollen, A., Waelbroeck, M., and Robberecht, P. (1995) Properties of chimeric secretin and VIP receptor proteins indicate the importance of the N-terminal domain for ligand discrimination. *Biochem. Biophys. Res. Commun.* **211**, 885–891.
13. Beechem, J.M. (1992) Global analysis of biochemical and biophysical data. *Methods Enzymol.* **210**, 37–54.
14. Hadac, E.M., Ghanekar, D.V., Holicky, E.L., Pinon, D.I., Dougherty, R.W., and Miller, L.J. (1996) Relationship between native and recombinant cholecystokinin receptors: Role of differential glycosylation. *Pancreas* **13**, 130–139.
15. Powers, S.P., Fourmy, D., Gaisano, H., and Miller, L.J. (1988) Intrinsic photoaffinity labeling probes for cholecystokinin (CCK)-gastrin family receptors. D-Tyr-Gly-[(Nle^{28,31},pNO$_2$-Phe^{33})CCK-26-33]. *J. Biol. Chem.* **263**, 5295–5300.

Chapter 21

Application of Fluorescence Resonance Energy Transfer Techniques to Establish Ligand–Receptor Orientation

Kaleeckal G. Harikumar and Laurence J. Miller

Summary

Fluorescence resonance energy transfer (FRET) has been utilized to determine distances between a fluorescence donor and a fluorescence acceptor having appropriately overlapping spectra. In this chapter, we utilize this approach to establish distances between a fluorescence donor situated in a distinct position within a docked ligand and a fluorescence acceptor situated in a distinct position within its receptor. This technique is applicable to receptor expressed in the environment of an intact cell containing the full complement of signaling and regulatory proteins. A number of controls are necessary, including those establishing the normal function of the modified ligand and receptor, the absence of energy transfer to non-receptor proteins, and the specificity of transfer between the donor of interest and the acceptor of interest. We have utilized the example of FRET between a secretin peptide incorporating $Alexa^{488}$ and a secretin receptor construct derivatized with $Alexa^{568}$. The latter was prepared by the derivatization of a mono-cysteine-reactive receptor construct with a fluorescent methanethiosulfonate reagent. This approach can provide important spatial information that can be useful in the meaningful docking of a ligand at its receptor.

Key words: Fluorescence, Fluorescence resonance energy transfer, G protein-coupled receptor, Ligand docking, Receptor conformation, Secretin receptor.

1. Introduction

Understanding the molecular basis of ligand binding and the conformational changes associated with receptor activation represents key insights for the rational design and refinement of candidates in the development of receptor-active drugs. However, crystallographic approaches that provide high-resolution structures of intact receptors have only been successfully applied to a few members of the G protein-coupled receptor superfamily

Wayne R. Leifert (ed.), *G Protein-Coupled Receptors in Drug Discovery, vol. 552*

Book doi: 10.1007/978-1-60327-317-6_21

(1, 2). Other high-resolution structural approaches have been more broadly applied to selected domains of these receptors *(3, 4)*. Lower resolution insights have come from resonance transfer techniques, photoaffinity labeling, and structure-activity series *(5–8)*.

Fluorescence approaches provide another useful technique for the examination of the environment of bound ligands, for the exploration of protein–protein interactions, and even for the quantification of intra- and inter-molecular distances between a fluorescence donor and a fluorescence acceptor *(9–13)*. The latter is the focus of this chapter, applying the technique that was initially described as a tool for spectroscopic measurement of distances by Stryer and Haugland *(14)* to determine the distances between positions with a receptor-bound ligand and residues within the receptor. This can theoretically provide relative distances to guide the meaningful docking of a ligand to its receptor.

In this chapter, we use as an example the prototypic Family B G protein-coupled receptor, the secretin receptor, occupied by a fluorescent analog of its natural hormonal ligand, the 27-amino acid peptide secretin *(15)*. Such studies require the incorporation of a fluorescence donor within an analog of the natural ligand that retains its high-affinity binding and full biological activity, to be certain that the distances will be most reflective of natural hormone binding. Additionally, this requires the ability to position fluorescence acceptors into distinct positions within the receptor, so as not to disrupt its ability to bind and respond appropriately to agonist ligands. This was achieved by developing a receptor template construct lacking any derivatizable free extracellular cysteine residues, representing a pseudo-wild type, null-cysteine-reactive receptor, and modifying it to develop mono-cysteine-reactive receptor constructs that can be selectively derivatized to produce sites of fluorescence acceptors in distinct extracellular domains *(12)*. These constructs can be stably expressed on Chinese hamster ovary (CHO) cell lines for derivatization and study.

Resonance energy transfer studies have been utilized extensively to explore bimolecular interactions and to determine distances between residues in soluble proteins that are easily over-expressed in their fully folded natural state and purified *(16–18)*. The application of this technique to membrane receptors that are expressed in their natural membrane environment along with relevant regulatory proteins provides more of a challenge. Nevertheless, this has been successfully applied to a number of G protein-coupled receptors, including the neurokinin-1 receptor *(11)*, cholecystokinin receptor *(19)*, secretin receptor *(12)*, and the β_2-adrenergic receptor *(9)*.

2. Materials

2.1. Cell Culture

1. CHO cell lines stably expressing pseudo-wild type, null-cysteine-reactive and mono-cysteine-reactive secretin receptor constructs *(12)* (*see* **Note 1**).
2. Tissue culture flasks.
3. Ham's F-12 medium (pH 7.0) (Invitrogen, Carlsbad, CA, USA).
4. Fetal clone II medium supplement (Hyclone Laboratories, Logan, UT, USA).
5. Penicillin-streptomycin (Invitrogen).
6. Trypsin-EDTA.
7. Phosphate-buffered saline (pH 7.0).
8. Non-enzymatic cell dissociation medium (Sigma, St Louis, MO, USA).
9. CO_2 incubator.

2.2. Synthesis of Alexa^{568}-MTS Reagent (Acceptor for Energy Transfer Studies)

1. 2-Aminoethyl-methanethiosulfonate hydrochloride (Toronto Research Chemical, North York, Ontario, Canada).
2. Alexa^{568}-succinimydyl ester (Molecular Probes, Eugene, OR, USA) (*see* **Note 2**).
3. Dimethyl sulfoxide.
4. *N*-diethyldiisopropyl amine (Aldrich Chemicals, St Louis, MO, USA).
5. High-performance liquid chromatography (Beckman Coulter).
6. Reversed-phase C-18 column (Beckman Coulter, Fullerton, CA, USA).
7. Acetonitrile.
8. Trifluoroacetic acid.

2.3. Labeling of Cells Expressing Cysteine Mutants

1. CHO cell lines stably expressing pseudo-wild type, null-cysteine-reactive secretin receptors.
2. CHO cell lines stably expressing mono-cysteine-reactive secretin receptors.
3. Alexa^{488}-secretin (Alexa^{488}-HSDGTFTSELSRLRDSARLQ-RLLQGLV). Fluorescent agonist ligand specific for secretin receptor *(15)* was chosen as a donor for fluorescence resonance energy transfer (FRET) studies (*see* **Note 3**).
4. Labeling of cells was performed in Krebs–Ringer–HEPES medium (pH 7.4) [25 mM HEPES, pH 7.4, 104 mM NaCl, 5 mM KCl, 2 mM $CaCl_2$, 1 mM KH_2PO_4, 1.2 mM

$MgSO_4$] (prepared freshly with protease inhibitors added) (*see* **Note 4**).

5. Alexa^{568}-MTS reagent (cell impermeant fluorescent sulfhydryl-reactive reagent chosen as acceptor for energy transfer studies) (*see* **Note 2**).
6. Bovine serum albumin (Equitech-Bio, Inc., Kerrville, TX, USA).
7. Soybean trypsin inhibitor (Invitrogen).
8. Low retention microfuge tubes (Fisher Scientific, Chino, CA, USA).
9. Refrigerated microcentrifuge (Beckman Coulter, Inc).

2.4. Fluorescence Measurements

1. Alexa^{488}-secretin bound to the Alexa^{568}-MTS-labeled secretin receptor-bearing cell suspension (freshly labeled cells in suspension).
2. SPEX Fluoromax-3 spectrofluorophotometer (SPEX industries, Edison, NJ, USA).
3. Datamax-3 software (SPEX Industries).
4. Quartz cuvette (Starna Cells, Inc., Atascadero, CA, USA).

3. Methods

FRET requires appropriate spatial approximation and geometry between donor fluorophore and acceptor fluorophore, with the pair having adequate overlap between the emission spectrum of the donor and the absorption spectrum of the acceptor. For this work, we have chosen Alexa^{488} (excitation peak at 480 nm, emission peak at 520 nm) and Alexa^{568} (excitation peak at 568 nm, emission peak at 603 nm) as the pair of donor and acceptor fluorophores, respectively. In the application of this technique to a ligand-bound receptor, the high affinity, highly selective binding of the ligand probe should make that part of the experimental system relatively easy to establish, assuming that structure-activity considerations allow the fluorescent modification of the ligand. This is demonstrated by the saturability of the signal, utilizing a molar excess of non-fluorescent ligand as competitor.

The major challenge for this experimental system is the development of pseudo-wild type, null-cysteine-reactive, and mono-cysteine-reactive receptor constructs. This may require extensive receptor mutagenesis and characterization. Alignment of structurally related receptors and those from other species can be quite helpful in the determination of what positions to utilize for insertion of cysteine residues. A number of controls are ultimately important to be certain that all of the resonance energy transfer reflects the specific cysteine within the receptor that was derivatized, and not the other membrane proteins that also contain reactive cysteine residues. These controls include the study of cells expressing null-cysteine-reactive receptor and non-receptor-bearing cell lines *(12)*. No significant FRET should be observed in the absence of derivatization of a receptor cysteine residue.

3.1. Cell Culture

1. Chinese Hamster ovary cells stably expressing the pseudo-wild type, null-cysteine-reactive, and mono-cysteine-reactive secretin receptors are cultured in Ham's F-12 medium supplemented with 5% Fetal clone II and 1% penicillin and streptomycin mixture (*see* **Note 5**).
2. Confluent cells are detached from the tissue culture plastic ware using 0.05% trypsin–EDTA (*see* **Note 6**).
3. Count the cells using a hemocytometer and reseed the cells into sterile tissue culture flasks at a density of 100,000 cells per flask in freshly prepared Ham's F-12 medium supplemented with 5% Fetal clone II and 1% penicillin and streptomycin.
4. Cells are grown in a humidified chamber with 5% CO_2 in air at 37°C.
5. After 3 days in culture, medium is aspirated and the cells are washed with phosphate-buffered saline (pH 7.0).
6. Cells are detached from the tissue culture flasks using the non-enzymatic cell dissociation medium.
7. Harvest the cells by centrifugation at 200 × *g* for 5 min at room temperature and resuspension of the cells in Krebs–Ringer–HEPES medium (pH 7.4) for fluorescent labeling.

3.2. Synthesis of Alexa^{568}-MTS Reagent

1. Weigh and dissolve the 2-aminoethyl-methanethiosulfonate hydrochloride in dimethyl sulfoxide.
2. Neutralize this solution with *N*-diethyldiisopropyl amine.
3. Weigh and dissolve the Alexa^{568}-succinimdylester in dimethyl sulfoxide (*see* **Note 7**).
4. Mix both reagents and allow the reaction to proceed for 2 h at room temperature.
5. Check the progress of the reaction in an analytical high-performance liquid chromatograph using 0.1% trifluoroacetic acid and acetonitrile.

6. Purify and collect the product in a reversed-phase high-performance liquid chromatograph using 0.1% trifluoroacetic acid and acetonitrile.
7. Collect the product peak at the appropriate retention time.
8. Lyophilize the product into a dry powder and resuspend in water when ready to use for labeling the cells (*see* **Note 8**).

3.3. Labeling of Cells Expressing Cysteine Mutants

1. Approximately 50,000 cells expressing the receptor constructs are suspended in a small microfuge tube in Krebs–Ringer–HEPES medium (pH 7.4).
2. Intact cells are incubated with Alexa^{568}-MTS reagent for 20 min at room temperature with constant gentle shaking to avoid sedimentation of any cells.
3. After incubation, the unreacted Alexa^{568}-MTS reagent is removed by centrifugation at 200 × *g* for 5 min (*see* **Note 9**).
4. The cells are washed once again with room temperature Krebs–Ringer Hepes medium (pH 7.4) and resuspend in the same buffer for Alexa^{488}-secretin ligand binding.
5. Alexa^{568}-MTS-labeled receptor-bearing cells are incubated with 100 nM Alexa^{488}-secretin ligand for 2 h at 4°C with occasional shaking.
6. The cell suspension is once again washed with ice-cold medium, centrifuged, and resuspended in cold medium for FRET measurements. Labeled cell suspensions are kept cold to avoid the dissociation of receptor-bound ligand and are completely resuspended to get a clear signal from the samples.

3.4. Fluorescence Spectroscopy

1. Steady-state fluorescence absorption and emission spectra are collected using a SPEX Fluoromax-3 spectrofluorometer (**Fig. 1**). Start the fluorometer and set up the excitation and emission wavelengths, slit width and acquisition conditions using a constant increment. This should provide a stable and reliable signal.
2. The Alexa^{488}-secretin bound to the Alexa^{568}-MTS-labeled secretin receptor-bearing cell suspension is transferred into a quartz cuvette and the fluorescence is promptly recorded. The cuvette must be clean, since impurities can affect the fluorescence characteristics, including intensity and spectral patterns (*see* **Note 10**).
3. Fluorescence energy transfer emission spectra (*see* **Note 11**) are collected as described below.

3.5. Fluorescence Energy Transfer Measurements

1. Steady-state energy transfer fluorescence emission spectra are collected using a SPEX Fluoromax-3 spectrofluorometer (**Fig. 2**).

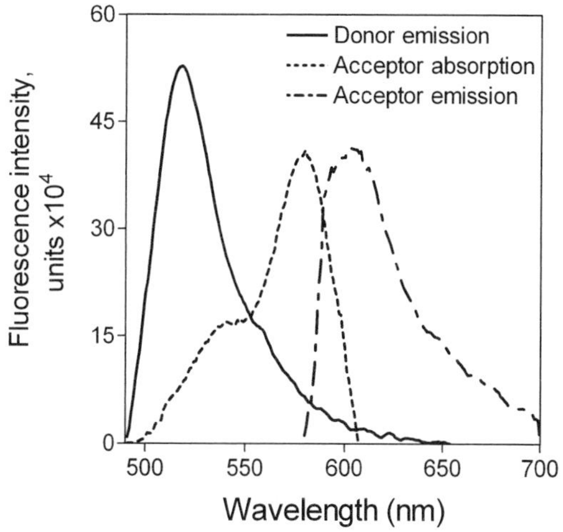

Fig 1. Fluorescence spectra of donor and acceptor. Shown is the fluorescence emission spectrum of the Alexa^{488}-secretin fluorescence donor when excited by 482 nm light. This same wavelength light elicited no significant emission from the fluorescence acceptor, Alexa^{568}. In contrast, this acceptor yielded strong emission when stimulated with 568 nm light. The absorption spectrum of this acceptor is also shown.

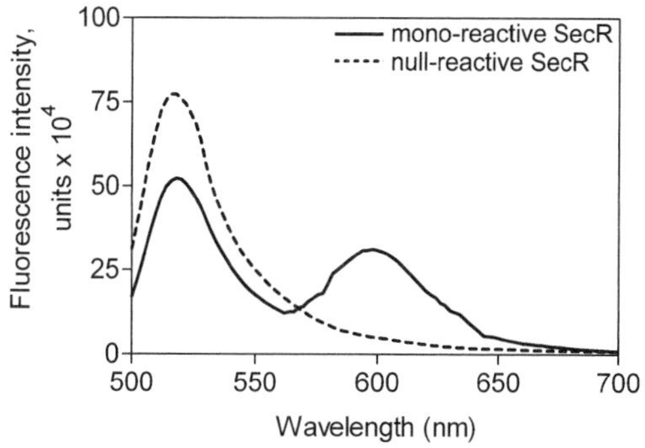

Fig 2. Fluorescence emission spectra of null-cysteine-reactive and mono-cysteine-reactive secretin receptor constructs. Shown are representative fluorescence emission spectra collected between 500 and 700 nm, after derivatizing the CHO cells expressing these constructs with the Alexa^{568}-MTS reagent, allowing the cells to bind the Alexa^{488}-secretin peptide, and stimulating the fluorescence by exposure to 482 nm light. There is a significant FRET signal at approximately 600 nm in the cells expressing the mono-cysteine-reactive construct, but not in those expressing the null-cysteine-reactive construct.

2. The Alexa^{488}-secretin bound to the Alexa^{568}-MTS-labeled secretin receptor-bearing cell suspension is transferred into 1 mL quartz cuvette and the fluorescence is recorded at room temperature.
3. The emission spectra are recorded from 500 to 700 nm by exciting samples at 482 nm. Emission is collected at a band pass of 4.0 with an integration time of 0.3 nm/s.

4. The spectra are collected using the Datamax-3 software attached to the Fluoromax-3 spectrofluorometer.
5. Similar emission profiles are collected with buffer as well as with cells which are not exposed to fluorescent ligand or derivatized, considered as background measurements. Corrected spectra are acquired by subtracting the relevant blank spectrum from each sample spectrum. This can be achieved by incorporating the blank spectral values in the correct application module.
6. Emission spectra are also collected from cells only labeled with $Alexa^{488}$-secretin (donor only) by exciting at 482 nm and the emission is collected from 500 to 650 nm, with a band width of 4.0 at an integration time of 0.3 nm/s.
7. Emission spectra are collected from cells only derivatized with $Alexa^{568}$–MTS reagent (acceptor only) by exciting at 568 and emission is collected from 570 to 700 nm with a bandwidth of 4.0 at an integration time of 0.3 nm/s.
8. Control energy transfer spectra are also collected by using 100-fold excess of non-fluorescent secretin peptide.

3.5.1. Deconvolution of Donor and Acceptor Emission Spectra

1. Establish the component of the FRET spectrum representing donor emission by matching the intensity of the donor emission peak from the donor-only emission spectrum to the peak in that portion of the collected FRET spectrum (*see* **Note 12**).
2. Establish the component of the FRET spectrum representing acceptor emission by matching the intensity of the acceptor emission peak from the acceptor-only emission spectrum to the peak in that portion of the collected FRET spectrum (*see* **Note 13**).
3. Check the validity of the deconvolution of the spectra by calculating the percentage difference between the summation spectrum and the FRET emission spectrum. This should be less than 3%, with close approximation of the region of the spectra near the peaks (*see* **Note 14**).

3.5.2. Quantum Yield Measurement

1. Quantum yield is the ratio of number of photons emitted to the number of photons absorbed by a fluorophore. Here, the quantum yield of the donor fluorophore, $Alexa^{488}$-secretin, is determined using the equation,

$$Q_d = Q_s(F_d/F_S)(A_S/A_d)$$

where s and d refer to standard and donor, F refers to integrated corrected emission spectra with constant slit opening, and A represents the absorbance at the excitation wavelength to avoid inner filter effect (see **Note 15**).

2. Sodium fluorescein in 0.1 N sodium hydroxide is used as a standard with the standard quantum yield value for this reagent of 0.92.

3.5.3. Calculations

1. The distance between the donor and the acceptor is calculated by using the Förster equation: $R_o = 9786(Jn^{-4}\kappa^2 Q_D)^{1/6}$ Å.

   This is used to determine the distance between a fluorescence donor and a acceptor at which 50% of the donor energy is transferred from donor to acceptor (*see* **Note 16**).
2. n indicates the refractive index for an aqueous medium (n = 1.4). This can reliably be utilized for hydrophilic fluorophores that label their targets through aqueous reactions.
3. κ^2 represents the orientation factor, describing the relative orientation of the transition dipoles of donor and acceptor fluorophores. This value is typically considered to be 2/3, when donor and/or acceptor fluorophores exhibit isotropic, dynamic orientations within the nanosecond time scale (lifetime) utilized in the studies (*see* **Note 17**).
4. The overlapping signal J is calculated using the equation,

$$J = \int F(\lambda)\varepsilon(\lambda)\lambda^4 d\lambda / \int F(\lambda) d\lambda \, \text{cm}^3\text{M}^{-1}$$

   where $F(\lambda)$ is the fluorescence intensity of the donor at wavelength λ, and $\varepsilon(\lambda)$ is the extinction coefficient of acceptor calculated based on the absorption of the acceptor (*see* **Note 18**).

3.5.4. Efficiency of Energy Transfer

1. The efficiency of energy transfer between donor and acceptor is calculated based on the changes in the donor fluorescence intensity in the absence and the presence of acceptor.
2. The efficiency of transfer is determined based on the equation

$$E = 1 - F_{DA}/F_D$$

   where the F_{DA} is the background-subtracted fluorescence intensity in the presence of acceptor, and F_D is the background-subtracted fluorescence intensity in the absence of acceptor.

3.5.5. Corrected Distance Measurements

The measured distances are corrected based on the efficiency of transfer and are calculated by the equation,

$$R = R_o[(1 - E)/E]^{1/6} \text{ Å}.$$

where R is the corrected distance, R_o is the Förster distance when the efficiency of transfer is considered to be 50%. E is the efficiency of transfer.

4. Notes

1. Monitor the morphology and degree of confluency of the cells before harvesting them for fluorescent labeling. Cells should be healthy and 70–80% confluent.
2. Alexa^{568}-MTS reagent is developed as a fluorescence acceptor for resonance energy transfer. This reagent is cell impermeant and can only derivatize free accessible cysteine residues present within the extracellular milieu. An advantage of this approach is the ability to perform the energy transfer studies in intact cells with receptors in a natural environment that includes regulatory proteins.
3. Fluorescent Alexa^{488}-secretin peptides are stored at –20°C in small aliquots wrapped in aluminum foil to protect them from light, avoiding multiple freezing and thawing cycles, which leads to losses in potency.
4. All buffers and solvents used for fluorescence measurements are degassed and bubbled with nitrogen to prevent any quenching due to dissolved oxygen.
5. The complete Ham's F12 medium supplemented with fetal clone II and antibiotic solution should be prepared freshly before adding to the cells for culture.
6. Working solution of trypsin-EDTA (0.05%) is made from the stock solution of 0.25% by dilution with sterile phosphate-buffered saline (pH 7.0).
7. For better efficiency in coupling reactions, the dimethylsulfoxide solution should be kept in the dark in a brown bottle, avoiding exposure to light and oxidation.
8. Fluorescent Alexa^{568}-MTS reagent is stored at –20°C in small aliquots wrapped in aluminum foil to protect them from light and to avoid multiple cycles of thawing and refreezing.
9. The cells should be centrifuged only at low speed to avoid breaking the cells and should be resuspended carefully in buffer for further labeling with Alexa^{488}-secretin.
10. The quartz cuvette is washed using concentrated nitric acid, water, and ethanol, followed by extensive washing with nanopure water to remove the impurities.
11. Choosing the donor and acceptor for energy transfer studies, one has to be keep in mind the spectral profiles of both donor and acceptor so that adequate overlap exists between the donor emission and the acceptor absorption spectra for effective energy transfer. Alexa^{488} and Alexa^{568} represent a good pair for energy transfer studies.

12. The emission spectrum of the donor to be used represents the normalized spectrum in which the relevant blank spectral values have been subtracted.
13. The emission spectrum of the acceptor to be used represents the normalized spectrum in which the relevant blank spectral values have been subtracted.
14. The difference between the summation of the deconvoluted donor and acceptor emission spectra relative to the FRET emission spectrum should be less than 3%.
15. The measurement of quantum yields of the probes in solution and receptor-bound state is carefully performed at room temperature and in deoxygenated medium to avoid oxygen quenching.
16. The overlap integral can be calculated using the fluorescence emission spectrum of the donor-only condition (with no acceptor) and the absorption spectrum of the acceptor-only condition (with no donor).
17. For the relative orientation of donor and acceptor, the range can be from 0 to 4. However, given the practical issues in this type of experiment and a reasonable amount of rotational mobility of the fluorophores, the error introduced by using 2/3 is relatively small, typically in the range of less than 10%. Fluorophore mobility can be established using measurements of steady state or time-resolved fluorescence anisotropy.
18. For calculating the overlapping signal, the emission spectra of the donor should be corrected using relevant blanks and integrated.

Acknowledgments

This work was supported by a grant from the National Institutes of Health, DK46577, the Fiterman Foundation, and Mayo Clinic.

References

1. Cherezov, V., Rosenbaum, D. M., Hanson, M. A., Rasmussen, S. G., Thian, F. S., Kobilka, T. S., et al. (2007) High-resolution crystal structure of an engineered human beta2-adrenergic G protein-coupled receptor. *Science* **318**, 1258–1265.
2. Palczewski, K., Kumasaka, T., Hori, T., Behnke, C. A., Motoshima, H., Fox, B. A., et al. (2000) Crystal structure of rhodopsin: A G protein-coupled receptor. *Science* **289**, 739–745.
3. Parthier, C., Kleinschmidt, M., Neumann, P., Rudolph, R., Manhart, S., Schlenzig, D., et al. (2007) Crystal structure of the incretin-bound extracellular domain of a G protein-coupled receptor. *Proc. Natl. Acad. Sci. USA* **104**, 13942–13947.
4. Runge, S., Thogersen, H., Madsen, K., Lau, J., and Rudolph, R. (2008) Crystal structure of the ligand-bound glucagon-like peptide-1

receptor extracellular domain. *J. Biol. Chem.* **283**, 11340–11347.

5. Ding, X. Q., Dolu, V., Hadac, E. M., Holicky, E. L., Pinon, D. I., Lybrand, T. P., et al. (2001) Refinement of the structure of the ligand-occupied cholecystokinin receptor using a photolabile amino-terminal probe. *J. Biol. Chem.* **276**, 4236–4244.
6. Dong, M., Lam, P. C., Gao, F., Hosohata, K., Pinon, D. I., Sexton, P. M., et al. (2007) Molecular approximations between residues 21 and 23 of secretin and its receptor: Development of a model for peptide docking with the amino terminus of the secretin receptor. *Mol. Pharmacol.* **72**, 280–290.
7. Park, C. G., Ganguli, S. C., Pinon, D. I., Hadac, E. M., and Miller, L. J. (2000) Cross-chimeric analysis of selectivity of secretin and VPAC(1) receptor activation. *J. Pharmacol. Exp. Ther.* **295**, 682–688.
8. Harikumar, K. G., and Miller, L. J. (2005) Fluorescence resonance energy transfer analysis of the antagonist- and partial agonist-occupied states of the cholecystokinin receptor. *J. Biol. Chem.* **280**, 18631–18635.
9. Granier, S., Kim, S., Shafer, A. M., Ratnala, V. R., Fung, J. J., Zare, R. N., et al. (2007) Structure and conformational changes in the C-terminal domain of the beta2-adrenoceptor: insights from fluorescence resonance energy transfer studies. *J. Biol. Chem.* **282**, 13895–13905.
10. Milligan, G., and Bouvier, M. (2005) Methods to monitor the quaternary structure of G protein-coupled receptors. *FEBS J.* **272**, 2914–2925.
11. Turcatti, G., Nemeth, K., Edgerton, M. D., Knowles, J., Vogel, H., and Chollet, A. (1997) Fluorescent labeling of NK2 receptor at specific sites in vivo and fluorescence energy transfer analysis of NK2 ligand-receptor complexes. *Receptors Channels* **5**, 201–207.
12. Harikumar, K. G., Lam, P. C., Dong, M., Sexton, P. M., Abagyan, R., and Miller, L. J. (2007) Fluorescence resonance energy transfer analysis of secretin docking to its receptor: Mapping distances between residues distributed throughout the ligand pharmacophore and distinct receptor residues. *J. Biol. Chem.* **282**, 32834–32843.
13. Milligan, G. (2004) Applications of bioluminescence- and fluorescence resonance energy transfer to drug discovery at G protein-coupled receptors. *Eur. J. Pharm. Sci.* **21**, 397–405.
14. Stryer, L., and Haugland, R. P. (1967) Energy transfer: A spectroscopic ruler. *Proc. Natl. Acad. Sci. USA* **58**, 719–726.
15. Harikumar, K. G., Hosohata, K., Pinon, D. I., and Miller, L. J. (2006) Use of probes with fluorescence indicator distributed throughout the pharmacophore to examine the peptide agonist-binding environment of the family B G protein-coupled secretin receptor. *J. Biol. Chem.* **281**, 2543–2550.
16. Brouillette, C. G., Dong, W. J., Yang, Z. W., Ray, M. J., Protasevich, I. I., Cheung, H. C., et al. (2005) Forster resonance energy transfer measurements are consistent with a helical bundle model for lipid-free apolipoprotein A-I. *Biochemistry* **44**, 16413–16425.
17. Liang, J. J., and Liu, B. F. (2006) Fluorescence resonance energy transfer study of subunit exchange in human lens crystallins and congenital cataract crystallin mutants. *Protein Sci.* **15**, 1619–1627.
18. Mansoor, S. E., Palczewski, K., and Farrens, D. L. (2006) Rhodopsin self-associates in asolectin liposomes. *Proc. Natl. Acad. Sci. USA* **103**, 3060–3065.
19. Harikumar, K. G., Pinon, D. I., Wessels, W. S., Dawson, E. S., Lybrand, T. P., Prendergast, F. G., et al. (2004) Measurement of intermolecular distances for the natural agonist Peptide docked at the cholecystokinin receptor expressed in situ using fluorescence resonance energy transfer. *Mol. Pharmacol.* **65**, 28–35.

Chapter 22

Detection of GPCR/β-Arrestin Interactions in Live Cells Using Bioluminescence Resonance Energy Transfer Technology

Martina Kocan and Kevin D.G. Pfleger

Summary

Bioluminescence resonance energy transfer (BRET) is a powerful and increasingly popular technique for studying protein–protein interactions in live cells and real time. In particular, there has been considerable interest in the ability to monitor interactions between G protein-coupled receptors (GPCRs) and proteins that serve as key regulators of receptor function, such as β-arrestin. The BRET methodology involves heterologous co-expression of genetically fused proteins that link one protein of interest (e.g., a GPCR) to a bioluminescent donor enzyme and a second protein of interest (e.g., β-arrestin) to an acceptor fluorophore. If the fusion proteins are in close proximity, resonance energy will be transferred from the donor to the acceptor molecule and subsequent fluorescence from the acceptor can be detected at a characteristic wavelength. Such fluorescence is therefore indicative of the proteins of interest linked to the donor and the acceptor interacting directly or as part of a complex. In addition to monitoring protein–protein interactions to elucidate cellular function, BRET also has the exciting potential to become an important technique for live cell high-throughput screening for drugs targeting GPCRs, utilizing ligand-induced interactions with β-arrestins.

Key words: Bioluminescence resonance energy transfer, BRET, G protein-coupled receptor, arrestin, *Renilla* luciferase, Rluc8, fluorophore, Venus.

1. Introduction

The various derivations of the bioluminescence resonance energy transfer (BRET) technique all involve a non-radiative transfer of energy between a bioluminescent donor enzyme, a variant of *Renilla* luciferase (Rluc), and a complementary acceptor fluorophore, a variant of green fluorescent protein (GFP), upon oxidation of a coelenterazine substrate *(1–4)*. BRET[1] is initiated by oxidation of the luciferase substrate coelenterazine *h* (benzyl-coelenterazine)

Wayne R. Leifert (ed.), *G Protein-Coupled Receptors in Drug Discovery, vol. 552*

Book doi: 10.1007/978-1-60327-317-6_22

resulting in light emission with a peak at ~480 nm. Following efficient energy transfer, the light emitted from the corresponding acceptor molecule such as Venus can be detected peaking at a characteristically longer wavelength of ~530 nm. In contrast, $BRET^2$ is initiated by oxidation of the luciferase substrate known as DeepBlueC (bisdeoxycoelenterazine, coelenterazine-*400a*, or di-dehydro coelenterazine). This results in an emission peak at about 400–420 nm upon Rluc-mediated oxidation and utilizes GFP10 or GFP^2 as acceptor, producing light emission peaking at ~510 nm *(1–4)*. A third form of the BRET technique, known as extended BRET (eBRET), has also been established utilizing a caged form of coelenterazine *h* known as EnduRen *(5)*. In brief, the relative strengths of $BRET^1$, $BRET^2$, and eBRET are higher BRET signals, lower background noise and a longer detection window, respectively *(3)*. BRET can be applied to study protein–protein interactions in live cells and real time following genetic fusion of proteins of interest with either donor or acceptor molecules *(1, 2, 6)*. This technology has exceptional utility for monitoring G protein-coupled receptor (GPCR) interactions with both membrane and cytosolic proteins *(2–4, 7–9)*, particularly the intracellular adaptor and scaffolding molecule, β-arrestin *(3, 5, 10, 11)*. β-arrestin plays an instrumental role in the desensitization and internalization of most GPCRs, in addition to providing a secondary signalling platform enabling the switch from G protein-dependent to G protein-independent signalling *(12)*.

2. Materials

2.1. Fusion Construct Generation and Validation

1. cDNA for proteins of interest (e.g., GPCR and β-arrestin).
2. cDNA for complementary BRET donor and acceptor in appropriate expression vectors (such as pcDNA3.1 from Invitrogen, Mount Waverley, VIC, Australia). Donor for $BRET^1$ and $BRET^2$: Rluc variant such as Rluc8 [from S. S. Gambhir, Stanford University, CA, USA *(13)*]. Acceptor for $BRET^1$: GFP variant such as Venus [from A. Miyawaki, RIKEN Brain Science Institute, Wako city, Japan *(14)*]. Acceptor for $BRET^2$: GFP variant such as GFP10 [from Michel Bouvier, Department of Biochemistry, Université de Montréal, Canada *(15)*] or GFP^2 (PerkinElmer, Waltham, MA, USA).
3. Assay reagents and instruments required for experiments to validate fusion proteins. These may include confocal microscopy, signalling assays, or other measures of protein function.

2.2. Cell Culture

1. Cell culture plates: 6-well clear plates (BD Falcon, North Ryde, NSW, Australia) and 96-well white plates (Nunc, Rochester, NY, USA).
2. Appropriate cell line for transfection, such as COS-7 or HEK293 cells.
3. Appropriate cell culture media, such as Dulbecco's modified Eagle's medium (DMEM; from Gibco BRL, Carlsbad, CA, USA) containing 0.3 mg/mL glutamine (Gibco), 100 IU/mL penicillin, 100 μg/mL streptomycin (Gibco), and 10% fetal calf serum (Gibco).
4. DMEM without phenol red (Gibco) containing 0.3 mg/mL glutamine (Gibco), 100 IU/mL penicillin, 100 μg/mL streptomycin (Gibco), 10% fetal calf serum (Gibco), and 25 mM HEPES (Sigma-Aldrich, Castle Hill, NSW, Australia).
5. Transfection reagent, such as Genejuice (Merck, Kilsyth, VIC, Australia).
6. 0.05% trypsin-0.53 mM ethylenediamine tetraacetic acid (EDTA) (Gibco).

2.3. BRET Detection

1. Luciferase substrate (coelenterazine): 5 mM coelenterazine *h* (benzyl-coelenterazine) dissolved in methanol (Invitrogen) for $BRET^1$; 1 mM DeepBlueC (bisdeoxycoelenterazine, coelenterazine-*400a*, di-dehydro coelenterazine) dissolved in anhydrous or absolute ethanol (PerkinElmer or Molecular Imaging Products Company, Bend, or, USA) for $BRET^2$.
2. Microplate luminometer capable of measuring light through two filters. Examples include the VICTOR Light (PerkinElmer), Mithras LB 940 (Berthold Technologies, Bad Wildbad, Germany) and FLUOstar Optima or POLARstar Optima (BMG Labtech, Offenburg, Germany).
3. Visualization of the spectral shift observed with BRET is optional, but certainly complements data generated using the dual-filter microplate luminometers. Examples of suitable scanning spectrometers include the Cary Eclipse (Varian, Palo Alto, CA, USA), the Spex fluorolog or fluoromax (Jobin Yvon, Edison, NJ, USA), and the FlexStation II (Molecular Devices, Sunnyvale, CA, USA).

3. Methods

There are currently three generations of BRET assay methodology ($BRET^1$, $BRET^2$, and eBRET). The procedures for $BRET^1$ and $BRET^2$ will be described in detail as they are the most widely used and illustrate recent advances in the BRET technology *(3, 13)*. The eBRET method is similar to these derivations, with the EnduRen substrate possessing the same spectral properties as coelenterazine *h*, the substrate for BRET[1] *(3)*. Variations to the protocol to enable the use of eBRET will be described in the "Notes" with cross-referencing from the relevant section.

3.1. Fusion Construct Generation and Validation

1. Fusion constructs are prepared by in-frame insertion of the cDNA for the protein of interest (GPCR or β-arrestin) into a suitable expression vector [such as pcDNA3.1 (Invitrogen)] containing the cDNA of the required donor (Rluc variant) or acceptor (GFP variant) *(7)*. Rluc8 *(13)* with Venus *(14)* is currently the best combination of donor and acceptor for BRET[1] (or eBRET), whereas the combination of Rluc8 with GFP10 *(15)* or GFP[2] (PerkinElmer) is most suitable for BRET[2] *(3)*.
2. Using DNA recombinant techniques, the stop codon between the cDNA sequences is removed and replaced with a linker region (*see* **Note 1**).
3. The fusion proteins are tested to ensure that appropriate levels of luminescence (using a luminometer following addition of coelenterazine substrate) or fluorescence (using a fluorometer following direct laser excitation) are observed (*see* **Note 2**).
4. The fusion proteins need to be validated to ensure that the addition of the donor or acceptor molecule does not alter normal function. GPCRs can be assessed using ligand binding and/or secondary signaling assays to test the ligand affinity/efficacy/potency of tagged versus untagged receptors. It may also be advisable to assess effects on internalization profiles. Confocal microscopy is recommended to ensure correct protein localization and this applies to both GPCRs and β-arrestins in the presence and absence of agonist stimulation (*see* **Note 3**).

3.2. Cell Culture

1. Cells are plated into 6-well clear cell culture plates so that they are 50–80% confluent after 24 h (or as appropriate for the selected transfection reagent).
2. Cells are maintained at 37°C, 5% CO_2 in a humidified incubator.
3. After 24 h, cells are transiently transfected with an appropriate concentration and ratio of donor to acceptor cDNA (*see* **Note 4**).
4. If BRET is to be detected in an adherent layer, the cells are detached (optionally using trysin-EDTA) after a further 24 h. The cells are resuspended in HEPES-buffered DMEM without phenol red and 40–100 μL distributed per well into a 96-well white cell culture plate (*see* **Note 5**).

5. The cells are maintained at 37°C, 5% CO_2 in a humidified incubator for a further 24 h to allow attachment.
6. Prior to BRET detection, the relative expression of fluorescent and luminescent fusion proteins can be assessed if desired. A separate aliquot of each sample is excited directly by a laser followed by measurement of fluorescence. A coelenterazine substrate is then added to the same sample followed by measurement of luminescence.
7. Scanning spectral analysis of luminescent proteins can also be performed with a separate aliquot of each sample.

3.3. BRET Detection

1. Coelenterazine *h* (Invitrogen) for $BRET^1$ is reconstituted in methanol and DeepBlueC (PerkinElmer or Molecular Imaging Products Company) for $BRET^2$ is reconstituted in anhydrous or absolute ethanol. These are agitated gently until resuspended and stored at –20°C protected from light (*see* **Note 6**).
2. Immediately prior to adding to cells, the luciferase substrate is diluted in Dulbecco's phosphate buffered saline (D-PBS; Gibco) with $CaCl_2$, $MgCl_2$, and D-glucose to produce a final concentration of 5 μM. The substrate continues to be protected from light (*see* **Note 7**).
3. The media on the cells is removed and replaced with D-PBS (plus $CaCl_2$, $MgCl_2$, and D-glucose) containing 5 μM substrate taking extreme care not to detach cells. The BRET assay is carried out immediately (*see* **Note 8**).
4. BRET measurements are taken at 37°C using a luminometer capable of measuring light through two filter windows. Filtered light emissions are measured in each of the "donor wavelength window" [400–475 nm for $BRET^1$ (or eBRET) or 370–450 nm for $BRET^2$] and "acceptor wavelength window" [520–540 nm for $BRET^1$ (or eBRET) or 500–525 nm for $BRET^2$]. Light from each well is measured through each filter (either simultaneously or sequentially) for 1–5 s before moving to the next well.
5. Measurements are repeated as required, and this process is ideally automated by using an instrument with appropriate kinetics software.
6. For real-time detection of ligand-induced interactions such as between GPCRs and β-arrestins (**Fig. 1**), measurements can be taken for a period prior to treatment. Subsequent ligand addition (by injection if time points are required immediately after treatment) is followed by measurements taken for a desired period of time in order to observe the effect. In parallel, duplicate samples are treated with vehicle only.

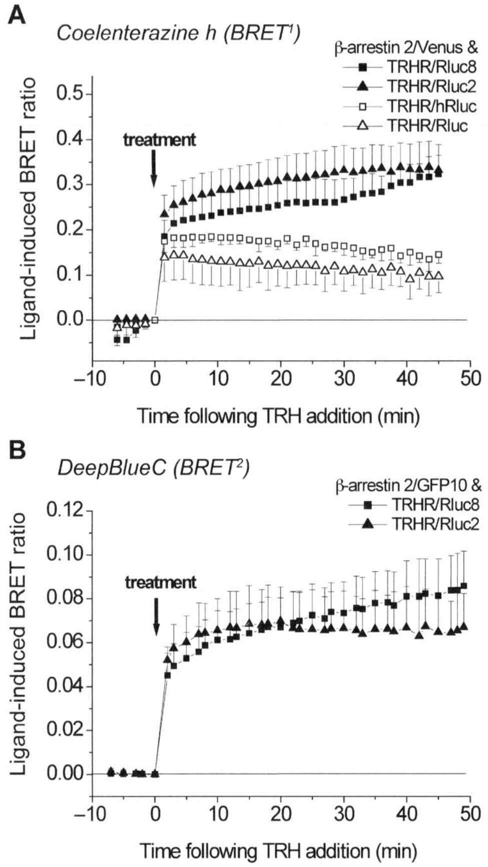

Fig. 1. Detection of protein–protein interactions by real-time BRET^1 (**A**) and BRET^2 (**B**) assays. Kinetic data comparing different thyrotropin-releasing hormone receptor (TRHR)/luminophore fusion proteins using TRH-induced interaction with β-arrestin 2/Venus (BRET^1) or β-arrestin 2/GFP10 (BRET^2). Transiently co-transfected HEK293 cells were assayed before and after treatment with TRH or vehicle. The luciferase substrate coelenterazine *h* for BRET^1 (**A**) or DeepBlueC for BRET^2 (**B**) was added immediately prior to real-time measurements at 37°C. Data shown are mean ± SEM of three independent experiments. Adapted from *(3)* with permission from SAGE and *Journal of Biomolecular Screening*.

7. A good complementary method to BRET detection by dual-filter luminometry is visualization of the spectral shift characteristic of BRET using scanning spectrometry (**Fig. 2**). A secondary peak or shoulder appears at a wavelength characteristic of the acceptor emission *(3, 16)* (*see* **Note 9**).

3.4. BRET Signal Calculation and Interpretation

1. The BRET ratio is calculated by dividing fluorescence over luminescence meaning the emission through the "acceptor wavelength window" [e.g., 520–540 nm for BRET^1 (or eBRET) or 500–525 nm for BRET^2] over emission through

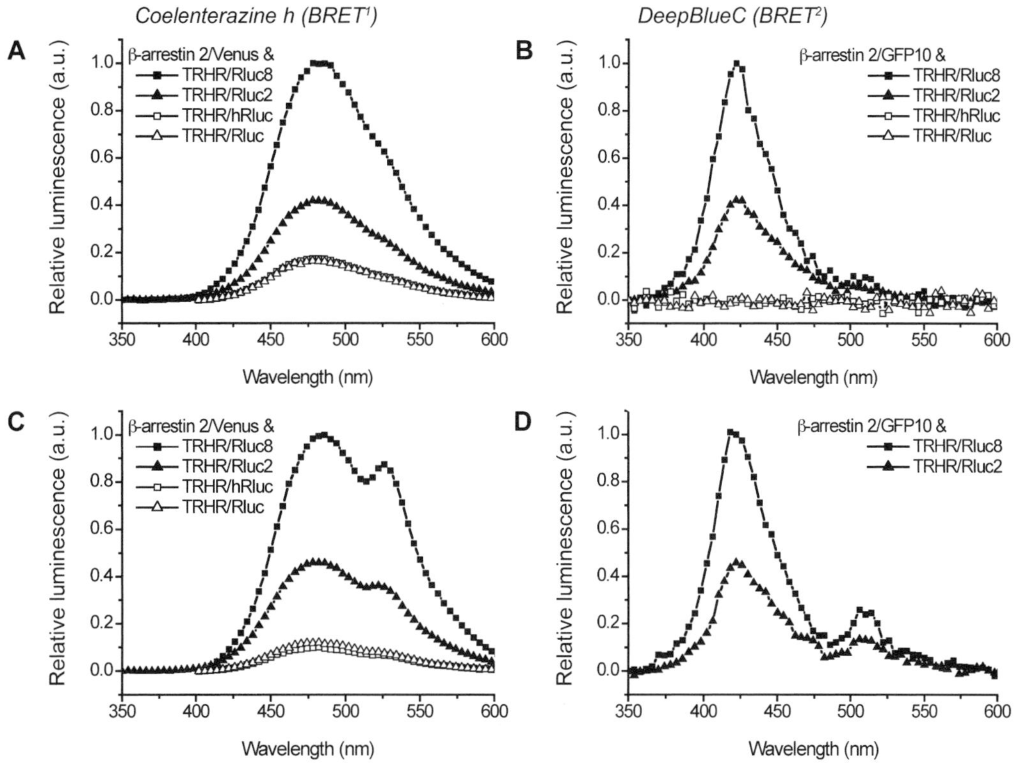

Fig. 2. Spectral analysis comparing luminescence intensities of different luciferase-tagged thyrotropin-releasing hormone receptor (TRHR) fusion proteins in untreated (**A**, **B**) and TRH-treated (**C**, **D**) HEK293 cells using coelenterazine *h* (**A**, **C**) or DeepBlueC (**B**, **D**) as luciferase substrate. Cells were co-transfected with β-arrestin 2/Venus (**A**, **C**) or β-arrestin 2/GFP10 (**B**, **D**) and TRHR tagged with one of various luciferase constructs. Emission spectra were recorded immediately after substrate addition. In untreated cells, an emission maximum of ~480 or ~420 nm corresponds to luciferase oxidizing coelenterazine *h* (**A**) or DeepBlueC (**B**), respectively. In treated cells, an additional emission peak appears at ~530 (**C**) or ~510 nm (**D**) that corresponds to emission from Venus or GFP10, respectively, thereby demonstrating BRET due to TRHR/β-arrestin 2 interactions. Data are representative of at least three independent experiments. Reprinted from *(3)* with permission from SAGE and *Journal of Biomolecular Screening*.

the "donor wavelength window" [e.g., 400–475 nm for $BRET^1$ (or eBRET) or 370–450 nm for $BRET^2$]. This in itself is not the "BRET signal" as the background signal needs to be taken into account.

2. The ligand-induced BRET signal is calculated by subtracting the ratio of emission through the "acceptor wavelength window" over emission through the "donor wavelength window" for a vehicle-treated cell sample from the same ratio for a second aliquot of the same cells treated with ligand *(2, 5)* (*see* **Note 10**). With this calculation, the vehicle-treated cell sample represents the background, eliminating the requirement for measuring a "donor-only" control sample *(2, 5)* (*see* **Note 11**).
3. Real-time kinetic BRET profiles are prepared by plotting the BRET signal against time (**Fig. 1**). Apparent association (or dissociation) rate constants can potentially be calculated from such data *(10)*.

4. BRET dose–response curves are prepared by replotting BRET data as BRET signal against the logarithm of ligand concentration (**Fig. 3**). The concentration eliciting a half-maximal response (EC_{50} value) can be calculated from such data following curve-fitting by non-linear regression *(3, 10)*.

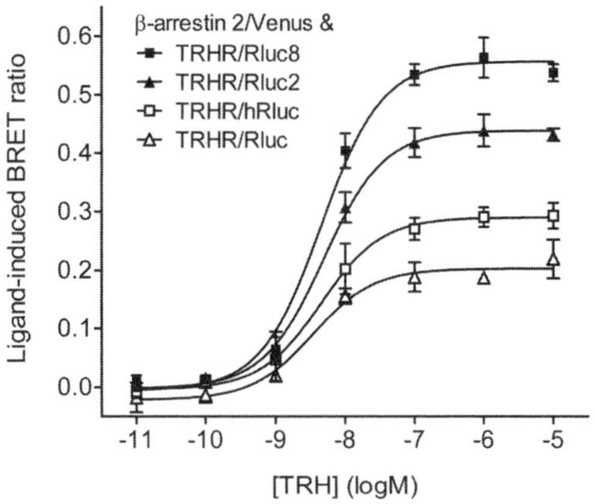

Fig. 3. Thyrotropin-releasing hormone (TRH) dose–response curves comparing TRH-induced interactions of different TRH receptor (TRHR)/luminophore fusion proteins with β-arrestin 2/Venus using BRET[1] assays. The luciferase substrate coelenterazine *h* was added to transiently co-transfected HEK293 cells immediately prior to commencing the assay at 37°C. Measurements were taken ~30 min after treatment with various concentrations of TRH or vehicle. Data shown are mean ± SEM of three independent experiments. Reprinted from *(3)* with permission from SAGE and *Journal of Biomolecular Screening*.

5. Alternatively, scanning spectrometry data can be used to quantify the BRET signal. Within wavelength windows corresponding to the filters in the luminometer, the area under the curve can be determined so that BRET is calculated in a similar manner to that described above for dual-filter luminometry (*see* **Note 12**).

6. To assess the potential suitability of the assay for high-throughput screening, the Z'-factor is calculated with respect to the mean and standard deviation (SD) of control data using the equation $Z' = 1 - [(3\ \text{SD of positive control} + 3\ \text{SD of negative control})/|\text{mean of positive control} - \text{mean of negative control}|]$ *(17)*. The "positive control" data should be the mean and SD of the fluorescence over luminescence (meaning emission through the "acceptor wavelength window" over emission through the "donor wavelength window") for the ligand-treated samples. The "negative control" data should be the mean and SD of the same ratio for the vehicle-only treated samples *(3)*. Presentation in this manner, without background subtraction, allows the variance in both of the ratios to be evaluated (**Fig. 4**; *see* **Note 13**).

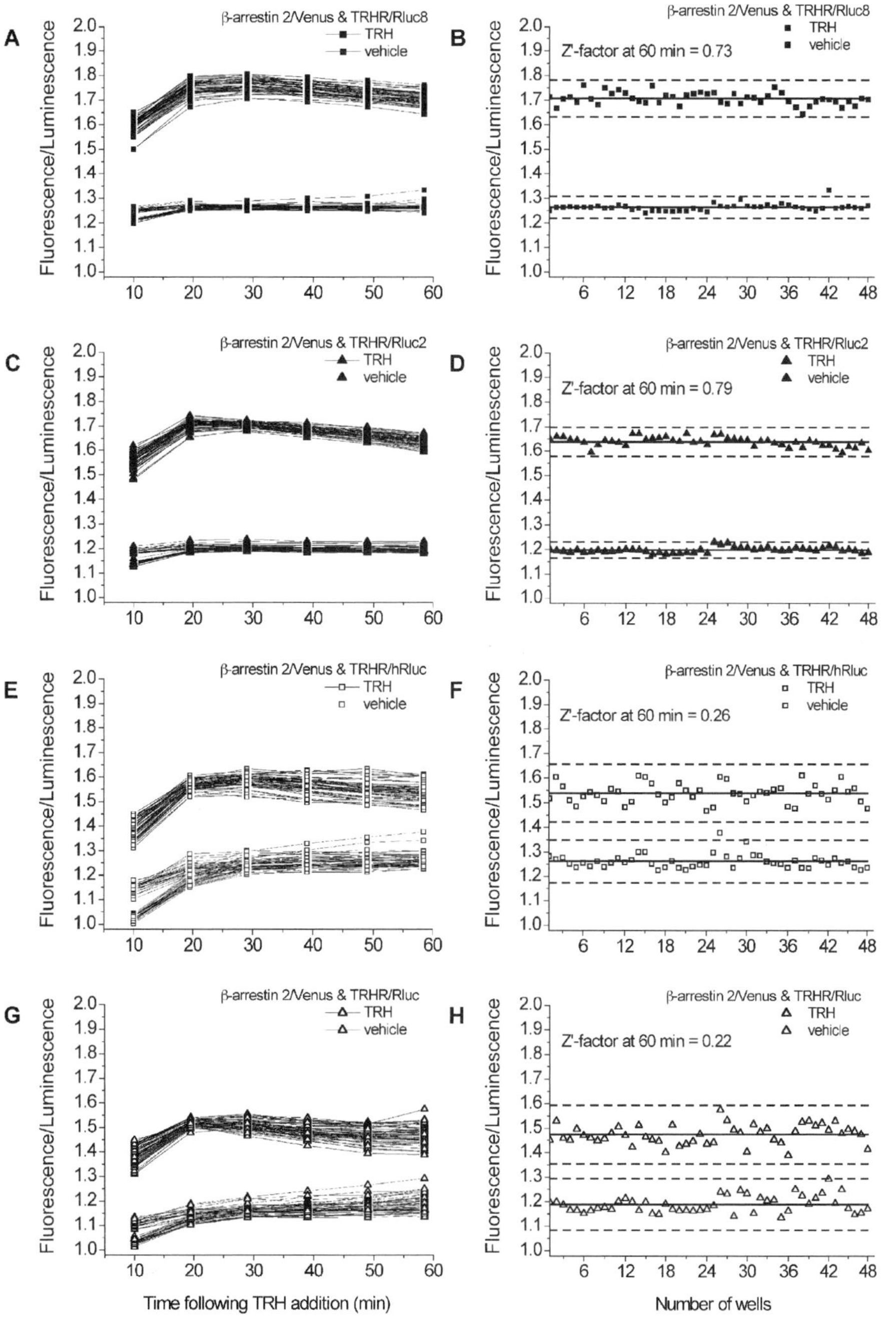

Fig. 4. BRET Z'-factor assay performance detecting thyrotropin-releasing hormone (TRH)-induced interactions of TRH receptor (TRHR)/Rluc8 (**A**, **B**), TRHR/Rluc2 (**C**, **D**), TRHR/hRluc (**E**, **F**), and TRHR/Rluc (**G**, **H**) with β-arrestin 2/Venus over time. Transiently co-transfected HEK293 cells were treated with TRH (positive control) or vehicle (negative control) and luciferase substrate coelenterazine *h* that were both added immediately prior to real-time measurements at 37°C. Fluorescence/luminescence values are presented against time (**A**, **C**, **E**, **G**) or well number at 60 min (**B**, **D**, **F**, **H**) following TRH/phosphate-buffered saline (PBS) addition. In **B**, **D**, **F**, and **H**, the solid horizontal lines show the means of the positive control (TRH) and negative control (PBS). Broken lines display 3 SD from the mean of each data set. Data shown are representative of three independent experiments. Reprinted from *(3)* with permission from SAGE and *Journal of Biomolecular Screening*.

4. Notes

1. The relative orientation of the donor and acceptor dipoles is an important factor in achieving efficient resonance energy transfer. Therefore, the probability of optimal relative orientation being achieved can potentially be increased by incorporating a linker region between the proteins of interest and the donor or acceptor to enable greater freedom of movement *(18)*. For example, when detecting thyrotropin-releasing hormone receptor (TRHR)/Rluc8 interacting with β-arrestin/Venus or β-arrestin/GFP10, we have used 5–7 amino acid linker regions *(3)*. Longer linker regions may be required for GPCRs with short or non-existent C-terminal tails, such as the mammalian type 1 gonadotropin-releasing hormone receptor *(8, 19)*.
2. Assessment of various parameters needs to be considered if low relative luminescence or fluorescence counts are observed. These include the cDNA sequence of fusion proteins, transfection optimization with respect to amount and ratio of cDNAs, cell number, substrate viability, presence of a reducing agent such as ascorbic acid, and instrument calibration.
3. If a protein of interest is not functioning correctly despite the cDNA sequence being confirmed, the donor or acceptor molecule may be compromising normal protein function. This may be alleviated by using longer linker regions (*see* **Note 1**) or changing donor and acceptor positioning. When studying GPCR interactions with β-arrestin using BRET, it is clearly advisable to position a donor or acceptor on the end of the GPCR C-terminus as this is cytosolic; however, both N- and C-terminal β-arrestin fusion proteins have been used successfully.
4. A titration should be carried out to establish the optimal ratio of donor to acceptor cDNA. The optimal ratio depends on expression efficiency as well as the type of donor and acceptor used. Please note that there is not necessarily a direct relationship between cDNA quantity and final concentration of functional protein expressed.
5. Cells can also be assessed in suspension, which is preferable for carrying out BRET cell titration assays for example *(3)*. In this case, cells are detached, resuspended in medium with appropriate coelenterazine substrate, and transferred to a white 96-well plate immediately prior to BRET detection.
6. For eBRET studies, EnduRen (Promega, Madison, WI, USA) is reconstituted in tissue culture grade dimethylsulfoxide (DMSO). Care is taken to ensure complete resuspension, which is likely to require extensive vortexing for up to 10 min and warming to 37°C. Aliquots are stored at –20°C protected from light.

7. When using EnduRen, this is diluted in HEPES-buffered DMEM without phenol red at 37°C immediately prior to adding to cells to produce a final concentration of 30–60 μM. The substrate continues to be protected from light.
8. When using EnduRen, media replacement is optional. The cells are incubated in media with substrate at 37°C, 5% CO_2 in a humidified incubator for at least 1.5 h prior to BRET detection.
9. Spectral analysis of luminescent proteins uses the identical cell culture preparation protocol as BRET detection by dual-filter luminometry. Therefore, it can be performed in parallel if a separate aliquot of each sample is prepared. Media in the plate is replaced with D-PBS-containing ligand (treated sample) or vehicle (untreated sample). Samples are incubated at 37°C, 5% CO_2 in a humidified incubator for a desired time to allow the ligand-induced interaction to occur. Substrate is added to a final concentration of 5 μM, and emission spectral scans are performed using a scanning spectrometer (*see* **Notes** 7 and **8**). For example, time-gated luminescence emission spectra are detected in the 350–600 nm wavelength range, with the time gate window set to 300 ms and emission slit to 10 nm (**Fig. 2**).
10. A negative ligand-induced BRET ratio following ligand treatment may indicate that there are fewer interactions and/or those occurring are weaker and/or more transient than those observed prior to ligand addition. This could result from inverse agonism of an interaction dependent upon active receptor conformation, for example. Alternatively, a conformational change may result in a greater distance or less favorable relative orientation between donor and acceptor.
11. Two alternatives for this calculation are as follows:
    (a) Subtraction of the ratio of emissions for a sample containing only the donor-linked fusion protein (background) from the ratio of emissions for a sample containing both donor- and acceptor-linked proteins. This method can be applied for both ligand-induced as well as non-ligand-mediated/constitutive interactions. It is assumed that the ratiometric nature of the BRET calculation accounts for differences in protein expression between samples with and without acceptor-linked fusion protein. However, it remains advisable to express similar amounts of this protein in both cell populations.
    (b) When investigating the effect of GPCR point-mutations, including upon the interaction with β-arrestin, the "BRET ratio above wild-type baseline" can be calculated as the ratio of emissions for each cell sample minus the same ratio for the vehicle-treated wild-type receptor cell

sample. This calculation is similar to the "ligand-induced BRET ratio" except that determination of the background in this manner enables observation of agonist-independent BRET signals compared to wild-type receptor.

12. A second method of calculating the BRET signal from scanning spectrometry data involves normalization of the Rluc emission peak to an intensity of 1 for each spectrum recorded. Subsequently, the BRET signal is calculated using the area under the curve between 500 and 550 nm for $BRET^1$ (or eBRET) or between 480 and 530 nm for $BRET^2$. If ligand-induced BRET signal is calculated, the background is taken as the area under the curve in this wavelength region from a vehicle-only treated sample. Alternatively, a sample containing only the donor-linked fusion protein *(16)* or a sample containing the vehicle-treated wild-type receptor (*see* **Note 11**) can also be used to calculate the background in the same way.
13. Statistical analysis of BRET assays comparing the variance in the ratios from ligand-treated and vehicle-treated samples can also be performed using ANOVA with suitable post-tests or Student's *t*-tests *(2)*.

Acknowledgments

The authors are grateful to Professor Sanjiv Sam Gambhir, Dr. Atsushi Miyawaki, and Professor Michel Bouvier for generously providing Rluc8, Venus, and GFP10 cDNA, respectively. The authors' work using the BRET methodology was funded by the National Health and Medical Research Council (NHMRC) of Australia (Project Grants #404087 and #566736, and Development Grant #513780). Kevin D. G. Pfleger was supported by an NHMRC Peter Doherty Fellowship (#353709).

References

1. Pfleger, K. D. G. and Eidne, K. A. (2006) Illuminating insights into protein-protein interactions using bioluminescence resonance energy transfer (BRET). *Nat. Methods* **3**, 165–174.
2. Pfleger, K. D. G., Seeber, R. M., and Eidne, K. A. (2006) Bioluminescence resonance energy transfer (BRET) for the real-time detection of protein-protein interactions. *Nat. Protoc.* **1**, 337–345.
3. Kocan, M., See, H. B., Seeber, R. M., Eidne, K. A., and Pfleger, K. D. G. (2008) Demonstration of improvements to the bioluminescence resonance energy transfer (BRET) technology for the monitoring of G protein-coupled receptors in live cells. *J. Biomol. Screen.*, **13**, 888–898.
4. Milligan, G. and Bouvier, M. (2005) Methods to monitor the quaternary structure of

G protein-coupled receptors. *FEBS J.* **272**, 2914–2925.

5. Pfleger, K. D. G., Dromey, J. R., Dalrymple, M. B., Lim, E. M. L., Thomas, W. G., and Eidne, K. A. (2006) Extended bioluminescence resonance energy transfer (eBRET) for monitoring prolonged protein-protein interactions in live cells. *Cell. Signal.* **18**, 1664–1670.
6. Xu, Y., Kanauchi, A., von Arnim, A., G., Piston, D. W., and Johnson, C. H. (2003) Bioluminescence resonance energy transfer: Monitoring protein-protein interactions in living cells. *Meth. Enzymol.* **360**, 289–301.
7. Pfleger, K. D. G. and Eidne, K. A. (2003) New technologies: Bioluminescence resonance energy transfer (BRET) for the detection of real time interactions involving G protein-coupled receptors. *Pituitary* **6**, 141–151.
8. Pfleger, K. D. G. and Eidne, K. A. (2005) Monitoring the formation of dynamic G protein-coupled receptor-protein complexes in living cells. *Biochem. J.* **385**, 625–637.
9. Milligan, G. (2004) Applications of bioluminescence- and fluorescence resonance energy transfer to drug discovery at G protein-coupled receptors. *Eur. J. Pharm. Sci.* **21**, 397–405.
10. Hamdan, F. F., Audet, M., Garneau, P., Pelletier, J., and Bouvier, M. (2005) High-throughput screening of G protein-coupled receptor antagonists using a bioluminescence resonance energy transfer 1-based beta-arrestin2 recruitment assay. *J. Biomol. Screen.* **10**, 463–475.
11. Pfleger, K. D. G., Dalrymple, M. B., Dromey, J. R., and Eidne, K. A. (2007) Monitoring interactions between G protein-coupled receptors and beta-arrestins. *Biochem. Soc. Trans.* **35**, 764–766.
12. Dromey, J. R. and Pfleger, K. D. G. (2008) G protein-coupled receptors as drug targets: The role of β-arrestins. *Endocr. Metab. Immune Disord. Drug Targets* **8**, 51–61.
13. De, A., Loening, A. M., and Gambhir, S. S. (2007) An improved bioluminescence resonance energy transfer strategy for imaging intracellular events in single cells and living subjects. *Cancer Res.* **67**, 7175–7183.
14. Nagai, T., Ibata, K., Park, E. S., Kubota, M., Mikoshiba K., and Miyawaki, A. (2002) A variant of yellow fluorescent protein with fast and efficient maturation for cell-biological applications. *Nat. Biotechnol.* **20**, 87–90.
15. Mercier, J. F., Salahpour, A., Angers, S., Breit, A., and Bouvier, M. (2002) Quantitative assessment of β1- and β2-adrenergic receptor homo- and heterodimerization by bioluminescence resonance energy transfer. *J. Biol. Chem.* **277**, 44925–44931.
16. McVey, M., Ramsay, D., Kellett, E., Rees, S., Wilson, S., Pope, A. J., and Milligan, G. (2001) Monitoring receptor oligomerization using time-resolved fluorescence resonance energy transfer and bioluminescence resonance energy transfer. *J. Biol. Chem.* **276**, 14092–14099.
17. Zhang, J.-H., Chung, T. D. Y., and Oldenburg, K. R. (1999) A simple statistical parameter for use in evaluation and validation of high throughput screening assays. *J. Biomol. Screen.* **4**, 67–73.
18. Wu, P. and Brand, L. (1994) Resonance energy transfer: Methods and applications. *Anal. Biochem.* **218**, 1–13.
19. Kroeger, K. M., Hanyaloglu, A. C., Seeber, R. M., Miles, L. E., and Eidne, K. A. (2001) Constitutive and agonist-dependent homo-oligomerization of the thyrotropin-releasing hormone receptor. Detection in living cells using bioluminescence resonance energy transfer. *J. Biol. Chem.* **276**, 12736–12743.

Chapter 23

Using Reporter Gene Technologies to Detect Changes in cAMP as a Result of GPCR Activation

Daniel J. Rodrigues and David McLoughlin

Summary

The measurement of cyclic adenosine monophosphate levels through reporter gene technology represents one of the most popular and cost-effective methods to assess changes in functional activity of G protein-coupled receptors (GPCRs). This chapter provides a generic protocol for the successful execution of a reporter gene assay for GPCRs, stably transfected within Chinese hamster ovary cell lines, signaling through the Gs pathway. It also highlights areas to investigate when developing reporter gene assays and additional factors to consider for assays that deviate from the protocol and cell line defined.

Key words: G protein-coupled receptor, cAMP, reporter gene, beta-lactamase, cell-based adherent assay.

1. Introduction

G protein-coupled receptors (GPCRs) represent one of the most popular therapeutic targets for pharmaceutical industry. They elicit their function through initial binding of ligands on the extracellular surface and subsequent activation of signaling pathways to invoke a cellular response. There are a range of signaling pathways mediated through GPCR activation, involving a variety of second messenger effectors. One of the most well known is cyclic adenosine monophosphate (cAMP), which is modulated through GPCRs that signal through either the Gs or Gi/o proteins (**Fig. 1**). Many GPCRs, which have therapeutic potential, signal via the cAMP effector. As such, this second messenger element has become a popular tool for measuring changes in functional response from GPCRs.

Wayne R. Leifert (ed.), *G Protein-Coupled Receptors in Drug Discovery, vol. 552*

Book doi: 10.1007/978-1-60327-317-6_23

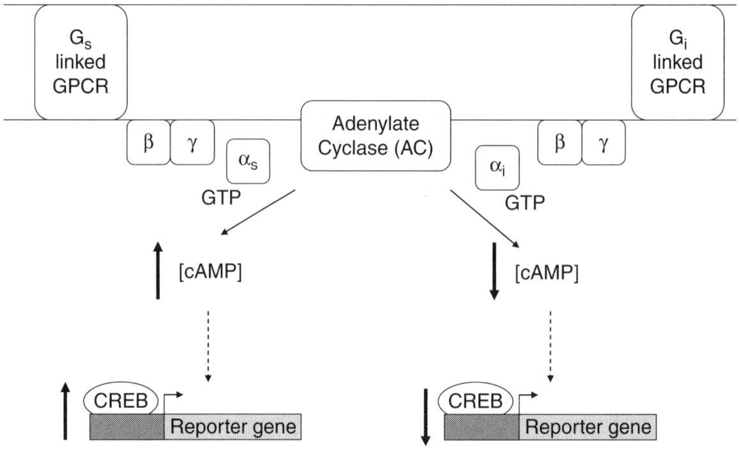

Fig. 1. Overview of the signaling cascade involving cAMP within reporter gene assays. Both G_S- and G_i-linked GPCRs activate signaling pathways through changes in concentration of intracellular cAMP. For G_S-linked GPCRs, the GTP-activated $G_{\alpha S}$ subunit modulates adenylate cyclase to increase cAMP concentrations and upregulate transcription of the reporter gene. In the case of G_i-linked GPCRs, adenylate cyclase activity is inhibited leading to downregulation of reporter gene transcription.

Over recent years, there has been a significant increase in the assay formats available to monitor changes in cAMP as a result of GPCR activation or antagonism *(1, 2)*. While each assay methodology carries its own merits, reporter gene assays still represent a popular format within pharma companies. One of the reasons behind this is that the format is highly sensitive to small changes in cAMP concentration, due to the amplification steps in the signaling cascade. This, in turn, facilitates lower cell numbers to be used which can increase the cost-effectiveness of the assay. The technology traditionally utilizes the endogenous signaling pathway of the receptor to affect transcription of a target reporter gene. The target gene is typically associated with an upstream regulatory component; in the case of cAMP signaling pathways, the cAMP response element binding (CREB) protein is responsible for regulating transcription of the reporter gene (**Fig. 1**).

Typically, the reporter gene regulated expresses an enzyme; perhaps the most well known is beta-lactamase although other enzymes have been used such as luciferase *(3)*. The intrinsic role of beta-lactamase is to cleave the beta-lactam rings, normally present within antibiotic compounds *(4)*. Based on this enzymatic function, beta-lactam derivatives have been synthesized that contain two extrinsic fluorescent probes and are commercially available. The most commonly known derivatives are CCF2-AM™ and CCF4-AM™, available from Invitrogen™ (Carlsbad, CA, USA). In both cases, the fluorescent groups are separated in space by the beta-lactam ring. The dyes are synthesized in an esterified form to enable the probe to permeate the cells *(5)*. Following cleavage by cellular esterases, the dye is converted to the negatively charged substrate which is retained within the cell with the aid of the anion channel blocker, probenicid.

The reporter gene technology can also be used to monitor changes in receptor activity through other signaling pathways such as the G_q-coupled pathways and in other systems beyond GPCR signaling *(6, 7)*. However, this chapter will focus on experimental methods to follow cAMP-modulated pathways using beta-lactamase as the reporter gene within Chinese hamster ovary (CHO) cells, stably transfected with a target receptor.

2. Materials

2.1. Cell Culture and Plate Preparation

1. Phosphate-buffered saline solution (PBS; Gibco, BRL, Bethesda, MD, USA).
2. Cell dissociation buffer (Gibco, BRL).
3. Dulbecco's Modified Eagles Medium (D-MEM) (Gibco, BRL) supplemented with 10% foetal bovine serum (PAA Laboratories, Somerset, UK), non-essential amino acids (NEAA) (Gibco, BRL), Glutamine (Gibco, BRL), and any additional nutrients and selection markers necessary for the growth of the cell line containing the transfected receptor. Typical selection markers used are Geneticin, Zeocin, Blasticidin, or Puromycin. Once prepared, media solution can be kept at 4°C. It is recommended to prepare fresh media every 2 weeks.
4. T225 flasks for cell growth (Corning Life Sciences, NY, USA).

2.2. Reporter Gene Assay

1. Tissue culture treated, black, clear-bottom, 384-well plates (Greiner, Kremunster, Austria).
2. CCF4-AM Geneblazer dye (Invitrogen): Prepare the dye solution by solubilizing in 100% dry DMSO to a concentration of 1 mg/mL. Once prepared, dispense the solution into brown microfuge tubes in 1 mL aliquots in store at –20°C to minimize freeze-thaw cycles. Frozen samples have been re-used for up to 10 freeze-thaw cycles with minimal change in assay signal.
3. 1 M sodium hydroxide solution: Weigh 40 g of NaOH and dissolve in 1 L of purified (e.g., distilled) H_2O. Store at room temperature. It is recommended to make fresh solutions every 2 weeks.

4. Probenicid: 200 mM solution prepared in 200 mM NaOH. To make a 5 mL solution, weigh 280 mg of Probenecid and dissolve in 1 mL of 1 M NaOH. Ensure that the probenicid is in solution by vortexing and, if necessary, incubating in a sonicating waterbath. If the probenecid still has not dissolved, the solution should be discarded and the process repeated until a clear probenecid solution is produced at this stage. Once in solution, add a further 4 mL of either PBS solution or deionized water to give a 5 mL solution of 200 mM probenicid in 200 mM NaOH.
5. Loading solution B consists of 100 mg/mL Pluronic-F127 in DMSO + 0.1% acetic acid and is commercially available (Invitrogen). Store at room temperature. The solution can go cloudy or the pluronic may come out of solution below room temperature. If this happens, heat the solution in a 37°C incubator for approximately 30 min or until the solution is clear.
6. Loading solution C consists of 24% PEG400, 18% Tamra Red 40 quencher v/v in water, and is commercially available (Invitrogen). Store in a darkened area or within a cupboard at room temperature wrapped in foil.
7. Dye loading solution: To make 5 mL of the beta-lactamase dye loading solution, add 56 μL CCF4-AM dye to 280 μL of loading solution B followed by the addition of 4.31 mL of loading solution C. Finally, slowly add 350 μL of 200 mM probenicid solution in 200 mM NaOH.

3. Methods

1. Stably transfected CHO cells are grown in T225 flasks up to a maximum confluency of 80%. It is possible to use cells at lower confluency levels. However, it is recommended not to allow the cells to grow beyond an 80% confluency as receptor expression can be affected.
2. The growth media is removed and the cells washed with 20 mL PBS buffer.
3. After removal of the PBS buffer, add 5 mL of cell dissociation buffer, incubate the cells in the flask at 37°C for 5 min to facilitate cell dissociation.
4. After 5 min, gently tap the closed flask to remove the cells; the solution should go cloudy indicating the cells are in solution. Once this is the case, add 10 mL of PBS to the flask to dilute

the cell dissociation buffer in the flask. Transfer the contents to a sterile falcon tube and centrifuge at approximately 500 × *g* for 5 min. Discard the supernatant, re-suspend the cells in 10 mL media, and calculate the cell number using either a hemocytometer or a Cedex™ counter.

5. Based on the cell density, prepare a solution to a concentration of 5×10^5 cells/mL in growth media, add 20 μL per well in a 384-well plate, and incubate at 37°C overnight (*see* **Notes 1, 2**and **3**).
6. The following day, inspect the plated cells using a microscope to ensure that they are adhered to the bottom of the plate (*see* **Notes 4** and **5**).
7. Test compounds are then prepared in PBS at the appropriate test concentration. For agonist assays, compounds are prepared at 5 × final concentration, added as 5 μL aliquots, and then incubated at 37°C for 4 h. For antagonist assays, the compounds are prepared at 6 × final concentration and added as 5 μL aliquots (*see* **Notes 6** and **7**). Following antagonist addition, the agonist is prepared at 6 × final concentration in PBS, added as 5 μL aliquots, and the stimulated cells are incubated for 4 h at 37°C to allow for receptor activation, downstream signaling, and transcription of the beta-lactamase reporter gene (*see* **Note 8**).
8. After 4 h of agonist stimulation, 6 μL of the 6 × CCF4/AM loading buffer is added to the cells and the plate is incubated at room temperature in the dark for 2 h.
9. In order to ensure that the dye concentration is consistent across assay types, the 6 × loading dye solution is added as 5 μL aliquots for agonist assays. The microplate is then read in a bottom-read, plate reader measuring fluorescence intensity with 405 nm excitation and 450 and 530 nm emissions. The data are plotted as a ratio of the emissions 450/530 nm (*see* **Notes 9** and **10**).
10. Following plate reading, the cellular response can also be observed by fluorescence microscopy with UV illumination. Stimulated cells will appear blue while unstimulated cells will appear green *(8)*.

4. Notes

1. The method above states that a cell density of 10,000 cells/well is required. As mentioned earlier, one of the advantages of the reporter gene technology is that it is possible to use a lower cell density and still achieve high-quality data (**Fig. 2**).

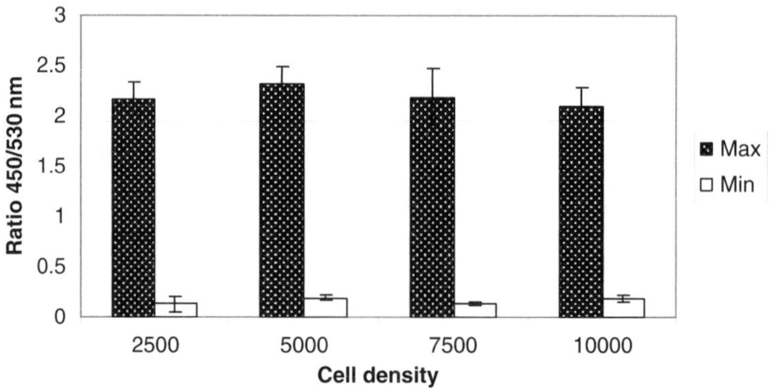

Fig. 2. Variations in assay signal as a function of the cell number. The data shown is from an agonist beta-lactamase assay using an aminergic GPCR. The fact that there is no change in either the maximum (100% effect) or the minimum (0% effect) controls demonstrates that lower cell densities can be used to run reporter gene assays. However, it should be noted that this should be investigated independently for each transfected cell line

As such, when developing a reporter gene assay, the recommendation is to assess the cell density required for each cell line.

2. The growth and plated media defined above represents a generic set of conditions. While the media uses non-dialyzed serum, it may be necessary to use either dialyzed, heat-inactivated or charcoal-stripped serum which can help reduce the presence of endogenous small ligands which may affect receptor expression (e.g., aminergic receptors).
3. In addition to being a cost-effective assay format, reporter gene assays can also be miniaturized to 1536-well plate densities *(9)*. The advantage of this is that the assay cost can be further reduced through the use of fewer reagents. Typical volumes used in 1536-plate densities are 4-μL cells with separate 1 μL additions of antagonist, agonist, and dye solutions to give a total volume of 7 μL.
4. It is crucial to ensure that the cells are adhered to the plate bottom as the signal is measured using a bottom-read, plate reader (**Fig. 3**). As mentioned above, it is recommended to visually inspect the plated cells using a microscope before starting the assay, to ensure that they have adhered. When running the assay for the first time, it would also be prudent to view the cells after each addition step to ensure that there is no change in cell adherence over the course of the assay. When using automated systems or equipment, it is imperative to check the dispense heights and dispense speed in the case of 384-well liquid dispensers to ensure that cell adherence is not affected.

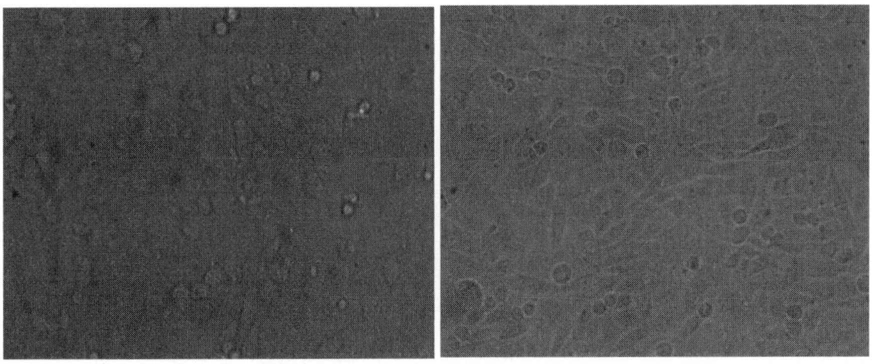

Fig. 3. Illustrative representations of cells plated within 384 well plates. *Right panel:* Cells incubated for 16 h after plating, showing that the cells are elongated and adhered to the bottom of the well. *Left panel*: Visualization of cells immediately after plating showing that the cells are circular suggesting that they are not adhered to the bottom of the well.

5. As mentioned above, the protocol describes the set-up of a reporter gene assay using a CHO cell line stably transfected with the target receptor. There may be times when an alternative cell line is used. The other common cell line used in reporter gene assays is human embryonic kidney (HEK) cells. While this cell line will give high-quality data, there are several additional factors that should be considered when developing an assay with this cell line:
   A. It is necessary to utilize poly-D-lysine-coated, tissue-culture-treated, black, clear bottom plates to enable these cells to adhere to the bottom of the wells.
   B. For the loading dye, it is not necessary to include probenicid as HEK cells are devoid of the ion channels that need to be blocked.
6. When testing compounds are prepared in a particular solvent, it is imperative to assess the tolerance level of the cells against the solvent concentration. Typically, this is performed by running dose–response curves of known compounds prepared at various solvent concentrations and following changes in the signal and pharmacology of the assay (**Fig. 4**).
7. The signaling cascade of G_i-coupled GPCRs involves a decrease of the basal levels of cAMP within the cell. Typically, the basal concentration of cAMP within cells is low. As such, when trying to monitor functional activity of G_i-coupled receptors in an assay, it is necessary to artificially elevate the cAMP levels within the cell to generate an assay window. The most common method used to achieve this is to treat the cells with Forskolin, which elevates the intracellular cAMP concentration through activation of the membrane-bound protein, adenylate cyclase. Typically, an EC_{50} concentration of

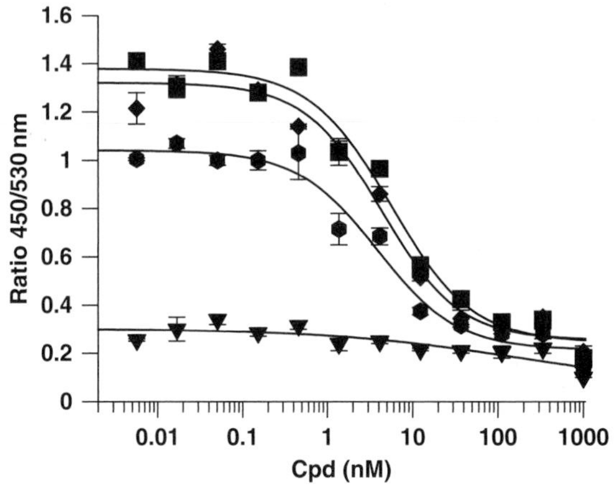

Fig. 4. Changes in pharmacology with differing concentrations of solvent. The data shown are from an antagonist beta-lactamase assay using an aminergic GPCR. An antagonist of known potency was prepared in the presence of differing concentrations of solvent. The concentrations tested are 0.12% v/v (■), 0.5% v/v (◆), 1% v/v (●) and 2% v/v (▼). The data demonstrate that the assay and cell line tested are tolerant up to solvent concentrations of 0.5% v/v.

Forskolin is added to retain assay sensitivity. However, it may be necessary to utilize a higher concentration depending on the window generated for the assay.

8. The protocol above recommends an incubation time of 4 h following agonist addition. While this is suitable for most assays, it is recommended to perform a time course to assess the optimal incubation time for each cell line as the coupling efficiency of the GPCR and the associated G protein can differ substantially between target receptors. As such, it would be worth investigating incubation times between 2 and 17 h following stimulation with the agonist.
9. One of the advantages of using a beta-lactamase reporter gene format is that the ratiometric data facilitate identification of potential fluorescent or cytotoxic compounds. Fluorescence intensity data for each wavelength should be comparable to that seen in the maximum and minimum control wells using a known agonist or antagonist of the receptor (**Fig. 5**). Raw data which are not consistent with this would suggest that the compound is either fluorescent or potentially cytotoxic to the cells.
10. Historically, a blank plate containing media with no cells has been run in parallel to the assay plate. The purpose of this plate was to subtract the data obtained from this plate from the assay plate to give a true reflection of the changes in fluorescence intensity from the assay. While this can still be

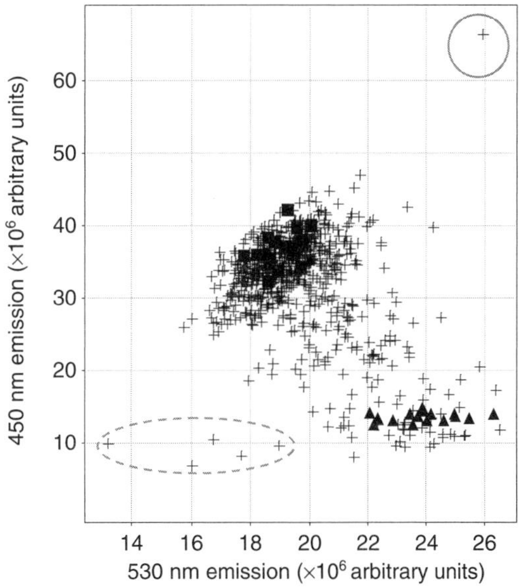

Fig. 5. Assessment and identification of potential fluorescent and cytotoxic compounds. The figure above illustrates the 450 nm emission readout against the 530 nm emission readout. Test compounds (+) should lie between the maximum (■) and the minimum (▲) controls. Any data outside of this region could be indicative of fluorescent compounds (*solid grey circle*) or could suggest the compounds are cytotoxic (*dashed grey circle*).

run, recent data generated in-house suggest that the "background subtract" has very little effect on either compound potency or data quality and as such is no longer necessary (**Fig. 6**).

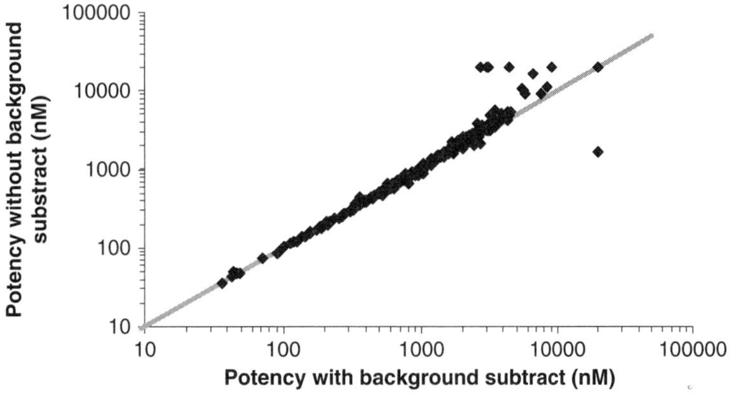

Fig. 6. Correlation of IC_{50} data with and without background subtract. Dose–response experiments were run in the presence and absence of a "background substract." IC_{50} values were calculated for both conditions and the data correlated for the compounds tested. The grey line represents equality between the IC_{50} estimates.

References

1. Williams, C. (2004) cAMP detection methods in HTS: Selecting the best from the rest. *Nat. Rev. Drug Discov.* **3**, 125–135.
2. McLoughlin, D., Bertelli, F., and Williams, C. (2007) The A, B, Cs of G protein-coupled receptor pharmacology in assay development for HTS. *Exp. Op. Drug Discov.* **2**, 603–619.
3. George, S.E., Bungay, P.J., and Naylor, L.H. (1997) Evaluation of a CRE-directed luciferase reporter gene assay as an alternative to measuring cAMP accumulation. *J. Biomol. Screen.* **2**, 235–240.
4. Wilke, M.S., Lovering, A.L., and Strynadka, N.C.J. (2005) β-Lactam antibiotic resistance: a current structural perspective. *Curr. Opin. Microbiol.* **8**, 525–533.
5. Hallis, T.M., Kopp, A.L., Gibson, J., Lebakken, C.S., Hancock, M., Van Den Heuvel-Kramer, K., and Turek-Etienne, T. (2007) An improved beta-lactamase reporter assay: Multiplexing with a cytotoxicity readout for enhanced accuracy of hit identification. *J. Biomol. Screen.* **12**, 635–644.
6. Kunapuli, P., Zheng, W., Weber, M., Solly, K., Mull, R., Platchek, M., Cong, M., Zhong, Z., and Strulovici, B. (2005) Application of division arrest technology to cell-based HTS: comparison with frozen and fresh cells. *Assay Drug Dev. Technol.* **3**, 17–26.
7. Bradley, J., Gill, J., Bertelli, F., Letafat, S., Corbau, R., Hayter, P., Harrison, P., Tee, A., Keighley, W., Perros, M., Ciaramella, G., Sewing, A., and Williams, C. (2004) Development and automation of a 384-well cell fusion assay to identify inhibitors of CCR5/CD4-mediated HIV virus entry. *J. Biomol. Screen.* **9**, 516–524.
8. Zuck, P., Murray, E.M., Stec, E., Grobler, J.A., Simon, A.J., Strulovici, B., Inglese, J., Flores, O.A., and Ferrer, M. (2004) A cell-based beta-lactamase reporter gene assay for the identification of inhibitors of hepatitis C virus replication. *Anal. Biochem.* **334**, 344–355.
9. Maffia III, A.M., Kariv, I.I., and Oldenburg, K.R. (1999) Miniaturization of a Mammalian Cell-Based Assay: Luciferase Reporter Gene Readout in a 3 Microliter 1536-Well Plate. *J. Biomol. Screen.* **4**, 137–142.

Chapter 24

A Quantum Dot-Labeled Ligand–Receptor Binding Assay for G Protein-Coupled Receptors Contained in Minimally Purified Membrane Nanopatches

Jody L. Swift, Melanie C. Burger, and David T. Cramb

Summary

A robust method to directly measure ligand–receptor binding interactions using fluorescence cross-correlation spectroscopy (FCCS) is described. The example receptor systems demonstrated here are the human mu-opioid receptor, a representative G protein-coupled receptor (GPCR), and Streptavidin, but these general protocols can be extended for the analysis of many membrane receptors. We present methods for the preparation of GPCR-containing membrane nanopatches that appear to have the shapes of nanovesicles, labeling of proteins in membrane vesicles, in addition to the coupling of quantum dots (QDs) to peptide ligands. Further, we demonstrate that reliable binding information can be obtained from these partially purified receptors.

Key words: Membrane nanopatches, Fluorescence correlation spectroscopy, Quantum dot.

1. Introduction

Most receptor–ligand (R–L) binding assays require the purification of receptor proteins in order to effectively measure binding constants. During purification, cell-membrane fractions are often solubilized with membrane detergents and washed with protein denaturants before the receptor is reconstituted into synthetic lipid bilayers. Membrane proteins possess hydrophobic domains residing in the lipid bilayer, and abstraction of integral proteins from their native lipid matrix can alter protein function *(1)*. Moreover, it is unlikely that membrane protein folding is recapitulated following protein purification, alterations in α-helix and β-strand content can occur even when reconstituted into bilayers *(2)*. In fact, studies of Na^+, K^+-ATPase ion channels reconstituted into

Wayne R. Leifert (ed.), *G Protein-Coupled Receptors in Drug Discovery, vol. 552*

Book doi: 10.1007/978-1-60327-317-6_24

synthetic lipid bilayer systems showed that Na^+, K^+-ATPase activity changed with lipid composition, and over different lipid ratios in binary mixtures *(3)*. Hydrophobic mismatch between the acyl chain length and the bilayer-spanning protein regions and changes in lateral pressure of lipids due to differential lipid packing and microdomain formation alter protein conformation, stability, and activity *(4)*. Hence, enzyme activity rates, ion transport, and ligand binding measurements for membrane proteins removed from their original lipid domain do not represent native activities. It is important to study membrane protein activity with minimal sample purification, ideally retaining integral proteins in native lipid mosaics.

Receptor–ligand interactions can be measured between a ligand and G protein-coupled receptor (GPCR) contained in crude cell-membrane nanopatches *(5)* **(Figs. 1** and **2)** readily prepared from cells expressing the membrane protein construct of interest (here, human mu-opioid receptor, aka hMOR) using a two-photon excitation fluorescence correlation/cross-correlation spectroscopy (TPE-FCS/FCCS) combined assay. We present a simple "one-pot" assay which has a number of advantages compared to conventional assays. The first advantage is that due to the zero background nature of FCCS, it is not necessary to do extensive purification of the receptor. This is particularly advantageous for GPCRs and other membrane receptors, allowing the receptor to be studied in a more natural lipid environment. Second, our assay is small (~200 μL) and thus does not require large volumes of purified material which can be time consuming and costly. The combined advantage of high signal-to-noise ratio and small sample

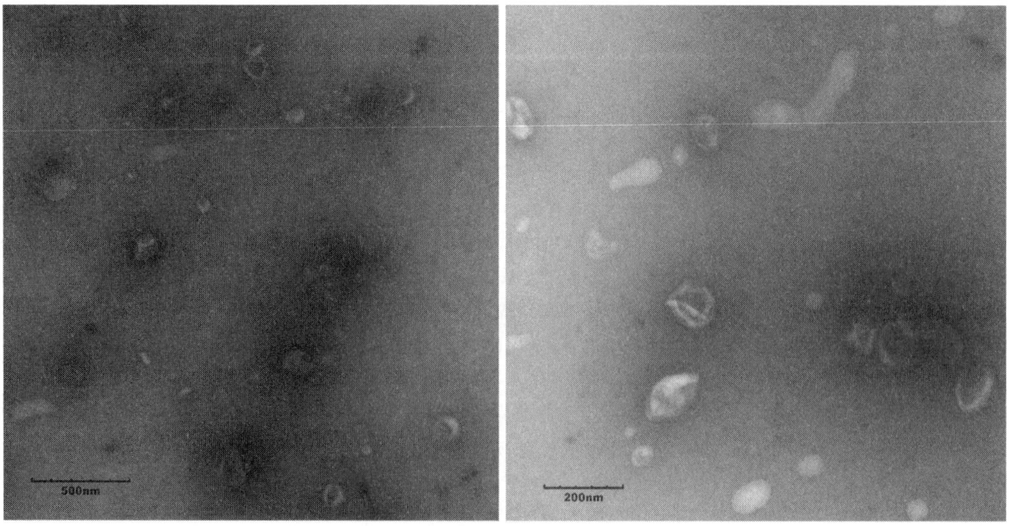

Fig. 1. TEM images of HEK 293 cell membrane patches expressing hMOR. Nanopatches appear as vesicles similar in shape to erythrocytes.

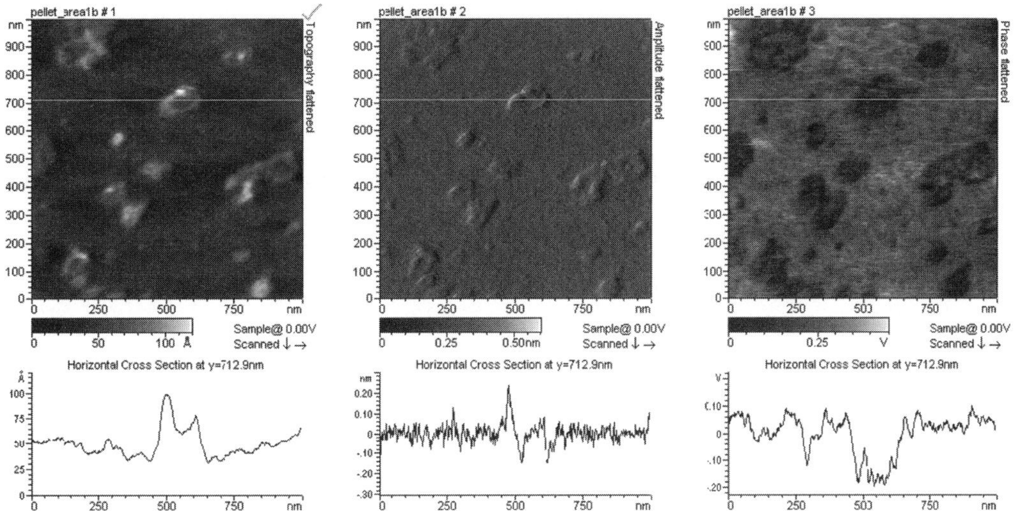

Fig. 2. Atomic force microscopy images of HEK-hMOR nanopatches deposited onto a mica surface. Images were collected of the sample in buffer.

volumes allow us to collect many data points over a narrow concentration range at low ligand concentrations. Working at low concentrations, one is less susceptible to non-specific binding interactions that plague typical radio-labeling assays. Finally, our assay examines a single population of receptors and thus reduces deviation within a single data set due to variations in the receptor populations in each sample.

In order to measure the relative concentrations of species needed to determine the ligand–receptor equilibrium constants, FCS and FCCS analyses of the titration solutions were employed. Autocorrelation decays were modeled assuming a Gaussian TPE volume using the following equation *(5, 6)*:

$$G(\tau) = G_{\mathrm{L(R)}}(0)\left(1 + \frac{8D_{\mathrm{L(R)}}\tau}{r_0^2}\right)^{-1}\left(1 + \frac{8D_{\mathrm{L(R)}}\tau}{z_0^2}\right)^{-1/2} \quad [1]$$

where the subscripts $L\,(R)$ indicate ligand or receptor, τ is the lag time, D is the diffusion constant, r_0 is the laser beam radius at its focus, and z_0 is the $1/e^2$ radius in the z direction. The diffusion coefficient in equation [**1**] represents the species' mobility.

Cross-correlation decays were modeled as above using the following equation *(5, 6)*:

$$G_{\mathrm{X}}(\tau) = G_{\mathrm{LR}}(0)\left(1 + \frac{8D_{\mathrm{LR}}\tau}{r_0^2}\right)^{-1}\left(1 + \frac{8D_{\mathrm{LR}}\tau}{z_0^2}\right)^{-1/2} \quad [2]$$

where the subscript *LR* represents labeled ligands and receptors which are physically bound together and thus dual-color labeled. The equations contain no terms to account for intersystem crossing or quantum dot (QD) blinking, the effects of which are minimized by keeping the excitation rates low.

It was previously demonstrated that the fractional occupancy, P_A, could be calculated simply using G(0)'s *(6)*. Briefly, in the absence of crosstalk between the two detection channels, the correlation and cross-correlation amplitudes are given by

$$G_{S(R)}(0) = \frac{\langle C_{L(R)} \rangle + \langle C_{LR} \rangle}{N_A\, V_{eff}\left(\langle C_{L(R)} \rangle + \langle C_{LR} \rangle\right)^2} \quad [3]$$

and

$$G_{LR}(0) = \frac{\langle C_{LR} \rangle}{N_A\, V_{eff}(\langle C_L \rangle + \langle C_{LR} \rangle)(\langle C_R \rangle + \langle C_{LR} \rangle)} \quad [4]$$

where, N_A is Avogadro's number, V_{eff} is the effective TPE volume, $\langle C_{LR} \rangle$ represents the time averaged concentration of dually labeled species, and $\langle C_{L(R)} \rangle$ represents the time averaged concentration of ligand (or receptor). To use this equation, one presumes that the correlation amplitude is free of crosstalk between the detection channels. Additionally, in the case of low concentrations, the autocorrelation G(0)'s were corrected for the contribution of background noise as necessary *(7)*.
Recall that fractional occupancy is

$$P_A = \frac{\langle C_{LR} \rangle}{\langle C_R \rangle + \langle C_{LR} \rangle} \quad [5]$$

This relation can be expressed in terms of G(0) values as follows:

$$P_A = \frac{\langle C_{LR} \rangle}{\langle C_R \rangle + \langle C_{LR} \rangle} = \frac{G_{LR}(0)}{G_L(0)} \quad [6]$$

Equation [**6**] shows that unlike the individual G(0)'s, P_A is not dependent upon the two-photon excitation volume (**Fig. 3**); however, where a precise calibration of this volume is available, more information about the system (such as the diffusion coefficients) can be gained.

Due to the possibility that there may be multiple receptors per nanopatch, one may need to consider a multiple-ligand equilibrium approach to binding. Thus, for *n* ligands (L) associating with a nanopatch (R) we have

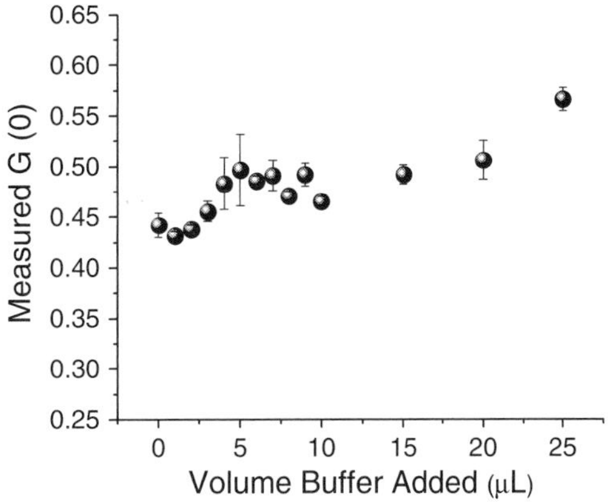

Fig. 3. Control titration of fluorescently labeled receptor, illustrating the relatively consistent concentration with small amounts of ligand added. The average *G*(0) value for the whole titration was found to be 0.48 ± 0.03. The initial sample volume was 200 μL. Note that once you add more than 10% of the initial volume, changes in the measured *G*(0) value are noted.

$$n\mathrm{L} + \mathrm{R} \Leftrightarrow (\mathrm{L})_n\mathrm{R} \qquad [7]$$

where n can be a whole number or a fraction. It can be shown that a standard analysis of this equilibrium produces the Hill equation for multi-ligand binding *(6)*:

$$\ln\left(\frac{P_A}{1 - P_A}\right) = n \ln(C_L) - \ln K'_d \qquad [8]$$

where P_A is the fractional occupancy of available binding sites on the nanopatch, C_L is the concentration of ligand, and K'_d is the dissociation constant for the equilibrium presented in Equation [7]. Additionally, in the absence of cooperativity, taking the nth root of the dissociation constant, K'_d, gives the dissociation constant, K_d, for the formation of an individual ligand–receptor complex.

2. Materials

2.1. Membrane Nanopatches

1. Minimum Essential Medium with L-glutamine (Fisher Scientific, Waltham, MA, USA) supplemented with 10% v/v fetal bovine serum (FBS, HyClone, Ogden, UT, USA).
2. If necessary, 0.25% trypsin-EDTA (Invitrogen, Carlsbad, CA, USA) in 2.0 mL aliquots and stored at –20°C.

3. Phosphate-buffered saline (PBS), 1 × solution: 137 mM NaCl, 2.7 mM KCl, 4.3 mM Na_2HPO_4, 1.4 mM KH_2PO_4, pH 7.4, 1-μm filter sterilized and stored at 4°C.

2.2. Quantum Dot-Labeled Peptides and Nanopatch Titration

1. Alexa Fluor 488 Penta His antibody (Qiagen Inc., Hilden, Germany).
2. QD streptavidin conjugate (Invitrogen).
3. Stock solution of biotinylated peptide, 0.1 mM Leu-enkephalin (BLEKYGGFL-biotin, MW 823.6) in ultrapure water, stored at 4°C. For storage over 1 week, 2 mM of sodium azide should be added to the stock solution to prevent the growth of unwanted material.
4. Mini-dialysis kit with appropriate molecular weight cutoff (Amersham Biosciences, Buckinghamshire, UK), for this application a kit with a 1-kDa cutoff is used.

3. Methods

Crude membrane nanopatches can be used as a platform for measuring receptor–ligand affinity. The key advantages of this technique are that membrane proteins are retained in their original lipid environment and the technically trivial preparation of the membrane nanopatches. To prepare patches, cell membranes are disrupted by sonication, and the resultant membrane fractions are isolated by ultracentrifugation with diameter ~100 nm *(5)*. The membrane fragments can then be stained with a lipophilic probe and the proteins antibody labeled. This simple method not only retains membrane receptors in their original lipid environment but also generates vesicles with diffusion profiles suitable for high-throughput FCCS assays. The method, however, does not allow for strict control of particle size or number of receptors per particle and samples can be very heterogeneous. It is also uncertain what proportion of membrane proteins is inverted with the ligand-binding domain opening to the vesicle lumen. These proteins are simply not included from the measured population as they would neither be antibody labeled at the extra-cellular terminus nor bound by a fluorescent ligand.

Biotinylated Leu-enkephalin is non-covalently linked to a QD via streptavidin, which is conjugated to the QD. On average, there are 10 streptavidin receptor sites per QD *(6)*. An over-labeling strategy is employed for both nanopatch and ligand preparation, ensuring that all fluorescent QDs contribute to both the autocorrelation amplitude and the overall expression of P_A participate in binding.

Binding curve titrations are carried out as previously described for a biotin–streptavidin model system *(6)*. A small amount of the labeled ligand is added to the labeled hMOR nanopatch sample, the system equilibrated (5 min), and autocorrelation and cross-correlation scans (average 60 s) collected for each addition of ligand. The fractional occupancy of receptors for each addition is determined at each TPE-FCCS data point. Plots of the fractional occupancy (P_A) versus ligand concentration are used to obtain the K_d for the system in question. For reliability, three titrations are averaged together to obtain the K_d for trial. Furthermore, the data from the averaged titrations are fitted using Equation [**8**] to obtain K_d and the average number of ligands per patch.

3.1. Preparation of Membrane Nanopatches

1. Harvest human embryonic kidney (HEK 293) cells for membrane vesicle preparation at peak levels of membrane protein expression, typically 3 days after human mu-opioid receptor transient transfection. Prior to harvesting, check cells for typical morphology and contamination. Number of plates harvested vary with the amount of sample required for assays; however, membrane vesicles can be stored at –80°C for at least 3 months.
2. Mechanically dislodge cells by washing plates with complete media, transferring the media to the next plate to dislodge cells, and finally placing the suspension in a sterile Falcon centrifuge tubes. Rinse dishes with a small amount of complete media and transfer to Falcon centrifuge tubes (*see* **Note 1**). Harvest cells by centrifugation (*see* **Note 2**). Discard the supernatant, and wash pellet three times with cold 1 × PBS: add PBS to the pellet, pipetting up and down to mix, and re-centrifuge. Discard supernatants and resuspend in 1 × PBS (*see* **Note 3**).
3. Cells are ruptured via microcavitation sonication. Keep cell suspensions on ice and place the pulse probe in cell suspension at a consistent tip-depth. For 8 mL volumes, ten 15-s pulses are typical, with 15-s breaks to avoid over-heating. During pauses in sonication, quickly cap the tube and invert to mix (*see* **Notes 4** and **5**).
4. Ultracentrifuge (10,000 × *g*, 40 min, 4°C) to remove large organelles and whole cells. Pour off supernatant into a new, autoclaved ultracentrifuge tube and ultracentrifuge (100,000 × *g*, 40 min, 4°C) to isolate membrane lysate. Re-suspend the pellet in a minimal volume of 1 × PBS. To resuspend, buffer solution will need to be forcefully ejected into the pellet and stirred with the pipette tip.

5. Pass the suspension through syringes of successively increasing needle gauge sizes (22, 25, 27) five times to disperse aggregates of membrane patches. Samples can be stored at –20°C for a few weeks or –80°C freezer for a few months. Prior to experiments, samples are thawed (15 min, 4°C) and gently vortexed (5 min) to disperse remaining aggregates. Average particle size can be rapidly determined with dynamic light scattering measurements.

3.2. Preparation of Quantum Dot-Labeled Peptides for Titrations

1. 40 nM QD streptavidin and 400 nM BLEK solutions in PBS with 0.1% BSA are made ready.
2. QD and BLEK are mixed together in a 1:1 ratio resulting in a solution with a final concentration of 20 nM QD. In this assay, it is assumed that each QD behaves as a single peptide, and for quantitative titrations the final concentration of ligand is calculated in the sample using this assumption. This assumption was validated in previous work illustrating that the steric bulk of the QD label prevents it from labeling or binding to multiple receptors *(6)*.
3. Place the total sample in a commercial mini-dialysis kit with a 1-kDa cutoff and dialyzed overnight or for a minimum of 12 h to remove any of the unbound enkephalin.
4. Once removing the sample from the dialysis tubing, it must be used immediately for titrations. This is due to the reduced stability of the biotin–streptavidin bond when either or both species is covalently attached to another molecule *(7)* (*see* **Note 6**).

3.3. Titrations of Nanopatches with Quantum Dot-Labeled Peptides

1. Place 200 μL of antibody-labeled nanopatches in a quartz sample chamber (*see* **Note 7**).
2. Add a small aliquot of the QD–streptavidin–BLEK solution (0.5–2 μL) to the sample, noting the exact volume of addition. Gently stir the sample with the tip of the pipette and equilibrate for 5 min.
3. After the equilibration time, obtain a dual autocorrelation scan and a cross-correlation scan. While the amplitude of the autocorrelation function of the labeled nanopatches does not contribute to the overall expression of P_A, keep track of this value to ensure that the concentration of patches does not change substantially during the course of the titration (*see* **Note 8**).
4. Add small aliquots of QD–streptavidin–BLEK, equilibrate, and continue to collect of auto/cross-correlation scans until a minimum of 10 data points (ligand concentrations) are obtained (*see* **Note 9**).

5. Calculate the fractional occupancy for each addition of ligand and plot against the concentration of ligand added.
6. Average a minimum of three separate titrations together in order to obtain a reliable K_d value for the ligand of interest. It is recommended that more titrations are carried out adding different volumes of ligand to ensure that a detailed plot is obtained. This is particularly important for concentrations close to the actual K_d value (*see* **Notes 10** and **11**).

4. Notes

1. Cells that are difficult to mechanically dislodge can be treated with 0.25% trypsin-EDTA for 1–2 min although it is preferable to avoid this step.
2. High centrifuge speeds will result in a cell pellets that are difficult to resuspend.
3. For convenience, transfer directly into an autoclaved ultracentrifuge tube to be used in later ultracentrifugation steps.
4. Sonication time for different cell types can vary. To determine if cells were successfully rupture, check sonicated samples under a microscope for whole cells.
5. Tubes should not be combined after sonication. Average size of vesicles differ between batches and mixing increases sample heterogeneity.
6. It is possible to rapidly remove unbound peptides by using microcentrifugation with the appropriate molecular cutoff. This method is recommended due to the labile nature of the biotin–streptavidin bond. For both dialyzed and microcentrifuged samples, the outer time limit found for using these samples is 3 h. The unlabeled or native biotin–streptavidin interaction has a reported dissociation rate constant of $5.4 \times 10^{-6}\ s^{-1}$ *(7)*. From previous experiments, we found that when both the biotin and the streptavidin molecules were coupled to other ligands/labels, the dissociation rate constant increases to $\sim 5.5 \times 10^{-5}\ s^{-1}$. While the dissociation rate is only increased by an order of magnitude, this has a profound effect on the dynamics of the equilibrium for the bond. In the case of the native biotin–streptavidin interaction (no labels or conjugated peptides), the half life of the bond calculated from the dissociation rate constant would be ~36 h compared to the labeled case, which we can estimate to be

~3.5 h. As the half-life of the bond refers to the time required for half of the ligand–receptors to dissociate this, it is worth noting that some of the biotinylated ligand may dissociate from the streptavidin QD prior to the end of the titration. At this point, the unlabeled ligand may occupy a receptor, and due to the lack of the fluorescent label would not contribute to the $G_{LR}(0)$, and result in an underestimated value for the P_A.

7. It is necessary to perform preliminary labeling studies to ensure the proper concentration of antibodies to use for labeling the particular receptor/protein of interest. Prepare a series of antibody solutions with a final concentration ranging from 0.5 to 10 μg/mL. Add this range of antibody concentrations to nanopatch solutions with various total protein concentrations (0.1–2 μg/mL) to produce a matrix of possible antibody–receptor/protein sample conditions. Following 5-min incubation period, place antibody-labeled nanopatches in a quartz sample chamber to examine using FCS. Compare the autocorrelation decay curves for free antibodies at each concentration (no patches added), with the autocorrelation decay curves for patch-antibody samples to determine if all the antibody added is bound to the patches or if there is an excessive amount of free antibody in solution. As the overall autocorrelation function will be dominated by the antibodies conjugated to the large patches, it is recommended to collect short scans which will bias for the smaller faster particles in solution. It is best to choose the regime (antibody vs. protein concentration) in which there is a slight excess of antibody so that all of the receptors which may interact with the ligand are labeled. For the gp-hMOR-C-His construct, it was found that 2 μg/mL Penta-His Alexa Fluor 488 conjugate was sufficient for labeling patches at concentrations of 0.5 μg/mL.
8. It may be necessary to adjust the concentration of the stock solution of the labeled ligand of interest to ensure that during the course of the titration you do not add more than 10% to the total volume (i.e., 20 μL to an initial 200 μL sample). For small volume additions, it is assumed that the concentration of the receptors remains relatively constant, and extra parameters do not need to be taken into account during data fitting.
9. To verify that no fluorescence resonance energy transfer or fluorescence quenching is occurring in the case of bound QD systems, ensure that no relative changes in the brightness (count rate per particle) of either species occur when both were present in solution.

10. A more detailed plot will ensure a more accurate determination of the true equilibrium constant. Typical radio-labeling ligand–receptor binding assays which examine only a few ligand concentrations over a large dynamic range and thus may not provide enough points for accurate K_d determination (**Figs. 4** and **5**).

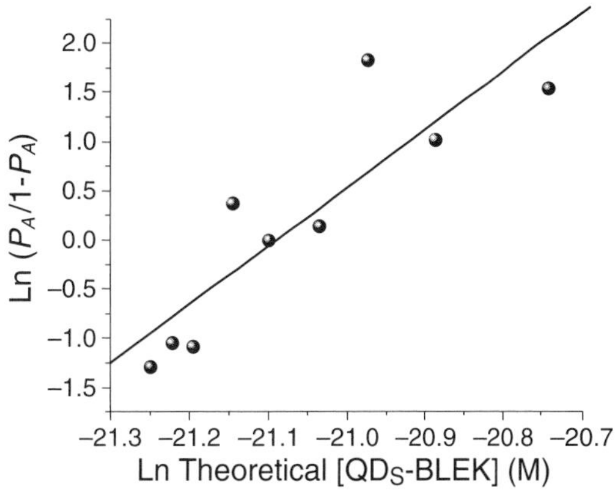

Fig. 4. HEK Nanopatches containing hMOR titrated with QD-BLEK. From the slope of the linear regression analysis, we calculate the Kd of 0.80 ± 0.1 nM and an average slope (*n*) of 3.0 ± 0.2.

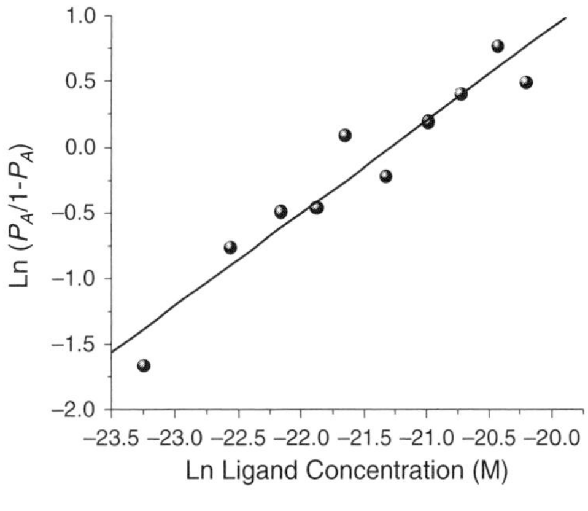

Fig. 5. Streptavidin–biotin binding titration. From the slope of the linear regression analysis, we calculate the K_d of 0.57 ± 0.2 nM and a slope $n = 0.70 \pm 0.07$. The slope of the linearized Hill plot can be used to determine the relative binding ratio of ligand to receptor.

11. It is recommended that blank titrations be run that contain no nanopatches or receptor of interest (**Fig. 6**). This will ensure that the concentration regime is within the dynamic range for which changes in the amplitude of autocorrelation function for the ligand ($G_L(0)$) are reflective of the concentration of

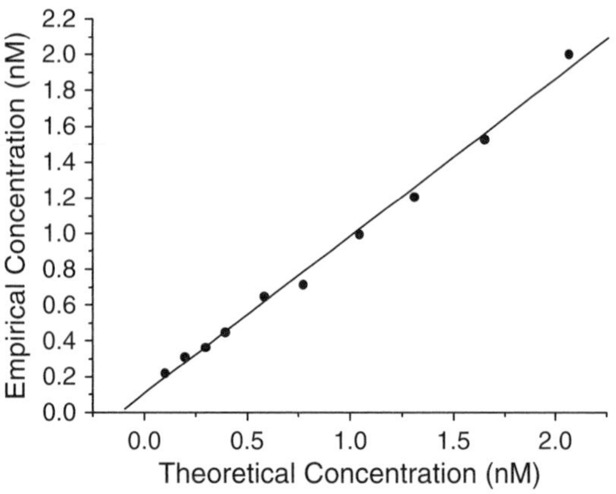

Fig. 6. Control titration of quantum dots. The circles represent the data which was fit to a standard linear regression. The resulting fit had a slope (*m*) of 0.88 ± 0.02 and an intercept of 0.11 ± 0.02.

ligand added (**Fig. 7**). If ligand is added but no changes in the amplitude of the autocorrelation function is observed, then assay parameters may need to be readjusted. It is possible to calculate the experimental concentration of the QD-labeled ligand with a well-calibrated focal volume. A plot comparing the empirically determined and theoretical concentrations should yield a straight line with a slope near unity. This is demonstrated in **Fig. 7**. We found that control titrations that were performed on the dialyzed QD-BLEK (**Fig. 7**) samples yielded linear relationships but did not have a slope that approached unity. It is possible to adjust the theoretical concentration of the ligand stock sample using this slope to ensure that the K_d is correctly identified.

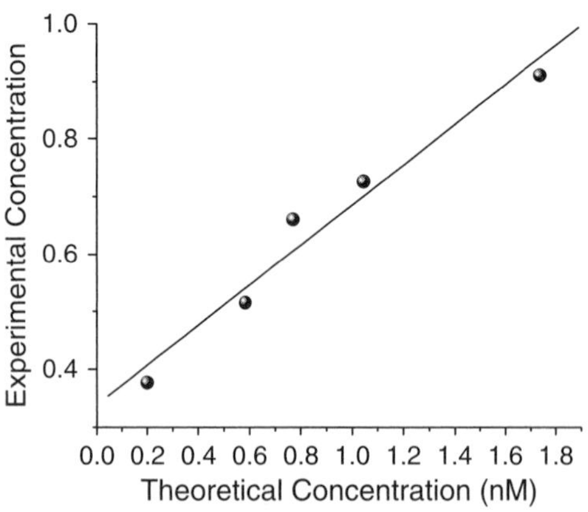

Fig. 7. Control titration of fluorescently labeled ligand. The *circles* represent the data which was fit to a standard linear regression. The resulting fit had a slope (*m*) of 0.35 ± 0.04 and an intercept (*B*) of 0.34 ± 0.04.

Acknowledgments

This work was supported by the National Sciences and Engineering Council of Canada, the Alberta Ingenuity Fund, the University of Calgary, and the Canadian Institute for Photonics Innovation.

References

1. Cooper, M.A. (2004) Advances in membrane receptor screening and analysis. *J. Mol. Recognit.* **17**, 286–315.
2. Shanmugavadivu, B., Apell, H.J., Meins, T., Zeth, K., and Kleinschmidt, J.H. (2007) Correct folding of the beta-barrel of the human membrane protein VDAC requires a lipid bilayer. *J. Mol. Biol.* **368**, 66–78.
3. Powalska, E., Janosch, S., Kinne-Saffran, E., Kinne, R.K., Fontes, C.F., Mignaco, J.A., and Winter, R. (2007) Fluorescence spectroscopic studies of pressure effects on Na^+, K(+)-ATPase reconstituted into phospholipid bilayers and model raft mixtures. *Biochemistry* **46**, 1672–1683.
4. Killian, J.A. (1998) Hydrophobic mismatch between proteins and lipids in membranes. *Biochim. Biophys. Acta.* **1376**, 401–415.
5. Swift, J.L., Burger, M.C., Massotte, D., Dahms, T.E., and Cramb, D.T. (2007) Two-photon excitation fluorescence cross-correlation assay for ligand-receptor binding: cell membrane nanopatches containing the human micro-opioid receptor. *Anal. Chem.* **79**, 6783–6791.
6. Swift, J.L., Heuff, R., and Cramb, D.T. (2006) A two-photon excitation fluorescence cross-correlation assay for a model ligand-receptor binding system using quantum dots. *Biophys. J.* **90**, 1396–1410.
7. Swift, J.L., and Cramb, D.T. (2008) Nanoparticles as fluorescence labels: Is size all that matters? *Biophys. J.* **95**, 865–876.

Chapter 25

Xenopus Oocyte Electrophysiology in GPCR Drug Discovery

Kasper B. Hansen and Hans Bräuner-Osborne

Summary

Deorphanization of the large group of G protein-coupled receptors (GPCRs) for which an endogenous activating ligand has not yet been identified (orphan GPCRs) has become increasingly difficult. A specialized technique that has been successfully applied to deorphanize some of these GPCRs involves two-electrode voltage-clamp recordings of currents through ion channels, which are activated by GPCRs heterologously expressed in *Xenopus* oocytes. The ion channels that couple to GPCR activation in *Xenopus* oocytes can be endogenous calcium-activated chloride channels (CaCCs) or heterologously expressed G protein-coupled inwardly rectifying potassium channels (GIRKs). We will describe a general approach for expression of GPCRs in *Xenopus* oocytes and characterization of these using electrophysiological recordings. We will focus on the detection of GPCR activation by recordings of currents through CaCCs that are activated by calcium release from the endoplasmic reticulum and thus the G_q signaling pathway.

Key words: *Xenopus laevis*, Oocyte, RNA, Transcription, Injection, GPRC6A, Intracellular calcium, Ligand.

1. Introduction

GPCRs comprise the largest superfamily of cell-surface receptors in mammals, and more than 1,000 different GPCRs have been identified since the first of these receptors were cloned more than 20 years ago *(1, 2)*. GPCRs signal through a wide range of effectors, and these receptors carry out a multitude of tasks in the central nervous system and the periphery *(3, 4)*. Numerous diseases and disorders have been linked to GPCRs and they therefore represent a major target for drug discovery *(4, 5)*. There is a remarkable chemical diversity among the diverse array of ligands that are known to activate GPCRs, including peptides, hormones, amino acids, ions, and photons of light *(3, 6)*. In the past decade,

Wayne R. Leifert (ed.), *G Protein-Coupled Receptors in Drug Discovery, vol. 552*

Book doi: 10.1007/978-1-60327-317-6_25

advances in bioinformatics have enabled the identification of open reading frames encoding putative GPCRs from public databases, and it has become clear that there is a large group of ~120 orphan non-olfactory GPCRs *(4, 6, 7)*. Not only will "deorphanizing" these GPCRs undoubtedly unveil new cellular substances and pathways that are important for mammalian physiology, but some of these orphan GPCRs may also represent future drug targets. The generic approach used for deorphanizing these receptors has been to co-express the receptors in mammalian cells with chimeric G proteins and then screen libraries of commercially available endogenous compounds in a calcium assay. However, this has become increasingly less successful as the low hanging fruits have been picked with this strategy, and it seems that the remaining orphan GPCRs will be much harder to deorphanize. Finding an activating ligand for the remaining orphan GPCRs will likely require a variety of specialized techniques that need to be picked for each target with its structural properties, expression profile, and expected physiological role in mind *(6, 8)*.

One of the specialized techniques that have been successfully applied to deorphanize GPCRs is two-electrode voltage-clamp recordings of currents through ion channels activated by GPCRs heterologously expressed in *Xenopus* oocytes (i.e., *Xenopus* oocyte electrophysiology) *(9–13)*. The ion channels that couple to GPCR activation in *Xenopus* oocytes can be endogenous CaCCs or heterologously expressed GIRKs. The main disadvantage of this system is the relatively low throughput. However, the system can provide high GPCR expression levels, which will give rise to large responses and enable robust detection of GPCR activation with high sensitivity. Many GPCRs are difficult to functionally express in mammalian cells due to their activation by constituents of sera and culture media or ligands excreted from the cells (causing desensitization and internalization following activation) *(4, 10, 14)*. One of the major advantages of *Xenopus* oocyte electrophysiology is that these problems are eliminated, since the oocytes are maintained in an inorganic buffer during expression of the GPCR and are constantly perfused during the measurements *(10, 15)*.

2. Materials

2.1. Linearization of Plasmid DNA and In Vitro RNA Transcription

1. 5–10 μg purified plasmid DNA and suitable restriction enzymes.
2. Buffer-saturated phenol, pH ≥ 7.4 (Invitrogen, Carlsbad, CA, USA), phenol : chloroform : isoamyl alcohol 25:24:1, pH 8.1–8.4 (Invitrogen), and chloroform stored protected from light at 4°C.
3. 3 *M* sodium acetate, pH 5.2: Prepare using RNase-free double-distilled water and adjust pH with 10% acetic acid.

4. 96–100% ethanol and 70% ethanol prepared using RNase-free double-distilled water.
5. TE buffer (DNA/RNA storage buffer): 1 m*M* EDTA, 10 m*M* Tris-HCl, pH 8.0 prepared using RNase-free double-distilled water.
6. mMESSAGE mMACHINE High Yield Capped RNA Transcription Kit (Ambion, Austin, TX, USA) that includes a suitable RNA polymerase (SP6, T3, or T7).
7. Microcentrifuge for all centrifuge steps.

2.2. Injection and Maintenance of Xenopus Oocytes

1. Zoom stereomicroscope with light source: Oocyte isolation, selection, micropipet preparation, and microinjection require a good zoom stereomicroscope with at least 10-fold magnification and a working distance of at least 10 cm.
2. Microinjector and micromanipulator: Cytoplasmic injections in oocytes can be performed in volumes between ~2–70 nL using either an automated injection device (e.g., Nanoject II, Drummond Scientific, Broomall, PA, USA) or 30 nL or more using a manual injection device (Drummond Scientific). Precise positioning of the microinjector requires a micromanipulator and an adaptor to secure the microinjector to the micromanipulator (Drummond Scientific).
3. Micropipet puller (e.g., PC-10 Puller, Narishige, East Meadow, NY, USA).
4. Glass capillaries with 1.19 mm O.D. and 0.5 mm I.D. (Drummond Scientific or World Precision Instruments, Sarasota, FL, USA) and mineral oil (e.g., light oil for molecular biology, Sigma-Aldrich, St. Louis, MO, USA) for back filling the glass capillaries using a back-filling needle (e.g., MicroFil, 34 ga., World Precision Instruments).
5. Incubator: *Xenopus* oocytes are for most purposes best maintained at 18°C. This normally requires a cooled incubator.
6. Injection chamber: Can be manufactured in several different ways using several different designs (*see* **Note 1**).
7. Pipettes for handling *Xenopus* oocytes: Can be prepared by breaking the tip of glass Pasteur pipettes (9 in., Fischer Scientific, Pittsburgh, PA, USA) to create a tip with an internal diameter of 1.5–2.5 mm. It is important to fire polish the tip to prevent damage to the oocytes.
8. Barth's solution: 88 m*M* NaCl, 1.0 m*M* KCl, 2.4 m*M* $NaHCO_3$, 0.91 m*M* $CaCl_2$, 0.82 m*M* $MgSO_4$, 0.33 m*M* $Ca(NO_3)_2$, 10 m*M* HEPES, pH 7.5 supplemented with 100 IU/mL penicillin, 100 μg/mL streptomycin (Invitrogen), and 100 μg/mL gentamycin (Fisher BioReagents).
9. Defolliculated *Xenopus* oocytes (*see* **Note 2**).

2.3. Electrophysiological Recordings from Xenopus Oocytes

1. Two-electrode voltage-clamp setup (*see* **Note 3**).
2. Extracellular recording solution: 115 m*M* NaCl, 2.5 m*M* KCl, 1.8 m*M* $CaCl_2$, 1.0 m*M* $MgCl_2$, 10 m*M* HEPES, pH 7.6 (*see* **Note 4**).

3. Methods

Xenopus oocyte electrophysiology with heterologously expressed GPCRs relies upon measurements of currents through ion channels using two-electrode voltage-clamp recordings (*see* **Fig. 1**). Activation of GPCRs that couple to the G_q signaling pathway

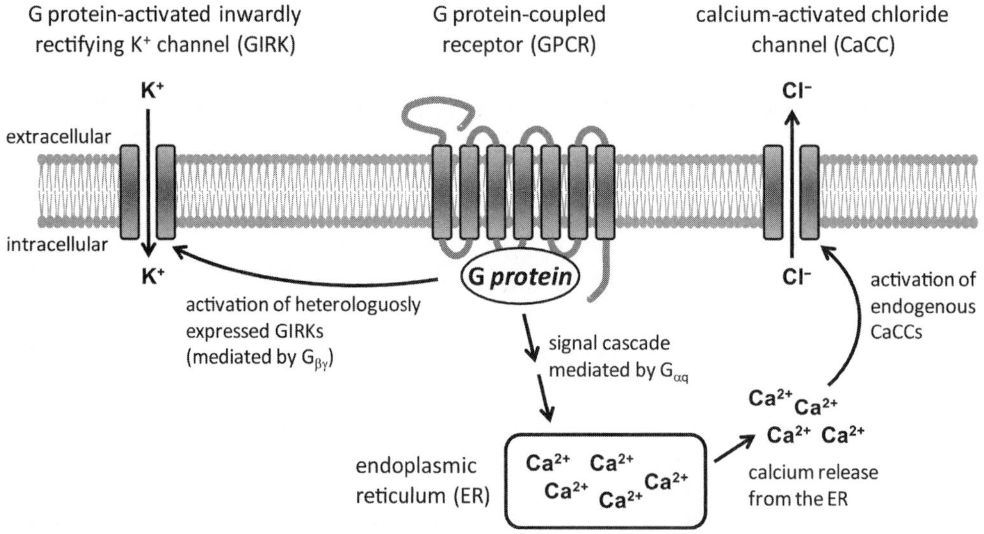

Fig. 1. GPCR-mediated activation of ion channels in *Xenopus* oocytes. GPCRs have been named based on their ability to recruit and regulate the activity of intracellular G proteins composed of three subunits; G_α, G_β, and G_γ. Briefly, the activated GPCR induces a conformational change in the G_α subunit of the associated G protein leading to release of GDP followed by binding of GTP *(36)*. Subsequently, the GTP-bound form of G_α dissociates from the receptor as well as from the stable $G_{\beta\gamma}$ dimer. Both the GTP-bound G_α and the released $G_{\beta\gamma}$ can modulate several cellular signaling pathways *(36–39)*. There are four main classes of G_α subunits; $G_{\alpha s}$ couples to stimulation of adenylyl cyclase; $G_{\alpha i}$ couples to inhibition of adenylyl cyclase; $G_{\alpha q}$ couples to the activation of phospholipase Cβ; and $G_{\alpha 12}$ couples to the activation of Rho guanine-nucleotide exchange factors *(38, 39)*. Activation of GPCRs that couple to the G_q signaling pathway will in turn result in release of calcium from the endoplasmic reticulum. The increased concentration of free calcium in the cytoplasm activates CaCCs that are endogenously expressed in *Xenopus* oocytes. Negatively charged Cl^- ions will then pass through the activated CaCCs, thereby producing a current across the membrane that can be monitored using two-electrode voltage-clamp electrophysiology. The released $G_{\beta\gamma}$ can directly activate GIRK channels that have been co-expressed with the GPCR of interest [only from G_i-coupled GPCRs *(39, 40)*]. However, GIRK only allow the positively charged K^+ ions to pass into the oocyte (i.e., inwardly rectifying), and therefore a specialized extracellular recording solution with high K^+ concentration is required in order to measure activation of these channels.

will result in release of intracellular calcium and in *Xenopus* oocytes; the increased concentration of free calcium in the cytoplasm will activate endogenous CaCCs. Negatively charged Cl^- ions will then pass through the activated CaCCs, thereby producing a current across the membrane that can be monitored using two-electrode voltage-clamp electrophysiology. It is possible to use *Xenopus* electrophysiology to study G_i-coupled GPCRs, if these are co-expressed with GIRK channels (*see* **Fig. 1**). The use of *Xenopus* electrophysiology in conjunction with GIRK channels will not be further discussed in this chapter; however, more information on this topic can be obtained from some of the several studies that have used GIRK expression in oocytes to study GPCRs (e.g., *16–20*).

The fact that only GPCRs that couple to the G_q signaling pathway are able to activate CaCCs in *Xenopus* oocytes does not necessarily limit the usefulness of this system as a general method for studying activation of GPCRs. It is now possible to direct the signal transduction pathway of most GPCRs to calcium release and thus activation of CaCCs using chimeric, mutated and/or promiscuous G proteins. G_i-coupled GPCRs have been successfully directed to calcium release in *Xenopus* oocytes by co-expression with a chimeric G_α subunit, $G_{\alpha q/i5}$ *(21)*. G_q-coupled GPCRs have also been successfully directed to the G_i signaling pathway and thus GIRK activation by co-expression with another chimeric G_α subunit, $G_{\alpha i3/q}$ *(17)*. To this end, co-expression with the bovine $G_{\alpha L2}$ subunit, a homologue of mouse $G_{\alpha 11}$, has been used in *Xenopus* oocytes to amplify GPCR signaling and thus increase electrophysiological responsiveness for some low expressing GPCRs *(22)*.

Expression in *Xenopus* oocytes is achieved by injecting *in vitro* transcribed RNA encoding the GPCR of interest (and, if necessary, the G protein) into the oocyte. Before synthesizing the RNA, the circular plasmid DNA is linearized by cutting with a restriction enzyme downstream of the open-reading frame encoding the GPCR. Prior to RNA transcription, this linearized DNA template is purified and cleansed from contaminants (e.g., RNases) preferentially using a phenol : chloroform extraction protocol (*see* **Note 5**). The principles of the *in vitro* RNA transcription described in this chapter have been carefully explained in several previous publications *(23–26)*. Finally, the RNA is injected into the cytoplasm of the oocyte *(23, 24, 27)*. Following incubation of the injected oocytes, the GPCR encoded by the injected RNA will usually be expressed at relatively high levels, allowing two-electrode voltage-clamp recordings of CaCC currents upon activation of the GPCR (*see* **Fig. 2**).

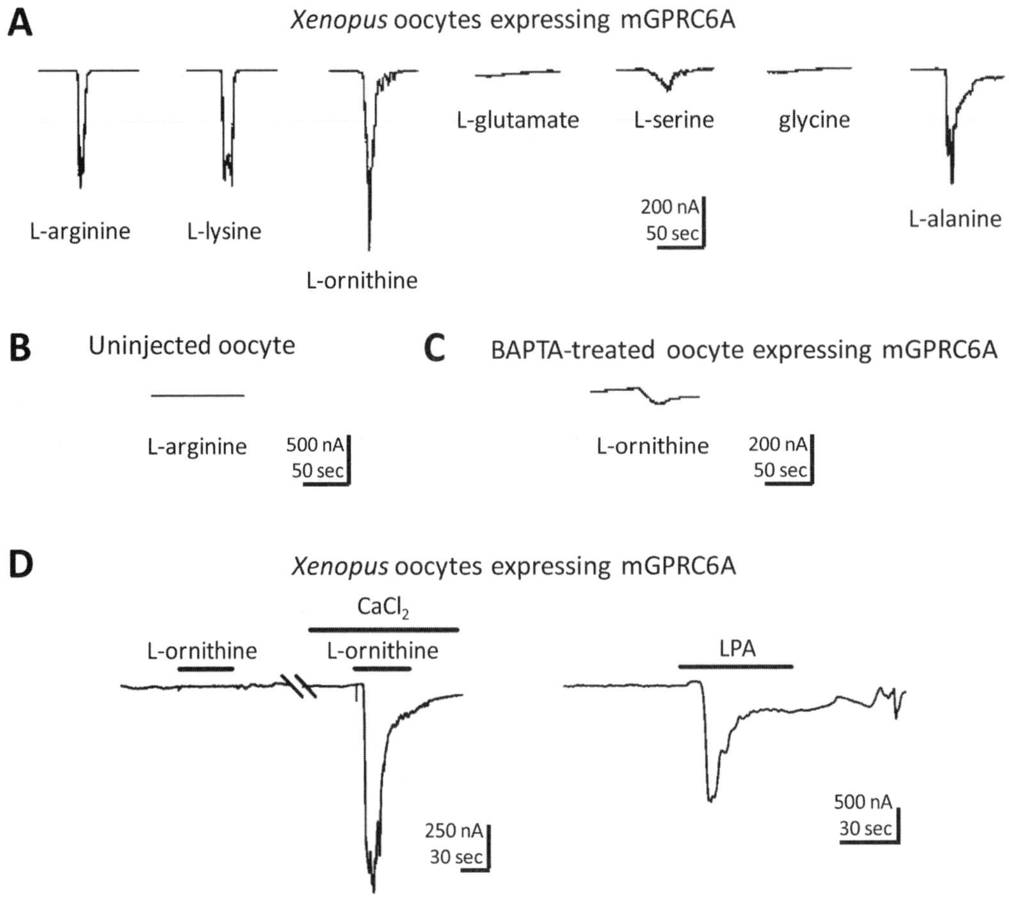

Fig. 2. Deorphanization and characterization of the GPCR termed GPRC6A from mouse (mGPRC6A) using *Xenopus* oocytes. (**A**) Traces of CaCC currents in *Xenopus* oocytes expressing mGPRC6A obtained using two-electrode voltage-clamping recordings at a holding potential of –80 mV. Strong activation of mGPRC6A was detected in response to application of L-arginine, L-lysine, and L-ornithine, whereas weaker activation was observed upon application of L-alanine and L-serine. No activation was observed upon application of L-glutamate and glycine. (**B**) Representative trace from an uninjected *Xenopus* oocyte showing that L-arginine does not activate CaCCs in the absence of mGPRC6A expression. In order to show that the responses shown in A) were indeed mediated by activation of mGPRC6A, all ligands were applied to uninjected oocytes. (**C**) Responsiveness to L-ornithine was severely attenuated when oocytes expressing mGPRC6A were treated with the calcium-chelator BAPTA-AM (100 μ*M*) prior to the recordings. This experiment demonstrates that intracellular calcium is necessary for mGPRC6A-mediated activation of CaCCs. (**D**) L-ornithine was unable to activate mGPRC6A in the absence of extracellular divalent cations (divalent cation-free extracellular recording solution was used). Co-application of L-ornithine and $CaCl_2$ restored mGPRC6A-mediated responses. Lysophosphatidic acid (LPA) was applied to mGPRC6A-expressing oocytes in the absence of extracellular divalent cations and was able to evoke responses at CaCCs through activation of endogenously expressed GPCRs. This demonstrates that the absence of extracellular divalent cations does not affect the function of CaCCs. All ligands in (A–D) were applied at 100 μ*M*, except $CaCl_2$ and LPA that were applied at 1.8 m*M* and 10 μ*M*, respectively.

3.1. Linearization of Plasmid DNA

1. Dilute 5–10 μg plasmid DNA in 200 μL of the suitable restriction enzyme buffer, add 20–40 units of restriction enzyme, and incubate 2–3 h at 37°C. Choose a restriction enzyme that leaves a 5′ protruding overhang (*see* **Note 5**).

2. Following the incubation at 37°C, add 1 volume (200 μL) buffer-saturated phenol to the 200 μL containing the linearized plasmid DNA. Shake for 5 min and centrifuge at 20,000 × *g* for 5 min.
3. Carefully remove the aqueous phase (top layer). Discard the organic phase. Add 1 volume (200 μL) phenol : chloroform : isoamyl alcohol to the 200 μL aqueous phase containing the linearized plasmid DNA. Shake for 5 min and centrifuge at 20,000 × *g* for 5 min.
4. Carefully remove the aqueous phase (top layer). Discard the organic phase. Add 1 volume (200 μL) chloroform to the 200 μL aqueous phase. Shake for 5 min and centrifuge at 20,000 × *g* for 5 min.
5. Carefully remove the aqueous phase (top layer) containing the linearized plasmid DNA and discard the organic phase. Add 1/10 volume (20 μL) 3 *M* sodium acetate, pH 5.2 (ice cold) and then add 2.5 volume (500 μL) 96–100 % ethanol (ice cold). Mix by vortexing (very briefly) and incubate 10 min on dry ice (or 30 min at –80°C).
6. Centrifuge at 20,000 × *g* for 30 min (4°C) and carefully remove the supernatant without disturbing the barely visible pellet containing the DNA. Add 200 μL 70% ethanol (ice cold). Do not resuspend. Centrifuge at 20,000 × *g* for 15 min (4°C).
7. Carefully remove the supernatant. Dry the pellet at room temperature or at 37–60°C for a couple of minutes. Do not over-dry, since this will make it difficult to resuspend the DNA.
8. Resuspend pellet in 5–10 μL TE buffer (*see* **Note 6**). Run 0.5 μL on an agarose gel to assess the concentration and the quality of the purified DNA. All plasmids should have been linearized and the DNA should appear as a single band on the gel (*see* **Note 7**). The concentration of DNA can be estimated by comparing band intensity with band intensities of a DNA ladder with known concentration. Store the linearized DNA template at –20°C.

3.2. In Vitro RNA Transcription

1. Prepare the reaction for RNA transcription using 2 μg linearized DNA template according to the instructions included in the mMESSAGE mMACHINE High Yield Capped RNA Transcription Kit (Ambion). Incubate the reaction at 37°C for 2 h.
2. Add 1 μL DNase (included in the transcription kit) to the reaction, mix carefully, and incubate at 37°C for 15 min. This step is required to remove the template DNA from the reaction prior to RNA precipitation.

3. Add 30 μL RNase-free water (included in the transcription kit) and 30 μL LiCl precipitation solution (included in the transcription kit), mix (do not vortex), and incubate at –20°C for ≥30 min.
4. Centrifuge for 15 min at 20,000 × *g* (4°C) to pellet the RNA. Carefully remove the supernatant. Carefully add 200 μL 70% ethanol (do not resuspend), and re-centrifuge for 15 min at 20,000 × *g* (4°C).
5. Carefully remove the 70% ethanol, briefly dry the RNA (37°C for a couple of minutes), and resuspend the RNA in 20 μL TE buffer (*see* **Note 6**). Run 1 μL on an agarose gel to assess the quality of the RNA. The RNA should appear as a single band on the gel (*see* **Note 7**). Keep RNA ice cold and RNase-free at all times and store at –80°C.

3.3. Expression of GPCRs in Xenopus Oocytes

1. Prepare injection pipettes using a standard pipette puller. The tips of the injection pipettes are broken under the stereomicroscope to an outer diameter of about 10–20 μm. Use gloves when handling injection pipettes and store the injection pipettes in an RNase-free environment.
2. Place the oocytes in the injection chamber containing Barth's solution. The oocytes can be manipulated using customized Pasteur pipettes.
3. Mount the injection pipette to the microinjector syringe according to the manufacturer's instructions. Back-fill the injection pipettes with mineral oil before mounting. The plunger will force oil out of the tip of the injection pipettes, which should result in a complete seal of oil between the tip and the plunger. Make sure there are no air bubbles in the injection pipette. The injection pipette can be moved and precisely positioned using a manual micromanipulator once it has been mounted to the microinjector syringe.
4. Transfer RNA to the injection pipette by placing a small volume, usually 2–3 μL, in the cap of a 1-mL microcentrifuge tube under the stereomicroscope and load it into the injection pipette using the microinjector. Watch the RNA solution as it is drawn into the injection pipette to ensure it has not been clogged and that there are no air bubbles in the injection pipette. Air bubbles in the injection pipette are constant hazards, since they will markedly increase variations in volume that is actually injected into the oocyte.
5. Place the injection chamber containing the oocytes under the stereomicroscope and inject the RNA by positioning the injection pipette over each oocyte and gently lowering the tip until it pierces the membrane. Some oocytes may leak after the injection pipette has been pulled back out of the

membrane. To allow proper diffusion of the RNA inside the oocyte, it is therefore advisable to wait 5–10 seconds after the RNA has been injected before retracting the injection pipette. Each oocyte can be injected with anywhere between 10 nL and as much as 100 nL RNA solution depending on the desired level of expression, which usually increase as more RNA is injected (*see* **Note 8**). We usually inject 50 nL, which means that 2 μL RNA solution is sufficient for injecting about 40 oocytes. Use a new injection pipette for each type of RNA to prevent cross-contamination and thus expression of the "wrong" protein.

6. Following the injection, place the oocyte in a petri dish containing Barth's solution and incubate at 18°C until the day of recording. Expression levels highly depend on the time and temperature of incubation (*see* **Note 8**).

3.4. Characterization of GPCRs using Electrophysiological Recordings

1. Make up ligand applications in extracellular recording solution. In order to perform the deorphanization experiment described in **Fig. 2A**, eight solutions were made. (1) wash (i.e., extracellular recording solution with no ligand), (2) 100 μ*M* L-arginine in extracellular recording solution, (3) 100 μ*M* L-lysine, (4) 100 μ*M* L-ornithine, (5) 100 μ*M* L-serine, (6) 100 μ*M* glycine, (7) 100 μ*M* L-alanine, and (8) 100 μ*M* L-glutamate. Apply the wash and ligand applications to the perfusion system of the two-electrode voltage-clamp setup and adjust the flow rates.
2. Place the injected oocyte in the recording chamber of the two-electrode voltage-clamp setup, penetrate the membrane with the two electrodes, and clamp the oocyte at the desired holding potential (i.e., membrane potential). Holding potentials in the range between –80 and –40 mV are suitable for recordings of GPCR-mediated activations of CaCCs.
3. Start the recording when the baseline current has stabilized and apply the ligand applications one at the time for a fixed time with a fixed interval between each application. GPCR-mediated activations of CaCCs are usually delayed by 10–20 seconds after the onset of the ligand application. About 30- to 60-second applications of each ligand should therefore be suitable to determine whether there is a response or not. It is recommended to allow 3–10 min intervals between each ligand application. In the event that a response is observed, the oocyte should be either replaced by a fresh oocyte or allowed to recover for at least 10 min, since GPCR-mediated activations of CaCCs exhibit strong desensitization (*see* **Note 9**). Independent of whether a response is observed or not, proper

control experiments must be designed in order to determine if the response is mediated by the GPCR of interest (*see* **Note 10**) or if the lack of response is caused by absence of GPCR expression (*see* **Note 11**).

4. Notes

1. An injection chamber is required in order to prevent oocytes from moving during injection. This can be achieved by gluing a polypropylene mesh to the bottom of a petridish. Alternatively, a chamber can be made by carving grooves in a silicone elastomer (e.g., Sylgard 184 silicone elastomer kit, World Precision Instruments), which has been applied to the bottom of a petridish.
2. Defolliculated healthy-looking stage V-VI oocytes are required for injection of RNA and subsequent expression of the receptor of interest. Oocytes are surgically removed from captive bred *Xenopus laevis* and treated with collagenase in order to remove the surrounding follicular layer. Maintenance and surgery of *X. laevis* as well as treatment, isolation, and selection of oocytes are described in, several publications that provide detailed protocols on these procedures *(23, 24, 27, 28)*.
3. In order to control the membrane potential, most electrophysiological recordings on oocytes are performed using a two-electrode voltage-clamp setup. The membrane potential is simply clamped to defined potentials using a feedback circuit, where an intracellular electrode records the actual intracellular potential and a second intracellular electrode passes the current needed to maintain the desired potential. The principles and design of the two-electrode voltage-clamp setup is described in detail elsewhere *(24)*.
4. The concentrations of divalent cations and the pH of the extracellular recording solution can be varied to meet special requirements of the receptor of interest *(15)*. Oocytes are stable during experiments using recording solutions without Mg^{2+} or without Ca^{2+}, but are unstable in the complete absence of divalent cations. Alternatively, Mg^{2+} and/or Ca^{2+} can be replaced by Ba^{2+}.
5. Several factors affect the ability to successfully express proteins in oocytes. In our experience, one of the more important factors is the choice of DNA template (i.e., vector, 5′ untranslated region (UTR), and 3′ UTR. The coding region should be cloned 3′ to an RNA polymerase promoter, either that

from SP6, T7, or T3 bacteriophage. The open-reading frame of most receptors can simply be inserted after the promoter for successful transcription and translation. However, expression may be increased by using a vector that has been designed specifically for expression in *Xenopus* oocytes, such as pGEMHE *(29)* or pXOOM *(30)*. These plasmids contain the *Xenopus* β-globin 5′ and 3′ UTRs, a T7 promoter on the 5′ end and a poly(A) tail on the 3′ end, which enhances stability and translatability of the RNA. The plasmid DNA should be linearized with a restriction enzyme that leaves a 5′ protruding overhang (or blunt end), since a 3′ protruding overhang can function as a primer for synthesis in the wrong direction, making antisense RNA that often interfere with translation. To increase the stability of the RNA, the site of linearization should be located after the poly(A) tail or 200–500 base pairs from the stop codon.

6. Resuspending dried DNA or RNA pellets may sometimes be difficult, especially if pellet has been over-dried. Patience and a great deal of pipetting are often required. If the DNA or RNA has not been properly resuspended, it may appear to be completely absent from the agarose gel.
7. The quality of the linearized DNA template critically affects the quality and the amount of transcribed RNA. It is important that the linearized DNA appear as a single band on the gel. The presence of higher order bands on the gel indicates that the DNA plasmid is not completely linearized. Using a partially linearized DNA template for RNA transcription will also produce higher order poorly-expressing RNA products, since the RNA polymerase will continue transcription on the DNA plasmid instead of producing several run-off transcripts. If the RNA does not appear as a single band on the gel, but rather appear as a smear, then there is likely breakdown of the RNA. This is often caused by the presence of RNases during transcription and/or in the RNA solution. To prevent contamination by RNases, it is important to always use cloves and preferentially filter tips when handling the template DNA and the RNA solutions.
8. Expression of GPCRs in *Xenopus* oocytes is influenced by several factors, and there are several ways to tweak the expression level to be more suitable for electrophysiological experiments. First of all, the time of incubation can be optimized. Some GPCRs are highly expressed already the day after injection and the following days, the expression level either declines rapidly or becomes too high for electrophysiological experiments. Other GPCR may require three or four days for sufficient expression. The time of incubation should therefore be optimized for each GPCR of interest. Secondly, the

temperature during incubation affects the GPCR expression. Expression may improve by leaving the oocyte at room temperature for a day and expression may come to a complete halt by incubation at 4°C. Thirdly, the level of expression usually increases as more RNA is injected. It is therefore highly recommended that the amount of injected RNA is optimized for each GPCR of interest (and for each batch of RNA). This optimization is usually achieved by keeping the injection volume constant and then titrating the amount of RNA by diluting the RNA solution with RNase-free water. Some GPCRs may require 10-fold or even 100-fold dilution of the RNA.

9. GPCR-mediated activations of CaCCs exhibit strong desensitization, presumably due to desensitization of the receptor itself, the CaCCs, and/or the proteins of the G_q signaling pathway proteins *(10, 31, 32)*. The strong desensitization, the random nature of the peak response, and the absence of steady state responses from CaCCs severely hamper quantification of the GPCR-mediated responses and thus generation of concentration-response relationships or comparison of responses from different ligands and oocytes (**Fig. 2**). Furthermore, the ability to detect GPCR activation highly depends on the expression level; activation of GPCRs that are expressed at very low levels may not result in intracellular calcium release of a sufficient magnitude as to activate CaCCs.
10. If CaCC activation is observed in response to application of a ligand, it is important to determine whether the response is indeed mediated by the GPCR of interest or an endogenous GPCR expressed in the oocyte. If no responses are observed upon application of the ligand to uninjected or water-injected non-expressing oocytes, then it can be safely concluded that the CaCC activation was mediated by the GPCR of interest (**Fig. 2**).
11. In the event that no CaCC responses are observed, it is important to determine whether the lack of response is caused by absence of GPCR surface expression, lack of functional CaCCs, or by lack of activity of the applied ligand. If a known activating ligand exists, then this ligand can be applied as a positive control for GPCR expression. If such a ligand has not yet been identified, then the only control for GPCR surface expressing may be Western blotting (*see 33, 34*). Application of 10 μM LPA will activate endogenously expressed G_q-coupled GPCRs in the oocyte *(35)*, and a response to this ligand will therefore demonstrate that functional CaCCs are present in the oocyte membrane (**Fig. 2**).

Acknowledgments

We would like to thank Associate Professor Petrine Wellendorph and Bolette Christiansen for sharing data from the deorphanization and characterization of GPRC6A. Our work has been supported by the Lundbeck Foundation, the Villum Kann Rasmussen Foundation, Fonden af 17-12-1981, and the Danish Medical Research Council.

References

1. Dixon, R. A., Kobilka, B. K., Strader, D. J., Benovic, J. L., Dohlman, H. G., Frielle, T., Bolanowski, M. A., Bennett, C. D., Rands, E., Diehl, R. E., Mumford, R. A., Slater, E. E., Sigal, I. S., Caron, M. G., Lefkowitz, R. J., and Strader, C. D. (1986) Cloning of the gene and cDNA for mammalian beta-adrenergic receptor and homology with rhodopsin. *Nature* **321**, 75–79.
2. Lefkowitz, R. J. (2004) Historical review: a brief history and personal retrospective of seven-transmembrane receptors. *Trends Pharmacol. Sci.* **25**, 413–422.
3. Wettschureck, N. and Offermanns, S. (2005) Mammalian G proteins and their cell type specific functions. *Physiol. Rev.* **85**, 1159–1204.
4. Wise, A., Jupe, S. C., and Rees, S. (2004) The identification of ligands at orphan G protein-coupled receptors. *Annu. Rev. Pharmacol. Toxicol.* **44**, 43–66.
5. Overington, J. P., Al-Lazikani, B., and Hopkins, A. L. (2006) How many drug targets are there? *Nat. Rev. Drug Discov.* **5**, 993–996.
6. Lagerström, M. C. and Schiöth, H. B. (2008) Structural diversity of G protein-coupled receptors and significance for drug discovery. *Nat. Rev. Drug Discov.* **7**, 339–357.
7. Chung, S., Funakoshi, T., and Civelli, O. (2008) Orphan GPCR research. *Br. J. Pharmacol.* **153**(Suppl 1), S339–S346.
8. Howard, A. D., McAllister, G., Feighner, S. D., Liu, Q., Nargund, R. P., Van der Ploeg, L. H., and Patchett, A. A. (2001) Orphan G protein-coupled receptors and natural ligand discovery. *Trends Pharmacol. Sci.* **22**, 132–140.
9. Speca, D. J., Lin, D. M., Sorensen, P. W., Isacoff, E. Y., Ngai, J., and Dittman, A. H. (1999) Functional identification of a goldfish odorant receptor. *Neuron* **23**, 487–498.
10. Wellendorph, P., Hansen, K. B., Balsgaard, A., Greenwood, J. R., Egebjerg, J., and Bräuner-Osborne, H. (2005) Deorphanization of GPRC6A: a promiscuous L-alpha-amino acid receptor with preference for basic amino acids. *Mol. Pharmacol.* **67**, 589–597.
11. Bächner, D., Kreienkamp, H., Weise, C., Buck, F., and Richter, D. (1999) Identification of melanin concentrating hormone (MCH) as the natural ligand for the orphan somatostatin-like receptor 1 (SLC-1). *FEBS Lett.* **457**, 522–524.
12. Lynch, K. R., O'Neill, G. P., Liu, Q., Im, D. S., Sawyer, N., Metters, K. M., Coulombe, N., Abramovitz, M., Figueroa, D. J., Zeng, Z., Connolly, B. M., Bai, C., Austin, C. P., Chateauneuf, A., Stocco, R., Greig, G. M., Kargman, S., Hooks, S. B., Hosfield, E., Williams, D. L., Jr., Ford-Hutchinson, A. W., Caskey, C. T., and Evans, J. F. (1999) Characterization of the human cysteinyl leukotriene CysLT1 receptor. *Nature* **399**, 789–793.
13. Birgül, N., Weise, C., Kreienkamp, H. J., and Richter, D. (1999) Reverse physiology in drosophila: identification of a novel allatostatin-like neuropeptide and its cognate receptor structurally related to the mammalian somatostatin/galanin/opioid receptor family. *EMBO J.* **18**, 5892–5900.
14. Kuang, D., Yao, Y., Wang, M., Pattabiraman, N., Kotra, L. P., and Hampson, D. R. (2003) Molecular similarities in the ligand binding pockets of an odorant receptor and the metabotropic glutamate receptors. *J. Biol. Chem.* **278**, 42551–42559.
15. Christiansen, B., Hansen, K. B., Wellendorph, P., and Bräuner-Osborne, H. (2007) Pharmacological characterization of mouse GPRC6A, an L-alpha-amino-acid receptor modulated by divalent cations. *Br. J. Pharmacol.* **150**, 798–807.

16. Corti, C., Restituito, S., Rimland, J. M., Brabet, I., Corsi, M., Pin, J. P., and Ferraguti, F. (1998) Cloning and characterization of alternative mRNA forms for the rat metabotropic glutamate receptors mGluR7 and mGluR8. *Eur. J. Neurosci.* **10**, 3629–3641.

17. Ohana, L., Barchad, O., Parnas, I., and Parnas, H. (2006) The metabotropic glutamate G protein-coupled receptors mGluR3 and mGluR1a are voltage-sensitive. *J. Biol. Chem.* **281**, 24204–24215.

18. Lingenhoehl, K., Brom, R., Heid, J., Beck, P., Froestl, W., Kaupmann, K., Bettler, B., and Mosbacher, J. (1999) Gamma-hydroxybutyrate is a weak agonist at recombinant GABA(B) receptors. *Neuropharmacology* **38**, 1667–1673.

19. Saugstad, J. A., Segerson, T. P., and Westbrook, G. L. (1996) Metabotropic glutamate receptors activate G protein-coupled inwardly rectifying potassium channels in Xenopus oocytes. *J. Neurosci.* **16**, 5979–5985.

20. Zhang, Q., Pacheco, M. A., and Doupnik, C. A. (2002) Gating properties of GIRK channels activated by $G_{\alpha 0}$- and $G_{\alpha i}$-coupled muscarinic m2 receptors in Xenopus oocytes: the role of receptor precoupling in RGS modulation. *J. Physiol.* **545**, 355–373.

21. Minami, K., Uezono, Y., Shiraishi, M., Okamoto, T., Ogata, J., Horishita, T., Taniyama, K., and Shigematsu, A. (2004) Analysis of the effects of halothane on G_i-coupled muscarinic M2 receptor signaling in Xenopus oocytes using a chimeric G alpha protein. *Pharmacology* **72**, 205–212.

22. Yamashita, S., Minakami, R., and Sugiyama, H. (1997) The G alpha protein GL2 alpha improves the ability to detect the subthreshold expressions of receptors linked to phospholipase C in Xenopus oocytes. *Jpn. J. Physiol.* **47**, 67–72.

23. Bossi, E., Fabbrini, M. S., and Ceriotti, A. (2007) Exogenous protein expression in Xenopus oocytes: basic procedures. *Methods Mol. Biol.* **375**, 107–131.

24. Stühmer, W. (1998) Electrophysiologic recordings from Xenopus oocytes. *Methods Enzymol.* **293**, 280–300.

25. Goldin, A. L. and Sumikawa, K. (1992) Preparation of RNA for injection into Xenopus oocytes. *Methods Enzymol.* **207**, 279–297.

26. Swanson, R. and Folander, K. (1992) In vitro synthesis of RNA for expression of ion channels in Xenopus oocytes. *Methods Enzymol.* **207**, 310–319.

27. Goldin, A. L. (1992) Maintenance of Xenopus laevis and oocyte injection. *Methods Enzymol.* **207**, 266–279.

28. Matten, W. T. and Vande Woude, G. F. (1995) Microinjection into Xenopus oocytes. *Methods Enzymol.* **254**, 458–466.

29. Liman, E. R., Tytgat, J., and Hess, P. (1992) Subunit stoichiometry of a mammalian K^+ channel determined by construction of multimeric cDNAs. *Neuron* **9**, 861–871.

30. Jespersen, T., Grunnet, M., Angelo, K., Klaerke, D. A., and Olesen, S. P. (2002) Dual-function vector for protein expression in both mammalian cells and Xenopus laevis oocytes. *Biotechniques* **32**, 536–538, 540.

31. Minakami, R., Katsuki, F., Yamamoto, T., Nakamura, K., and Sugiyama, H. (1994) Molecular cloning and the functional expression of two isoforms of human metabotropic glutamate receptor subtype 5. *Biochem. Biophys. Res. Commun.* **199**, 1136–1143.

32. Quick, M. W., Lester, H. A., Davidson, N., Simon, M. I., and Aragay, A. M. (1996) Desensitization of inositol 1,4,5-trisphosphate/Ca^{2+}-induced Cl^- currents by prolonged activation of G proteins in Xenopus oocytes. *J. Biol. Chem.* **271**, 32021–32027.

33. Everts, I., Petroski, R., Kizelsztein, P., Teichberg, V. I., Heinemann, S. F., and Hollmann, M. (1999) Lectin-induced inhibition of desensitization of the kainate receptor GluR6 depends on the activation state and can be mediated by a single native or ectopic N-linked carbohydrate side chain. *J. Neurosci.* **19**, 916–927.

34. Strutz, N., Villmann, C., Thalhammer, A., Kizelsztein, P., Eisenstein, M., Teichberg, V. I., and Hollmann, M. (2001) Identification of domains and amino acids involved in GluR7 ion channel function. *J. Neurosci.* **21**, 401–411.

35. Guo, Z., Liliom, K., Fischer, D. J., Bathurst, I. C., Tomei, L. D., Kiefer, M. C., and Tigyi, G. (1996) Molecular cloning of a high-affinity receptor for the growth factor-like lipid mediator lysophosphatidic acid from Xenopus oocytes. *Proc. Natl. Acad. Sci. USA* **93**, 14367–14372.

36. Hamm, H. E. (1998) The many faces of G protein signaling. *J. Biol. Chem.* **273**, 669–672.

37. Clapham, D. E. and Neer, E. J. (1997) G protein beta gamma subunits. *Annu. Rev. Pharmacol. Toxicol.* **37**, 167–203.

38. Kristiansen, K. (2004) Molecular mechanisms of ligand binding, signaling, and regulation within the superfamily of G protein-coupled receptors: molecular modeling and mutagenesis approaches to receptor structure and function. *Pharmacol. Ther.* **103**, 21–80.

39. Pierce, K. L., Premont, R. T., and Lefkowitz, R. J. (2002) Seven-transmembrane receptors. *Nat. Rev. Mol. Cell Biol.* **3**, 639–650.

40. Clapham, D. E. (1994) Direct G protein activation of ion channels? *Annu. Rev. Neurosci.* **17**, 441–464.

Chapter 26

Immunoprecipitation and Phosphorylation of G Protein-Coupled Receptors

Walter G. Thomas

Summary

G protein-coupled receptors (GPCRs) are integral membrane proteins with seven transmembrane-spanning α-helices. Following ligand activation, many GPCRs are rapidly phosphorylated on serine/threonine residues in their cytoplasmic domains, principally the carboxyl-terminus. GPCR phosphorylation recruits arrestin proteins to the activated receptor leading to receptor internalization and desensitization. Arrestins also act as scaffolds to recruit other regulatory and signaling molecules to the receptor. The low level of expression of GPCRs in tissues, the difficulty in developing antibodies that can specifically detect and harvest receptor protein, and the hydrophobic and heterogeneric nature of GPCRs makes examination of their structure, function, and biology an interesting challenge. Receptor phosphorylation is typically performed in cells transfected with wild and mutated receptors usually bearing an epitope tag and equilibrated with [^{32}Pi] to radiolabel cellular ATP pools. Following ligand stimulation, receptor protein is extracted using a detergent lysis buffer and immunoprecipitated with antibodies raised against the epitope tag; following separation on SDS-polyacrylamide gel electrophoresis, phosphorylated receptors are quantified using phosphorimaging.

Key words: G protein-coupled receptors (GPCRs), Phosphorylation, GPCR kinases (GRKs), Immunoprecipitation, Phosphorimaging.

1. Introduction

G protein-coupled receptors (GPCRs) are the largest superfamily of receptors in the human genome with about ~900 genes predicted *(1, 2)*. These receptors impinge on most aspects of human physiology by responding to an amazing variety of stimuli – including, ions, light, bioamines,

Wayne R. Leifert (ed.), *G Protein-Coupled Receptors in Drug Discovery, vol. 552*

Book doi: 10.1007/978-1-60327-317-6_26

nucleotides, lipids, odors, tastes, amino acids, peptides, and proteins. Perception and binding of a specific ligand leads to conformational changes in the GPCR that allows it to activate heterotrimeric guanine-nucleotide binding proteins (G proteins), which in turn activate various signal transduction pathways *(3)*. It is now appreciated that these receptors also function via alternative, complex protein–protein interactions, by trans-activating and modulating other receptors and channels and potentially by homo- and hetero-dimerization *(4)*.

Following activation, initial receptor signaling is usually quickly desensitized by a series of events at the levels of the receptor. Principal among these is the rapid phosphorylation of the receptor in its cytoplasmic regions by serine/threonine kinases that are activated by the signal generated by the receptor (e.g., protein kinase C or protein kinase A) or by recognizing the agonist-occupied, activated GPCR conformation (the GPCR kinases or GRKs) *(5)*. Phosphorylated receptors are bound by regulatory proteins termed arrestins, which sterically hinder further G protein activation and also interact with the cellular internalization machinery to mediate receptor endocytosis *(5–7)*. Arrestins are also now well recognized as scaffolding protein to activate secondary and tertiary receptor activities during the process of receptor trafficking *(8)*. Thus, receptor phosphorylation is central to determining the timing and co-ordination of GPCR signals and activities. Many GPCRs contain clusters of serine and threonine residues within their third cytoplasmic loop or carboxyl-terminus with multiple possible phosphorylation events, yet examples where the exact site and hierarchy of phosphorylation has been elucidated for a GPCR are relatively few. Also uncommon is the demonstration of agonist-driven phosphorylation of endogenously expressed GPCRs – the diminishingly low level of GPCR expression coupled with inherent difficulties in raising antibodies of high affinity, selectivity, and avidity has hindered progress in this area.

Demonstrating GPCR phosphorylation requires the following: labeling of the phosphorylated receptor, its isolation from the membrane, and purification and separation on SDS-polyacrylamide gel electrophoresis (SDS-PAGE). Antibodies capable of specific and quantitative detecting and harvesting the receptors and capable of detecting are not universally available and so techniques have developed for expressing epitope-tagged versions, which allow immunoprecipitation (using commercially available antibodies) and phosphorylation of wild-type and mutated receptors. Most studies have utilized transiently transfected receptors in cultured cells, where receptors are labeled with [^{32}P] and resolved and detected following SDS-PAGE.

2. Materials

2.1. Cell Culture, Transfection/Infection, and [^{32}P] Labeling

1. Dulbecco's Modified Eagle's Medium (DMEM, Invitrogen, Carlsbad, California, USA) supplemented with 10% fetal bovine serum (FBS, Invitrogen) and antibiotic/antimycotic (× 100 stock, Invitrogen).
2. Opti-MEM serum-free medium (Invitrogen).
3. Lipofectamine (Invitrogen).
4. 12-well culture plates (Falcon 3043 Multiwell 12-well polystyrene).
5. DMEM (phosphate-free) ((-Pi)DMEM) (MP Biomedicals, Solon, Ohio, USA).
6. ortho-^{32}P: 10 μCi/μL (MP Biomedicals) (*see* **Note 1**).

2.2. Agonist Stimulation, Cell Lysis, and Sample Handling

1. Phosphatase inhibitors: 0.5 m*M* okadaic acid (Invitrogen); 1 *M* sodium fluoride (0.42 g in 10 mL H_2O, store 1 mL aliquots at –20°C); 10 m*M* sodium pyrophosphate (*see* **Note 2**).
2. Angiotensin II: (Auspep, Melbourne, human AngII) 1 m*M* solution is prepared by dissolving 1 mg of AngII in 956 μL of 10 m*M* acetic acid. 50 μL aliquots stored frozen at –20°C.
3. Prepare a Styrofoam tray (~50 × 25 × 10 cm) filled with crushed ice on top of which is placed a perforated metal tray (40 × 20 cm × 2 mm thick) used to cool and support wads of water-soaked Whatman paper No. 1 (0.5 mm thick, cut to 12 × 8 cm).
4. An aspirator (water- or pump-driven) attached to a piece of flexible plastic tubing. We break a 2-mL plastic serological Pipette (Falcon BD Biosciences, San Jose, California, USA) and discard the plugged end and insert into the tubing. This is only used to aspirate non-radioactive material (*see* **Note 3**).
5. Disposable 3-mL plastic Pasteur pipettes (Fusion Scientific Melbourne, Victoria, Australia).
6. Standard phosphate buffered saline (PBS) for washing cells.
7. Plastic bags (30 × 15 cm).
8. Radioactive monitor (e.g., Cypher Survey instrument Model 5000, Health Physics Instruments).
9. Cell lysis buffer: 50 m*M* Tris-HCl pH 7.5, 150 m*M* NaCl, 5 μg/mL leupeptin, 1 μg/mL aprotinin, 1 m*M* phenylmethylsulfonyl fluoride (PMSF), 1 μg/mL pepstatin, 4 mg/mL n-dodecyl μ-maltoside (Sigma) and 0.5 mg/mL cholesteryl hemisuccinate (Sigma), store in aliquots at –20°C (*see* **Note 4**).

10. Wash buffer 1: 50 m*M* Tris-HCl, pH 7.5, 150 m*M* NaCl, 1% Triton X-100, 0.5% sodium deoxycholate, 5 μg/mL leupeptin, 1 μg/mL aprotinin, 1 m*M* PMSF, 0.7 μg/mL pepstatin, 1 m*M* ethylenediaminetetraacetic acid.
11. Wash buffer 2 (high salt): 50 m*M* Tris-HCl, pH 7.5, 500 m*M* NaCl, 0.1% Triton X-100, 0.05% sodium deoxycholate.
12. Wash buffer 3 (low salt): 50 m*M* Tris-HCl, pH 7.5, 0.1% Triton X-100, 0.05% sodium deoxycholate.
13. Immunoprecipitation wash buffers – wash buffers 1, 2, and 3 are modified from those described in Roche Applied Science protein A-agarose specification sheet describing immunoprecipitation using protein A-agarose.

2.3. SDS-PAGE and Phosphoimaging

1. Prepare or purchase 10% running/4% stacking SDS-PAGE gels and prepare standard SDS-PAGE running buffer: × 5 stock, 15.1 g Tris base, 72.0 g glycine, 5.0 g sodium dodecyl sulfate (SDS) to 1,000 mL with H_2O (*see* **Note 5**).
2. UREA-based SDS sample buffer (*see* **Note 6**). Weigh out 18.02 g of urea, add 10 mL of 10% SDS, 200 μL of bromophenol blue solution (20 mg/mL), 6.25 mL of 0.5 *M* Tris-HCl, pH 6.8. Add H_2O to give 35 mL total volume and dissolve. Add 5 mL β-mercaptoethanol and 10 mL glycerol. Mix and store as 1 mL aliquots at –20°C. This sample contains 62.5 mM Tris-HCl, pH 6.8, 2% SDS, 10% mercaptoethanol, 6 *M* urea, and 20% glycerol.
3. Gel-fixing solution: 10% acetic acid, 20% methanol in H_2O; to 700 mL of water add 200 mL of methanol and 100 mL of acetic acid; mix and store at room temperature.
4. Vacuum-based Gel dryer (e.g., Hoefer GD2000 Vacuum gel-drying system).
5. Western blotting apparatus (e.g., Biorad Transblot or Hoefer SE600-15-15).
6. A phosphorimager is required to quantify the incorporation of [^{32}P] into the receptor protein. Originally, we used a FUJIX Bio-imaging Analyzer BAS 1000 (Fuji Photo Film Co., Ltd., Tokyo, Japan) with Fuji-type BAS-IIIs phosphor-imaging plates but we have also used a Molecular Dynamics Typhoon 9200 Variable Mode Imager (Sunnyvale, CA, USA). Alternatively, radioactive proteins can be visualized by exposing dried gels to X-ray film (e.g., Kodak BioMax MS 8294985), although this is not quantitative.
7. TST (× 5 stock): 60.6 g Tris, 292.2 g NaCl in 2000 mL H_2O, pH to 8.8 with HCl and add 2 mL Tween-20. Final concentrations are 50 m*M* Tris, 500 m*M* NaCl, 0.1% Tween-200.

3. Methods

The method for determining phosphorylation of GPCRs is a three-part process. Firstly, cells are transfected with epitope-tagged receptors by standard protocols; secondly, cells are incubated with radioactive inorganic phosphate to produce cellular [^{32}P]ATP and then stimulated with ligand to activate the receptor and promote its phosphorylation; and finally, labeled receptors are extracted, immunoprecipitated, resolved on SDS-PAGE, and quantified using a Phosphorimager.

We routinely use the angiotensin type 1 receptor (AT1R) as a positive control for expression, immunoprecipitation, and phosphorylation *(9, 10)*. AT1R is rapidly and robustly phosphorylated following AngII stimulation *(11, 12)*; the receptor contains 13 serine/threonine residues in its carboxyl-terminus, and we have shown using site-directed mutagenesis *(9)* that the central region of the carboxyl-terminus (residues 332–338) is the major, if not sole, site of ligand-driven phosphorylation *(13)*. In our experience, commercial antibodies against the AT1R (and for GPCRs generally) need to be used with a degree of caution. We have successfully immunoprecipitated the AT1R using epitope-tagged version (HA, FLAG, Myc epitopes at either the N- or the C-terminus), but we are unable to replicate this with commercial antibodies raised against portions of the receptor amino acid sequence. In regard to epitope-tagging GPCRs, we test empirically whether one epitope tag or multiple concatenated tags are required for efficient immunoprecipitation – with the AT1R, one HA tag at either the N- or the C-terminus is sufficient. As we prefer to epitope-tag at the N-terminus [to avoid affecting the phosphorylation/regulatory event(s) at the carboxyl-terminus], we also mutated one of three N-linked glycosylation sites in the receptor (i.e., Asn^4 was mutated to glutamic acid) to provide unhindered access to the epitope tag by antibody *(10, 11)*. It is important to test that the modified receptor retains a capacity to be efficiently expressed at the cell surface and retains an appropriate pharmacology and functional activity compared to the untagged wild-type receptor.

3.1. Transfection

1. Receptors can be transfected into a variety of cell lines (HEK293, CHO-K1, COS-7). The choice is made based on the relevance to the receptor being studied. Ideally the expression of endogenous receptor should be low and transfected receptors should display features consistent with the receptor in its natural setting (e.g., affinity, signaling). We routinely use CHO-K1 cells for transfecting the AT1R.

2. We maintain stock cultures of CHO-K1 cells in 100 mm plates and passage them via standard trypsinization procedures. For phosphorylation experiments, we plate the cells into 12-well culture plates to give 80–90% confluence the following day with each well giving one data point.
3. Cells are transfected with either vector alone (negative control) or plasmid encoding the epitope-tagged receptor by standard procedures and allowed to express receptor for 36–48 h prior to starting the experiment (*see* **Notes** 7 and **8**).
4. 24–30 h post-transfection cells are washed with serum-free DMEM and incubated in 1 mL/well serum-free DMEM overnight.

3.2. [^{32}P] Loading of ATP Pools and Receptor Stimulation

When using radioactivity, work behind perspex screens at all times (*see* **Note 1**). To prepare for experiment, get ice tray ready; check storage container for liquid radioactivity; place Benchroll (Kleenex 2911, 41.5 cm wide) in areas where radioactivity will be handled; Perspex incubation box should be wiped down with ethanol and placed in incubator with lid ajar to allow equilibration with temperature, humidity, and CO_2. Scan all areas and equipment with monitor to ensure that it is non-contaminated.

Preparing radioactivity: to 4.8 mL (-Pi) DMEM in a 50-mL Falcon tube placed in a Perspex-holding box, add 96 μl (960 μCi) of ortho-[^{32}Pi] to get 80 μCi per 0.4 mL. This is enough for loading one 12-well plate.

Preparing lysis buffer: thaw one 5 mL vial of lysis buffer, add 50 μL 1 *M* sodium fluoride, 22.5 mg sodium pyrophosphate. Allow to dissolve (~15 min) with a gentle rocking motion. Place on ice.

1. On the morning of the experiment (36–44 h post-transfection), wash cells once with 1 mL (-Pi) DMEM.
2. Aspirate and add 0.4 mL (-Pi) DMEM containing 80 μCi ortho-[^{32}P] freshly diluted as above to each well.
3. Remove perspex box (pre-equilibrated in cell culture incubator) and place the 12-well plate in it. Return to incubator for 2 h.
4. Dilute AngII stock (10^{-3} *M*) 10 μL into 990 μL (-Pi) DMEM to give 10^{-5} *M* working solution. Just prior to stimulation, to add 4 μL of 0.5 m*M* okadaic acid stock to 4 mL of chilled lysis buffer (containing sodium fluoride/sodium pyrophosphate), final okadaic acid concentration equals 0.5 μ*M*. Mix and return to ice.
5. Remove Perspex box and plate from incubator and stimulate cells as required (e.g., add 44 μL of 10^{-5} *M* AngII working solution per well to give 10^{-6} *M*, final concentration) and return to Perspex box in incubator for 10 min at 37°C (*see* **Note 9**).

3.3. Cell Lysis, Receptor Extraction, Immunoprecipitation, and SDS-PAGE

1. Place plate(s) to wet paper pads chilled on ice and rapidly remove supernatants using disposable 3 mL Pasteur pipettes and wash twice with 1 mL ice-cold PBS. Remove solutions from AngII-stimulated wells first to minimize differences in stimulation.
2. Add 300 μL of ice-cold lysis buffer to each well on ice.
3. Rock gently in cold room behind dedicated Perspex screen for 1 h.
4. Transfer lysates to Sarstedt screw-capped, sealed Sarstedt microtubes (*see* **Note 10**).
5. Centrifuge full speed (10,000 × g) for 15 min in cold room.
6. Transfer supernatants to fresh tubes containing 10 μl of Protein-A Agarose and 10 μl of 6 % BSA stock (final concentration = 0.2%) (*see* **Note 11**).
7. Rock tubes for 1 h in cold room (*see* **Note 12**).
8. Centrifuge 20 sec 10,000 × g to pellet agarose beads.
9. Transfer the supernatants to fresh tubes containing anti-HA antibody (we use affinity purified 12CA5 monoclonal antibody to a peptide epitope derived from the hemagglutinin protein of human influenza virus (Roche Applied Science, Castle Hill, NSW, Australia; 1–2 μg/tube) and 20 μL of protein-A Agarose (Roche Applied Science).
10. Rock overnight in cold room. Remove tubes to small esky filled with ice.
11. Pellet agarose beads by centrifugation (20 sec, 10,000 × g) and carefully remove supernatant with a 1-mL pipette. Be careful not to disturb the beads which can be hard to see; typically ~50 μL of solution is left above the beads. Add 1 mL wash buffer 1 (4°C), recap tubes, and rock for 5 min; repeat wash step with another 1 mL of wash buffer 1.
12. Wash beads twice with 1 mL wash buffer 2 (4°C)
13. Wash beads once with 1 mL wash buffer 3 (4°C) and remove the supernatant as above. After this, recap and recentrifuge the tubes to pellet beads. The remaining solution (~50 μL) is carefully removed using a gel-loading tip (Quality Scientific Plastics Petaluma, California, USA) (*see* **Note 13**).
14. To final pellet, add 55 μL of urea-based SDS sample buffer; heat at 60°C for 15 min; pellet beads; and load 50 μl per lane being careful not to include beads.
15. Run 10% SDS-PAGE under standard condition to separate proteins until dye front is 1–2 cm from bottom of plate.

16. Fix gel for 1 h by gentle agitation in 200 mL of gel-fixing solution; replace after 30 min.
17. Dry the gel onto Whatman filter paper using a vacuum gel dryer for 2 h.

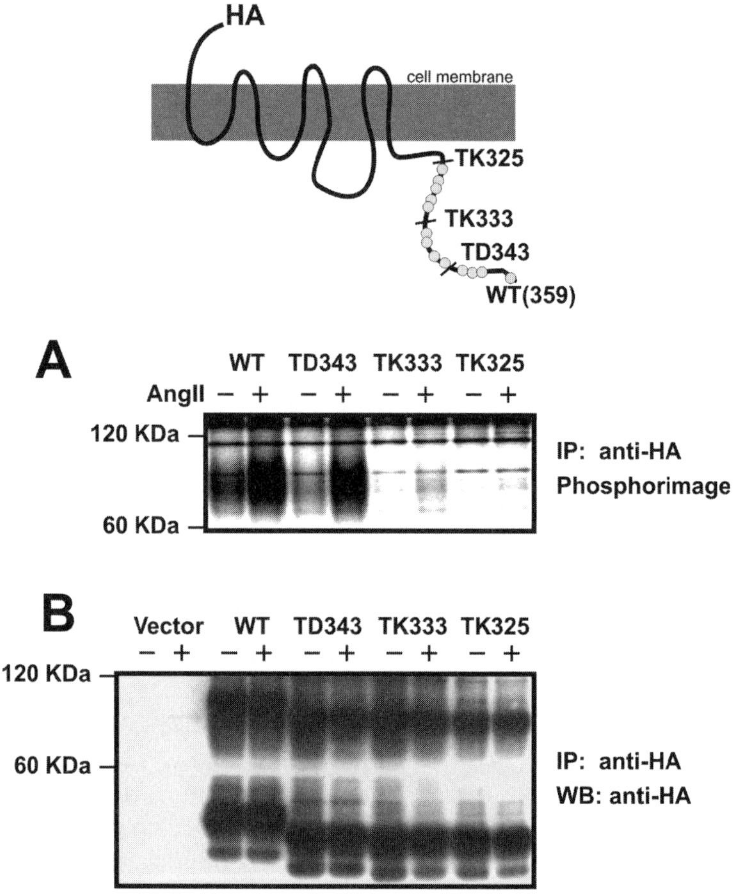

Fig. 1. The AT1R carboxyl-terminus is the site of AngII-mediated phosphorylation. The wild-type AT_{1A} receptor is 359 amino acids and shown (at top) is this receptor with an HA-epitope tag at the N-terminus to permit immunoprecipitation. Thirteen carboxyl-terminal serine and threonine residues are shown as circles and the position of truncations after Asp^{343} (TD343), Lys^{333} (TK333), and Lys^{325} (TK325) are indicated. (**A**) Receptor phosphorylation – CHO-K1 cells were co-transfected with HA-tagged wild-type AT_{1A} receptor (WT) or various truncated versions of the receptor (TD343, TK333, and TK325) and receptor phosphorylation determined by incorporation of ^{32}P into receptors following AngII-stimulation (100 n*M*, 10 min) and immunoprecipitation, SDS-PAGE and phosphorimaging. (**B**) Immunoprecitation and Western blot – cells were transfected with vector, WT or truncated receptor mutants, immunoprecipitated for the HA tag using 12CA5, and probed with 3F10 to detect receptor expression. The receptor protein is resolved as a faster migrating immature form and the mature glycosylated form ((60–120 KDa), which is expressed at the cell surface and phosphorylated following AngII stimulation (100 n*M*, 10 min) (see part A). Reproduced and modified from Qian *et al.* *Molecular Endocrinology* 15:1706–1719, 2001 (**Fig. 4**) *(9)* with permission of The Endocrine Society.

3.4. Phosphorimaging and Quantification

1. Wrap gel in thin plastic wrap (this is to protect moisture-sensitive phosphorimaging plates) and oppose against phosphorimaging plate overnight.
2. Protecting plate from light, develop phosphorimaging plate and follow software directions for locating radioactive bands and quantifying.
3. As a guide, we usually set an area outside the lanes of the gel as background and subtract from values obtained for receptor bands. Receptor bands are often broad reflecting a high degree of glycosylation (**Figs. 1** and **2**).

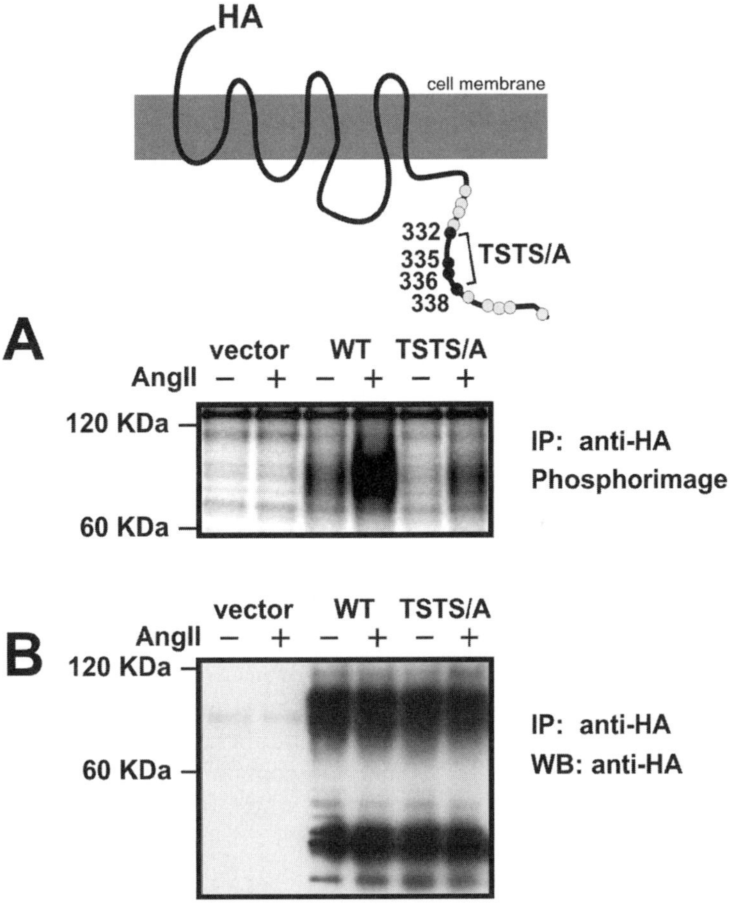

Fig. 2. Phosphorylation of the central region of the AT1R carboxyl-terminus. CHO-K1 cells were transfected with vector, HA-tagged wild-type AT1R (WT) or a mutated version of the receptor where serine and threonine residues at positions 332, 335, 336, and 338 were substituted with alanine (TSTS/A). (**A**) Receptor phosphorylation was determined by incorporation of ^{32}P into receptors following AngII-stimulation (100 n*M*, 10 min) and immunoprecipitation, SDS-PAGE and phosphorimaging. Quantification revealed >80% reduction in phosphorylation for TSTS/A, despite equivalent receptor expression compared to WT (**B**). Reproduced and modified from Qian *et al. Molecular Endocrinology* 15:1706–1719, 2001 (**Fig. 5**) *(9)* with permission of The Endocrine Society.

3.5. Alternative Western Blotting to Confirm Receptor Expression

1. After Step 15 of **Section 3.3** (above), alternatively, the gels can be Western transferred to PVDF membrane (Millipore Immobilin-FP transfer membrane) using standard protocols.
2. We block for 2 h at room temperature in 5% milk powder and 1% Tween-20 in TST. Add extra tween-20 and milk powder fresh.
3. Wash blot 3 times 15 min with agitation in × 1 TST.
4. For detecting 12CA5 immunoprecipitated HA-tagged receptors, we probe with an anti-HA antibody raised in a species other than mouse. We routinely use a rat monoclonal anti-HA high-affinity antibody (clone 3F10, Roche Applied Science). Dilute 1:1,000 to 1:3,000 in TST-5%Milk/1%Tween-20. Add to blot in a sealed plastic bag and incubate at 4°C overnight.
5. Wash blot 3 times 15 min with agitation in × 1 TST.
6. Add anti-rat IgG-HRP 1:5,000–1:10,000 in × 1 TST; incubate 45 min at room temperature.
7. Wash blot 3 times 15 min with agitation in × 1 TST.
8. Develop using standard Enhance Chemiluminescence (**Figs. 1** and **2**).

4. Notes

1. [^{32}P] should be handled under standard radioactive procedures mandated by the relevant Institution. As a general guide, only licensed and trained personnel should undertake the experiment; inexperienced staff should be closely supervised at all times; double-glove and check outer glove regularly for contamination using a monitor specific for beta emitters; where possible work behind a perspex screen and contain cell culture plates in a perspex box when incubating and transporting; replace gloves as required; check workbench, hood, pipettes, centrifuges, and other areas prior to commencing the protocol; monitor constantly during procedures and again at the end of the experiment. Decontaminate any work surface or equipment immediately using tissues soaked in Decon90 (Decon Laboratories Ltd., Hove, Sussex, England). We dedicate a set of pipettes and a bench centrifuge for radioactivity work. All tips, tissues, and other consumables contaminated with radioactivity are contained within a double plastic bag (30 × 15 cm) held in a Perspex holder. All

radioactivity in liquid form is contained in a 2.5-L plastic screw top bottle contained within a Perspex holder. Once full, it is stored behind Perspex for 1 year (~30 half-lives) and then disposed of down sink in fumehood.

2. Water refers to milliQ grade water (resistivity 18.2 MΩ-cm).
3. Only non-radioactive solutions are removed from plates using the aspirator. All radioactive solutions are pipetted by hand to prevent the generation of radioactive aerosols.
4. We mainly use two types of detergent-based cell lysis solutions – one is standard RIPA lysis buffer and the other is based on the detergents, n-dodecyl β-maltoside, and cholesteryl hemisuccinate. Both lysis buffers work well for extracting GPCRs and seem compatible with many antibodies. Nevertheless, they need to be tested empirically for a specific receptor and immunoprecipitating antibody. PMSF stock solution is prepared in methanol.
5. It is assumed SDS-PAGE gel rigs and powerpacks are available. We routinely use 1.5 mm thick gels in the large gel format (15 × 15 cm) plates with well-forming combs capable of holding the 55-μL sample. Smaller gel formats can be used but volumes need to be scaled to fit well sizes.
6. This sample buffer is critical for successful resolution of the highly hydrophobic GPCRs in SDS-PAGE. Samples should be heated at 60°C for 15 min (never boil samples which aggregates hydrophobic proteins), briefly centrifuged to retrieve the sample and pellet agarose beads, and loaded immediately without storage or freeze-thawing.
7. Before embarking on phosphorylation experiments, which require exposure to radioactivity, we confirm that the procedures described will efficiently extract and immunopurify the receptor. To test this, we undertake the immunoprecipitation without radioactivity and perform a Western transfer and probe this to detect the receptor protein. As an example, with our HA-tagged AT1R, we immunoprecipitated with the 12CA5 mouse monoclonal antibody and probed the Western with the anti-HA rat monoclonal (clone 3F10, Roche Applied Science) and an anti-rat IgG-horseradish peroxidise-based ECL detection. We include untransfected controls to ensure transfected receptor can be specifically immunoprecipitated and detected (**Figs. 1** and **2**).
8. Typically, we transfect 0.6 μg plasmid per well using 4.8 μL Lipofectamine. For this, 0.6 μg plasmid is diluted in 60 μL OPTI-MEM and mixed with 4.8 μL Lipofectamine also diluted in 60 μL OPTI-MEM. After 20 min, the complexes are dilute with the addition of 480 μL OPTI-MEM and the 600 μL total volume added to wells containing cells (wash

once with 1 mL OPTI-MEM to remove serum-containing media). After 5 h, the transfection reaction is aspirated and cells are then grown in 1 mL of DMEM+10%FBS.

9. Various doses and times of ligand stimulation are required to determine the kinetics of phosphorylation and optimal conditions for maximal phosphorylation.
10. Sarstedt o-ring sealed centrifuge tubes are absolutely required to prevent radioactive contamination during centrifugation and handling.
11. To accurately pipette agarose beads, mix beads frequently while pipetting and use pipette tips that have had 2–3 mm of the tip cut off to prevent blocking.
12. This step reduces non-specific binding of radiolabeled cell proteins in subsequent steps of immunoprecipitation procedure.
13. A steady hand is required to remove the last traces of wash buffer without disturbing the pellet of agarose beads. The technique we use is to steady the pipetting arm by resting the elbow on bench and using the index finger from the hand holding the tube to rest against the barrel of the pipetter and assist with control. By gently tipping the tube and locating the tip just above the beads residual solution can be accurately and consistently removed.

Acknowledgments

The author would like to thank Dr Hongwei Qian for his expertise in developing and optimizing the procedures described in the chapter. This work was supported via a project grant (418921) and Senior Research Fellowship (317814) from the National Health and Research Council of Australia.

References

1. Takeda S., Kadowaki S., Haga T., Takaesu H., Mitaku S. (2002) Identification of G protein-coupled receptor genes from the human genome sequence. *FEBS Lett.* **520**, 97–101.
2. Zhang Y., Devries M.E., Skolnick J. (2006) Structure modeling of all identified G protein-coupled receptors in the human genome. *PLoS. Comput. Biol.* **2**, e13.
3. Luttrell L.M. (2008) Reviews in molecular biology and biotechnology: transmembrane signaling by G protein-coupled receptors. *Mol. Biotechnol.* **39**, 239–264.
4. Pin J.P., Neubig R., Bouvier M., et al. (2007) International Union of Basic and Clinical Pharmacology. LXVII. Recommendations for the recognition and nomenclature of G protein-coupled receptor heteromultimers. *Pharmacol. Rev.* **59**, 5–13.
5. Reiter E., Lefkowitz R.J. (2006) GRKs and beta-arrestins: roles in receptor silencing,

trafficking and signaling. *Trends Endocrinol. Metab.* **17**, 159–165.

6. Lefkowitz R.J., Rajagopal K., Whalen E.J. (2006) New roles for beta-arrestins in cell signaling: not just for seven-transmembrane receptors. *Mol. Cell* **24,** 643–652.
7. Lefkowitz R.J., Whalen E.J. (2004) beta-arrestins: traffic cops of cell signaling. *Curr. Opin. Cell Biol.* **16**, 162–168.
8. Shenoy S.K., Lefkowitz R.J. (2005) Seven-transmembrane receptor signaling through beta-arrestin. *Sci. STKE.* **2005**, cm10.
9. Qian H., Pipolo L., Thomas W.G. (2001) Association of beta-Arrestin 1 with the type 1A angiotensin II receptor involves phosphorylation of the receptor carboxyl terminus and correlates with receptor internalization. *Mol. Endocrinol.* **15**, 1706–1719.
10. Thomas W.G., Motel T.J., Kule C.E., Karoor V., Baker K.M. (1998) Phosphorylation of the angiotensin II (AT1A) receptor carboxyl terminus: a role in receptor endocytosis. *Mol. Endocrinol.* **12**, 1513–1524.
11. Oppermann M., Freedman N.J., Alexander R.W., Lefkowitz R.J. (1996) Phosphorylation of the type 1A angiotensin II receptor by G protein-coupled receptor kinases and protein kinase C. *J. Biol. Chem.* **271**, 13266–13272.
12. Qian H., Pipolo L., Thomas W.G. (1999) Identification of protein kinase C phosphorylation sites in the angiotensin II (AT1A) receptor. *Biochem. J.* **343 Pt 3**, 637–644.
13. Oro C., Qian H., Thomas W.G. (2007) Type 1 angiotensin receptor pharmacology: signaling beyond G proteins. *Pharmacol. Ther.* **113**, 210–226.

Index

E

F

G

H

I

J

K

L

M

N

O

P

Q

R

S